Ninth Edition

An Outline of
Psychiatry

Clarence J. Rowe, M.D.
Clinical Professor Emeritus of Psychiatry
University of Minnesota
Minneapolis, Minnesota

Vice-President/Medical Affairs
Constance Bultman Wilson Center
Faribault, Minnesota

Walter D. Mink, Ph.D.
Professor of Psychology
Macalester College
Saint Paul, Minnesota

wcb
Wm. C. Brown Publishers
Dubuque, Iowa

To Shirley Holt Mink, Ph.D.

It could be said of me that in this book I have only made up a bunch of other men's flowers, providing of my own only the string that ties them together.

Montaigne 1533–1592

Library of Congress Catalog Card Number: 88–70844

ISBN 0–697–06453–0

Printed in the United States of America by Wm. C. Brown Publishers
2460 Kerper Boulevard, Dubuque, IA 52001

10 9 8 7 6 5 4 3 2 1

Contents

Introduction to the Ninth Edition

This Ninth Edition marks the thirty-fifth year of the Outline. In each edition the authors have tried to keep abreast of changes in psychiatry. As in the past, the contents of this book reflect our experiences in teaching, consulting, and clinical practice. It presents in outline form material that can be found more elaborately treated in other standard textbooks, many of which are listed as references at the ends of the chapters. We subscribe to the *biopsychosocial* model of disorders where applicable and try to use that scheme in the chapters that follow.

Classification of mental disorders follows the American Psychiatric Association's Diagnostic and Statistical Manual of Mental Disorders, Third Edition Revised (*DSM*-III-R) (1987). *DSM*-III-R follows the multiaxial classification established in *DSM*-III. The authors, in consort with others in the field, expect that *DSM*-IV is in the not too distant offing.

The authors acknowledge their gratitude to: Kay Crawford, Jan Trusso, and Linda Pangborn, for preparation of the manuscript; Jean Jagger Rowe, for many of the quotations; Sharon Weitzel, for assembling the glossary and a myriad of other matters essential to the finalizing of the manuscript; Sandra Tarman, and her staff of the Boeckmann Medical Library, St. Paul; Nancy Soth, and her staff of the Wilson Center, Faribault, Minnesota; and to Patricia McNulty Rowe, for unwitting contributions to the manuscript.
Clarance J. Rowe, M.D.
Walter D. Mink, Ph.D.

Etiology of Mental Disorders

The mind of men is a mystery; and, like the plant, each one of us naturally appropriates and assimilates that about him which responds to that which is within him.

Joseph Roux: "Prelude," *Meditations of a Parish Priest* (1886)

I. Introduction

A. Definition

Webster's Third New International Dictionary (1971) defines etiology as

1. A science or doctrine of causation or the demonstration of causes.
2. A branch of science dealing with the causes of particular phenomena.
3. All the factors that contribute to the occurrence of a disease or abnormal condition; cause; origin.

B. Actually, the essential causes of most mental disorders are unknown or incompletely understood. It is thus necessary for us to consider all the factors that could play a role in the development of any particular mental disorder.

C. One view is that mental disorder results from the interaction of the person (personality) with predisposing and precipitating factors. Subsumed in this view are the following:

1. Predisposing factors are those that render the personality susceptible or vulnerable and are present over a long period of time (subclinical).
2. Precipitating factors are events that precede the clinical onset of the disorder.
3. The severity of the predisposing factors determines the person's vulnerability or susceptibility to precipitating factors.
4. Precipitating factors of varying severity may produce disorder in mildly predisposed persons. For example:
   a) A loosely disorganized schizophrenic may be inordinately upset by a mild social rebuff.
   b) A well-integrated person may develop a mild anxiety reaction to a catastrophe, such as a fire or a flood.
5. Predisposing factors endure throughout the life of the individual. They may be cumulative or connected. Precipitating factors occur intermittently throughout the individual's lifetime. They may be related to special developmental tasks (see p. 3–6).

D. As a matter of fact, human behavior at any time is determined by the individual's physical and psychological status and his or her capacity, at that moment, to adapt to the immediate environment.

E. In the past, two major hypotheses have been advancd to account for mental illness: the psychogenic hypothesis and the somatogenic hypothesis.

1. Proponents of the *psychogenic hypothesis* regard mental disorder as the effect of environmental factors that affect the psychological integration and social adequacy of the individual, particularly the effectiveness of the management of individual needs in relation to the demands of the world.

2. Proponents of the *somatogenic hypothesis* regard mental disorder as resulting from the malfunction of the central nervous system in a way that affects cognitive, emotional, and expressive processes. Such malfunction may arise from physical influences or reflect genetically transmitted conditions.

F. The psychogenic and somatogenic hypotheses have been viewed as conflicting alternatives. This view is unnecessarily dualistic. All factors interact, whether they are categorized as "psychosocial" or "organic." It is the interaction of the factors that must be considered in any etiology.

G. One way of ranking factors is to separate those that contribute to vulnerability or susceptibility to stress (predisposing) from those that are stressors (the precipitating factors or psychosocial stressors as listed in the *Diagnostic and Statistical Manual of Mental Disorders, Third Edition, Revised [DSM-III-R]*). A partial listing of predisposing factors and precipitating factors that are frequently considered in etiological studies is contained in the following sections.

H. The diathesis-stress model views mental disorders as the product of a predisposition toward the development of a particular disorder (diathesis) and conditions operating on the person that require an adjustive response (stress).

II. **Predisposing factors**

A. Vulnerability

Vulnerability is a function of predisposing factors, which include but are not limited to the following:

1. Genetics

a) Genetic influences control both the characteristic development of members of a species but also are a source of individual differences. The influence of genes begins at conception and may be expressed at any time throughout life.

b) Chromosomal aberrations and faulty genes may result in metabolic or biochemical irregularities, which predispose individuals to particular disorders.

c) In the past, evidence for genetic factors in mental disorders came primarily from studies of the occurrence of disorders in families and of concordance rates in identical twins, but advances in molecular biology are producing discoveries of genetic markers for mental disorders.

d) Some examples of disorders with clear or strong presumptive evidence for the role of genetically transmitted influences are:

(1) Huntington's chorea (a degenerative disorder of the basal ganglia and cortex characterized by progressive intellectual loss and motor dysfunction) is related to a dominant inherited gene.

(2) Bipolar disorder (manic-depression), in one of its forms, has been related to a dominant gene but the disorder is not expressed in all people who inherit the gene.

(3) Alzheimer's disease (a progressive dementia, with diffuse brain deterioration, occurring in later life) has been linked in some studies to a genetic marker.[1]

(4) Support for a genetic cause of schizophrenia has been suggested by the incidence in children of schizophrenics and the concordance in identical twins (if one twin develops schizophrenia, in over 50% of the cases the other twin does, too), but at present no accurate genetic model has been developed and no genetic marker has been discovered.

   e) It should be kept in mind that pathological feelings and ways of thinking may be transmitted by parents to children by the parents' pathological behavior and example rather than through genetic inheritance. In such examples it is appropriate to talk of familial disorders that are not necessarily hereditary.

2. Age

   a) Certain periods of life are considered times of special stress, not only because of the physical changes that occur but also because of specific psychological stresses that are encountered during such periods.

   b) Adolescence, middle life (sometimes called the involutional period), and the senium (the geriatric age, the period of old age) are often thought of as periods of special stress.

B. Gender

1. Statistical studies indicate sex differences in the frequency of diagnosis of some disorders.

   a) More women than men with emotional problems consult physicians.

   b) Affective disorders are more common among women.

   c) Alcoholism is much more frequent among men.

   d) More attempts at suicide are made by women in the United States, but more men are successful.

2. It is difficult to separate factors that are role related from those that are constitutional or dimorphic.

C. Early childhood deprivations

1. Although environmental conditions are usually viewed as precipitating factors, some conditions in infancy and early childhood, if unrelieved, can have prolonged and immutable effects that can be considered predisposing factors.

2. Chronic malnutrition may retard physical and mental growth and produce lowered resistance to stress.

---

[1]Referred to as primary *dementia* of the Alzheimer type in DSM-III-R.

3. Extreme isolation from human contact during early childhood appears to produce chronic deficits in cognitive and social functioning.
4. Some recent studies suggest that extreme physical or sexual abuse in childhood may predispose adults to some deviant behaviors.

III. Precipitating factors
A. Environment
Environment includes the emotional as well as the physical milieu. Among environmental factors are the following:
1. Various family interactions (engagement, marriage, discord, separation, death, becoming a parent, conflict with a child, illness in a child).
2. Other interpersonal relationships (difficulties with friends, neighbors, or associates).
3. Living circumstances (change in residence, immigration).
4. Financial affairs (inadequate finances, financial reverses).
5. Legal affairs (being arrested, suing, being sued).
6. Occupation
   a) Stress related to the job (e.g., conflict with a supervisor, competition for promotion, but *not* overwork, which is usually a symptom rather than a cause of an emotional problem).
   b) Special occupational hazards (e.g., environmental hazards, such as asbestos, coal dust).
   c) Women's occupations in which they have to contend with sexist attitudes, including less pay, difficulty in moving into certain roles, and expected stereotypic feminine behavior in certain positions.
7. Poverty

B. Physical illness
Physical illness may pose both practical and emotional problems. Among these are the following:
1. Personal (pain, discomfort, enforced idleness)
2. Financial (cost of treatment, inability to make a living)
3. Emotional (reactivation of repressed conflicts, especially those related to feelings of dependency)
4. Body image (mutilative surgery, e.g., breast amputation, may cause certain disturbances of body image)
5. Endocrinal (e.g., hyperthyroidism may lead to tension and anxiety; hypothyroidism may lead to apathy and lethargy)

C. Physical handicaps
Physical handicaps may or may not give rise to emotional disturbances.
1. They may serve as a focus of inferiority feelings and result in such undesirable defenses as overcompensation (see chapter, "Adaptations to Anxiety").

2. However, many persons with physical handicaps do not manifest any significant emotional problems.

D. Exogenous factors

Exogenous factors include drugs, chemicals, infections, and trauma.

    1. Drugs and chemicals (e.g., alcohol, sedatives, narcotics, and industrial toxins cause organic mental disorder, or organic brain syndrome, or otherwise affect the individual's adaptive response (see chapter, "Organic Mental Syndromes and Disorders").

    2. Certain infectious diseases may lead to delirium. Syphilis may produce changes in the central nervous system with or without mental diseases.

    3. Trauma may lead to reversible or irreversible changes, with accompanying personality disorders, or to post-traumatic disorders.

E. Deprivations and deficiencies

    1. Starvation, for example, may lead to personality changes (meanness, suspiciousness, withdrawal).

    2. Sensory deprivation, of sight, for example, may lead to delirium with hallucinations (following cataract extraction when the eyes are kept covered postoperatively or the hallucinations described by lone explorers or sailors).

    3. Deprivation of sleep may lead to mental and personality changes (inability to concentrate, restlessness, apathy).

IV. Stages in development

A. Although development is a continuum, it is often divided into stages for convenience of description and discussion. (For a description of Freud's well-known stages of psychosexual development see chapter, "Psychodynamic Concepts.")

B. The developmental stages can serve as a background against which to consider any developmental sources of stresses and tasks whose resolution may contribute to vulnerability.

C. Jean Piaget proposed the following stages from his pioneer studies of cognitive development.

    1. Sensorimotor stage, from birth to eighteen months (preverbal).

    2. Preoperational stage, eighteen months to seven or eight years, with the beginnings of organized language.

    3. Stage of concrete operations, seven to eight years through eleven to twelve years.

    4. Formal operation stage, from eleven to twelve years to adulthood (capacity for abstract thought develops).

D. Arnold Gesell has outlined developmental milestones in the normally developing child from two weeks to six years.

    1. An infant smiles at one to two weeks.

    2. An infant follows an object with his or her eyes at two to four weeks.

3. The infant smiles meaningfully at a person (social smiling) at four to eight weeks.
4. The infant vocalizes at sixteen to eighteen weeks.
5. The infant sits by six to eight months.
6. The infant stands by nine to twelve months, and by twelve to fifteen months walks and talks.

E. Following is an outline of Erik Erikson's psychosocial stages of life as elaborated by Lawrence R. Allman and Dennis T. Jaffee.*

Life State	Approximate Age Period	Developmental Tasks
Infancy	0–2	Social attachment; object permanence; sensorimotor intelligence; maturation of motor functions
Toddlerhood	2–4	Self-control; language development; fantasy and play
Early childhood	5–7	Sex role identification; early moral development; group play
Middle childhood	8–12	Social cooperation; self-evaluation; skill learning; team play
Early adolescence	13–17	Peer group membership; heterosexual relationships
Later adolescence	18–22	Autonomy from parents; sex role identity; career choice values
Early adulthood	23–30	Marriage, childbearing, work, life-style
Middle adulthood	31–40	Management of household and career; child raising
Middle life	40–55	Coming to terms with achievements; career revision; consolidation of identity
Aging	55+	Redirection of energy to diminishing role; perspective of death; acceptance of own life

*Abridged and adapted from table 2.1 "Expanded outline of Erik Erikson's psychosocial stages of life" (p. 32) in *Abnormal Psychology in the Life Cycle* by Lawrence R. Allman and Dennis T. Jaffe. General Editor Phillip Whitten. Copyright © 1978 by Lawrence R. Allman and Dennis T. Jaffe and Phillip Whitten. By permission of Harper & Row, Publishers, Inc.

F. Adult development
 1. Influenced particularly by the ideas of Erikson, considerable attention has been paid in the past decade to stages of adult development (for a popular account, see *Passages* by Gail Sheehy).
 2. Accounts of adult development generally agree on the following issues:
  a) Adulthood is not static but in a state of change toward greater self-definition and organization of functions in a pattern of life.
  b) Adult development is continuous with childhood development.
  c) Adult development displays the interaction of individual needs and the requirements and opportunities of a natural and social environment.
  d) Adults must come to terms with the limitations of their span of life and their individual mortality.
 3. An example of current approaches to the study of adult development can be found in the work of Daniel Levinson and associates. (It should be noted that this approach is based on a study of men.)
  a) The life cycle consists of a series of roughly twenty-year eras: preadulthood (0–20), early adulthood (20–40), middle adulthood (40–60), late adulthood (60–80), and late, late adulthood (80+).
  b) Each era includes transition stages and periods of relative stability that display the development of, and commitment to, a life structure, a patterning of key choices, goals, and values.
  c) Transition stages, which occur at the beginning of each adult era and at the beginning of the middle decade as well (around 30 and 50), are times for assessment and modification of life structures.
  d) The transition periods of evaluation may also be periods of crisis for some persons (e.g., the "mid-life crisis" in the early 40s).
G. For additional developmental perspectives see the chapter, "Psychodynamic Concepts."
V. Etiology of mental disorders
A. The etiology of emotional disorders should be regarded as a complex interaction of genetic, psychosocial, and physical factors.
 1. Some of these factors are probably inborn, some develop so early that they become an integral part of the "basic" personality structure, and others come into play later on.

2. These statements can be represented schematically, but first let us define our terms again.
   a) Hereditary factors include the presence or absence of mental disorder in the family, the innate capacity to cope, physical endowment, and so forth.
   b) Early environmental influences include parental attitudes, family interaction, and sociocultural factors.
   c) Well-developed defenses (see chapter on adaptations to anxiety).
   d) Stress (physical trauma, loss of love object) (see chapter on anxiety).
   e) Mental disorder (e.g., anxiety, affective disorder, various psychotic disorders).
3. Thus, hereditary factors + early environmental influences (lead to) → the production of well-developed defenses + subsequent stress (may lead to) → mental disorder.

B. Therefore, mental disorders may result from the interaction of predisposing and precipitating factors with the personality.
C. This is sometimes referred to as the bio/psycho/social model.
D. Some aspects of psychosocial concepts are reviewed in the chapters, "Psychodynamic Concepts" and "Behavioral and Cognitive Concepts." Biological concepts are discussed in chapters on the various clinical syndromes and the chapter on pharmacological and somatic treatment.

References

American Psychiatric Association. *Diagnostic and Statistical Manual of Mental Disorders*. 3d ed., rev. Washington, D.C., 1987.

Bosselman, B. *Neurosis and Psychosis*. 3d ed. Springfield, Ill.: Charles C. Thomas, 1969.

Coleman, J. C., J. N. Butcher, and R. C. Carson. *Abnormal Psychology and Modern Life*. 7th ed. Glenview, Ill.: Scott, Foresman, 1984.

Kaplan, H. I., and B. J. Sadock. *Comprehensive Textbook of Psychiatry/IV*. 4th ed. Baltimore: Williams & Wilkins, 1985.

Kolb, L. C., and H. K. H. Brodie. *Modern Clinical Psychiatry*. 10th ed. Philadelphia: W. B. Saunders Co., 1982.

There is occasions and causes why
and wherefore in all things.

Shakespeare: *King Henry V*

Psychodynamic Concepts

I. Introduction
   A. Physical development

   The human organism undergoes a process of physical development from the moment of conception (fusion of sperm with ovum) until it reaches maturity. In part, this process is influenced by genetic determinants, but it also is affected by subsequent forces that may impair its goal, produce malfunctions, or limit the functioning of all or part of the organism. These forces derive largely from the experience of the organism in the environment.

   B. Psychological development

   Similarly, the same person undergoes a process of psychological development (maturation) that is also influenced by hereditary background and various environmental influences. Included in the latter are parental relationships, peer relationships, and cultural and social experiences.

II. Personality development
   A. Personality
      1. Personality has been defined in various ways. Simply stated, personality is the sum total of the individual's internal and external patterns of adjustment to life.
      2. Personality is, in part, determined by one's genetically transmitted organic endowment and in part by one's life experiences.
      3. As the individual develops, his or her behavior also changes. Thus, a newborn reacts differently to a given environmental stimulus than an adolescent or adult.
      4. For the various stages of personality development, see page 7 in the chapter, "Etiology of Mental Disorders" and page 138 in the chapter, "Personality Disorders."
   B. In this chapter, we will discuss various psychosocial conceptions of human behavior and the motivation as well as the psychosocial forces operant in mental disorders.

III. Psychodynamic concepts
   A. Definition

   Psychodynamics is the study, explanation, or interpretation of behavior or mental states in terms of mental or emotional forces or processes. It recognizes the role of *unconscious* motivation and assumes that one's behavior is determined by past experience, genetic endowment, and current reality. It is the science of mental forces in action (see Campbell, *Psychiatric Dictionary,* 5th ed. and the APA *Psychiatric Glossary,* 6th ed.)

B. History
1. Sigmund Freud (1856–1939)

Most of the current psychiatric conceptions of behavioral development and psychopathology originated with the work of Sigmund Freud, who created psychoanalysis. Psychoanalysis is

   a) A theory of how the mind works: including attempts to comprehend and explain both normal and abnormal functioning at all ages.
   b) An investigative or research method: basically using the free association technique to gain access to the patient's conscious and unconscious thoughts.
   c) A specific form of therapy using free association to obtain data in the form of thoughts, feelings, memories, fantasies, and dreams. It also involves "working through" and the development of insight (for additional information see the chapter, "Treatment in Psychiatry: Psychotherapy").

2. Origins

Psychoanalysis developed out of the teachings and opinions that prevailed at the time of Freud's work. Its basic elements (including dynamics of psychic processes, the classification of these processes into primary and secondary processes and into the unconscious and conscious [topography], and their economy [pleasure/displeasure]) were prefigured in Herbart, Fechner, Helmholtz, and Meynert.

3. Among the early theorists were the following:

   a) Gottfried Wilhelm Liebniz (1646–1716), the German philosopher and mathematician, believed that perception of elements occurred unconsciously. He presented the first systematic statement of degrees of consciousness.
   b) Johann Fredrick Herbart (1776–1841), developed the dynamic theory of unconscious mental processes some seventy years before Freud. Herbart's central thesis was that it must eventually be possible to describe mental processes in terms of scientific laws. And he dreamed of the "mathematical psychology."
   c) Gustav Theodor Fechner (1801–1887) referred to "negative sensations" that occurred below the threshold of consciousness. He employed not only a concept of inhibition but also repression. He also worked toward a "mathematical psychology."

d) Hermann Helmholtz (1821–1894), a nineteenth-century scientist who made contributions to physiology and other scientific fields, coined the terms "unconscious inference" and explained the associations of perception to past experience.

e) Theodore Meynert (1833–1892) was a German neurologist and psychiatrist who advocated the localization theory (mental and emotional life is dependent on the brain). Like Freud, he accorded a position of central importance to associations.

f) Joseph Brueur (1841–1925), a Viennese neurologist, published (1895) with Freud the classic, "Studien Uber Hysterie" (which Freud said were the "products of Brueur's mind").

g) Eduard von Hartman (Karl Robert) (1842–1906) was a metaphysical philosopher, who was called "the philosopher of the unconscious." He authored a book entitled *Philosophy of the Unconscious,* published in Berlin in 1869. He based his philosophical system on the premise that the unconscious permeates both will and reason.

h) Perhaps one could also include the great philosopher, Immanual Kant (1724–1804), who stated, "Innumerable are the sensations and perceptions where of we are not conscious. . . . The clear ideas indeed are but an infinitely small fraction of the same exposed to consciousness."

4. Psychoanalysis derived from two great antithetical traditions: nineteenth-century science contributed the framework under which Freud tried to fit his psychological discoveries. This framework was deterministic and materialistic, strongly oriented toward physics and evolutionary biology (from the rationalism of the Enlightenment); and the vision of the romantic poets and philosophers of the nineteenth-century (a cultural movement that rejected and undermined the dominant ideas of the Enlightenment and explored the "night side of life"). For example, Samuel Taylor Coleridge referred to the "unconscious" and "twilight realms of consciousness." Schopenhauer's concept "unconscious will" was roughly equivalent to the "id" as seen by psychoanalysts. For Freud the importance of psychoanalysis lay in its contribution to knowledge and not in its therapeutic benefits.

Although Freud was dependent on other contributions, he remains the first cartographer of the unconscious.

C. A comprehensive resume of psychoanalytic theories is beyond the scope of this outline. However, a few of the basic psychoanalytic concepts that have been found useful in general psychiatry will be listed.

IV. Sigmund Freud (1856–1939)

A. Thinking

Freud viewed thinking as composed of primary and secondary processes. This differentiation is viewed by many of his followers as his greatest accomplishment.

1. Primary processes

These are the psychological expressions of the underlying basic drives. They are assumed to be largely unconscious, present at birth, and thus can be considered innate. They are the more primitive modes of thinking. They are manifested in dreams but are also present during waking life. Thinking at this level follows the *pleasure principle*—the seeking of pleasure and the avoidance of pain.

2. Secondary processes

These are the reasonable and acceptable ways in which the underlying basic drives are controlled and permitted expression according to the demands of the outside world. They are characteristic modes of preconscious and conscious thinking and follow the *reality principle*.

B. Drives

There are certain significant desires and drives that are repressed. These constitute the *dynamic unconscious*, and they resist conscious expression because of their basic unacceptability (see "repression" in the chapter, "Adaptations to Anxiety").

C. Resistance

An individual resists attempts to make these repressed forces conscious through the use of defenses (see "Adaptations to Anxiety"). This constitutes what Freud called *resistance*.

D. Transference

Transference is the displacement of feelings for significant people in one's earlier life onto the physician or therapist.

E. Mind

To help explain all of these phenomena, Freud postulated a mind composed of the conscious, the preconscious (foreconscious), and the unconscious.

1. *The conscious* is composed of ideas, feelings, drives, and urges of which the person is aware. It is the scene of purposeful behavior.

2. *The preconscious,* which is midway between the conscious and the unconscious, comprises feelings, ideas, drives, and urges that are out of the individual's continuous awareness but that can be readily recalled. For example, you may not think about what you ate for supper last night, but you could easily recall the menu if asked.

3. *The unconscious* is made up of drives, feelings, ideas, and urges that are outside of the individual's awareness. One does not acknowledge or label them.

F. Divisions of personality
    Structurally, Freud divided personality into three parts. This tri-
    partite division included the id, ego, and superego.
    1. Id
        The *id* is the unconscious reservoir of primitive drives (in-
        stincts). The id is dominated by the primary process manner
        of thinking and the pleasure principle. It exists in all humans
        and in modified forms in all other animal life. Components of
        the id are:
        a) *Eros,* the name Freud gave to the creative forces, the life
            instinct. (Eros was the Greek god of love and originally
            represented the primeval power that created order and
            cohesion out of chaos.)
        b) *Thanatos,* Freud's term for the aggressive, destructive,
            or death forces. (Thanatos was the Greek god who per-
            sonified death and was the twin brother of Hypnos, or
            sleep.)
        c) *Homeostasis,* the individual's tendency to maintain a rel-
            atively stable psychological condition with respect to con-
            tending drives, motivations, and other psychodynamic
            forces. Freud felt that psychological growth depended on
            a proper balance between the creative and aggressive
            forces, with somewhat of a preponderance of the former.
        d) *Libido,* Freud's term for the emotional energy broadly
            derived from these underlying instincts (psychosexual
            energy) and presumably present at birth. The id serves
            as a reservoir for the libido, which has two general forms.
            (1) *Ego libido* is libido concentrated on the self, or nar-
                 cissism. *Primary narcissism* is the original state of
                 the newborn. (Narcissus was a Greek youth who fell
                 in love with his own reflection in the water.)
            (2) *Object libido* is libido that is directed outward
                 toward another person or thing.
        e) *Cathexis,* the name Freud gave to the process by which
            the unconscious primitive drives are vested with psychic
            energy.
    2. Ego
        The *ego* is the part of the personality that meets and interacts
        with the outside world; the "integrator" or "mediator" of the
        personality.
        a) The ego functions to help the individual deal with the
            world and yet to satisfy the underlying needs of the id
            through coping and problem-solving (see "Adaptations to
            Anxiety").
        b) It functions at all three levels of consciousness (conscious,
            preconscious, and unconscious).

c) The adaptive functions of the ego are the defenses against anxiety (see "Adaptations to Anxiety").

d) The opposition of ego energy to id energy is called *countercathexis.*

e) The ego is the executive function of the personality.

f) The part of the ego devoted to the development of parental substitutes (parental imagoes) is called the *ego ideal.* This is a part of a developing ego that is set aside, so to speak, to contain the mental images of the parents—for identification.

3. Superego

The *superego* is the censoring force of the personality. It is composed of the morals, mores, values, and ethics of the individual and is largely derived from one's parents.

a) The conscious part of the superego is called *conscience,* but it operates at all three levels of consciousness.

b) Most of us are conscious of our moral and ethical beliefs but remember only a portion of the training and experience that contributed to the formation of those beliefs.

c) If the ego contemplates violation of the superego's code, anxiety results; if the person carries out the contemplated violation despite the anxiety, guilt feelings ensue.

d) The infant's superego is primitive and undeveloped. It begins to develop in the second year and takes definite form at the age of four or five.

e) The punitive aspect of superego concerns itself with prohibitions, self-criticism, and guilt feelings (bad conscience).

f) The nonpunitive, positive aspect of the superego is sometimes separately designated as the *ego ideal.*

g) An overly strict superego usually leads to the development of a rigid, compulsive, unhappy person. A weak, defective superego permits a person to express hostile and antisocial strivings without anxiety or guilt.

G. Libido development (stages of psychosexual development)

Freud believed that the major development of adult personality takes place in infancy and early childhood.

1. The oral phase

a) The first twelve to eighteen months of life are characterized chiefly by preoccupation with feeding. Pleasure is derived mainly through the mouth. This period is called the *oral phase.*

b) The early part of the oral phase, the *sucking stage,* is passive.

c) The later oral phase, or *biting stage,* is aggressive (oral-sadistic).

2. The anal phase
   a) From the eighteenth month until the end of the third year, the infant's attention is centered on excretory functions. This is the *anal phase*.
   b) This is the first time the infant must adjust his or her behavior to the demands of others.
   c) This stage is also the foundation for the development of the superego.
   d) *Expulsive and retentive phases* are part of the anal phase, just as passive and aggressive ones are part of the oral phase.
3. The narcissistic or pregenital phase
   The oral and anal phases considered together are called the *narcissistic or pregenital phase* because the child's libido is satisfied within his or her own body.
4. The phallic phase
   The *phallic phase* extends from the end of the third year to the seventh year. The child becomes aware of his or her genitalia. During this stage, for the first time, the child's libido is directed outward and requires others for its satisfaction. It is characterized, psychosexually, by:
   a) *Castration anxiety,* which results from the boy's fear of damage to or loss of his genitals. It includes the childhood fantasy that female genitals result from the loss of the penis.
   b) *Penis envy,* which is the girl's desire to possess a penis and, thus, to become masculine.
   c) *The Oedipus complex,* which is the attachment of the child to the parent of the opposite sex, accompanied by envious and aggressive feelings toward the parent of the same sex.
      (1) This complex of aggressive feelings in the girl is called the *Electra complex.*
      (2) The resolution of this complex is usually accomplished by subsequent identification with the parent of the same sex.
5. Latency
   Latency is the stage between the Oedipal period and the adolescent years. In general, during this period, the person learns to recognize and cope with reality.
6. The genital phase
   The *genital phase* is the final stage of psychosexual development.
   a) It begins with puberty, with the physiological capacity for orgasms as well as the capacity for object love and mature heterosexuality.

      b) The early adolescent stage is narcissistic in that selfish interests predominate.

      c) Following this, there is a temporary homosexual phase in which adolescents prefer to meet in gatherings of the same sex.

      d) As adolescence progresses, attraction to the opposite sex begins to assert itself more strongly and the capacity for object love and mature heterosexuality emerges.

H. Adult character structure

  1. Adult character includes the ego's usual mode of dealing with the id, the superego, and the external world. It is patterned on an individual's experiences during the above stages.

  2. Character types

    According to Freudian theory, adults could be certain character types, based on fixations (from unresolved conflicts) at any of the stages.

      a) Oral character. This person has a passive-receptive orientation toward life and has oral preoccupations (eating, drinking, smoking, etc).

      b) Anal character. This frugal, orderly, obstinate person needs to feel in control of himself or herself in the environment.

      c) Phallic character. In the male, overcompensatory behavior is a reaction against underlying castration fears and grows out of a need to demonstrate his masculinity. In the female, the reaction to penis envy would be to assume "masculine" roles.

      d) Genital character. This concept is "an ideal." Such a person has successfully passed through all the developmental stages and is able to maturely participate in meaningful relationships with members of the opposite sex.

V. Alfred Adler (1870–1937)

A. Individual psychology

Adler founded the school of *individual psychology*—each person has his or her own special goals and unique manner of achieving them.

B. Organ inferiority

Adler placed more emphasis on the ego than on sexuality.

  1. He regarded organ inferiority as the most important etiological factor.

  2. He believed that the individual's development was determined by the adaptive push for superiority, or the drive to power. (The specific type of superiority depends upon the individual's biological background and early environment.)

3. In this quest for power, a particular *life-style*—the individual's stepwise, active, unique adaptation to the social milieu—evolves.

C. Personality

Adler regarded personality as developing out of the individual's attitudes toward herself or himself, toward other people (especially family), and toward society.

D. Inferiority complex

1. Adler coined the term *inferiority complex* to describe the conflict, partly conscious and partly unconscious, that impels the individual to attempt to overcome the distress accompanying feelings of inferiority (which are derived from the helplessness of the infant).

2. He believed that a neurotic disposition is caused by overprotection, neglect, or both, during childhood.

3. The person with strong feelings of inferiority may, however, compensate by trying to become superior in some special area.

4. The struggle for superiority may be successful, if modified by the demands of reality.

5. Thus, in the Adlerian formulation, neurosis represents the various psychological processes by which the individual seeks to cope with his or her inferiority.

E. Masculine protest

1. *Masculine protest* is Adler's term for the individual's (male/female) attempt to escape from the feminine submissive role. Women become tomboys or tyrannical wives or mothers. Men become Don Juans. This concept can be regarded as the main motive force in neurotic disorder. It is tied in with self-esteem: the neurotic purpose is the enhancement of self-esteem, the simplest form of which can be recognized in the exaggerated masculine protest.

2. Masculine protest may derive from the subject's own uncertainty of his or her role.

VI. **Carl G. Jung (1875–1961)**

A. Analytic psychology

Jung's modification of psychoanalysis was called *analytic psychology.*

B. Introversion and extroversion

Jung stressed life goals and the role of introversion and extroversion in personality development.

1. He defined *introversion* as inwardly directed libido, reflected in the tendency to be preoccupied with oneself.

2. *Extroversion* was his term for outwardly directed libido.

C. The libido
 1. Like Adler, Jung minimized the role of sexuality in personality dynamics.
 2. He believed that the libido was broadly derived from all life energy (not just from sex).
D. The unconscious
 1. In addition to the *personal* unconscious, Jung postulated a *collective* unconscious (racial or archaic unconscious), believing that there was an inheritance of primitive racial ideas and impulses.
 2. He believed the personal unconscious to be superficial and hence more accessible than the collective unconscious.
 3. The collective unconscious was later called the *objective psyche.* It included both
   a) *Autochthonous ideas,* ideas originating within the psyche without external stimuli.
   b) *Primordial images,* a phylogenetic memory heavily laden with mythological reference.
E. The shadow
 This is the term Jung gave to the objective counterpart of the underlying personal unconscious and collective unconscious. Coming to terms with it requires maturity and perspective (which usually emerge during the second half of life).
F. The persona and anima
 1. The *persona* is the social facade assumed by an individual (so named from the mask worn by actors in ancient Greek drama, which characterized the mood portrayed). The individual behaves in conformity with what is expected of him or her.
 2. The *anima* is the true inner self, or soul. In addition,
   a) The *animus* is the masculine component of the female personality.
   b) The *anima* is the female component of the male personality.
G. Self
 According to Jungian psychology, the self does not really come into awareness until the individual has dealt with his shadow and anima or animus.
H. Basic psychological functions
 1. Jung described four basic psychological functions: feelings, thinking, sensation, and intuition. (The first two are usually conscious; the second two are usually unconscious.)
 2. In addition, he saw people as having two general attitudes: extroversion and introversion.
 3. Thus, there were eight possible combinations.

I. Therapy

Jung believed that psychiatric treatment should deal with current problems and plans for the future as well as attempts to uncover past causal experiences.

VII. **Otto Rank (1884–1939)**

A. The birth trauma

Rank proffered the theory that the *birth trauma* was central to the individual's experience.

1. The process of birth produces primal anxiety in response to feelings of helplessness.
2. Separation from the mother is the original trauma, a sudden, violent change from the security of intrauterine existence to the uncertainties of the outer world.
3. Subsequent separations of any type are also traumatic.
4. Every pleasure is a seeking of the reestablishment of intrauterine primal pleasure.

B. Conflict and therapy

1. As the child becomes conscious of himself as separate from his mother, he develops conflict.
2. The desire for separation leads to guilt feelings.
3. According to Rank, a person has difficulty asserting his or her will.
4. In adulthood, a person possesses "a good" portion (approved by his parents and society), and a "bad" portion, called *counterwill* (which is disapproved).
5. Relieving guilt feelings is the central focus of treatment.

C. Personality

Rank described three character types:

1. The normal or average person (who accepts the will of the group)
2. The creative person (who sets his or her own ideals and governs himself or herself accordingly)
3. The neurotic person (who is not free to express his or her own will, but cannot conform to the group).

D. As the only nonmedical member of Freud's inner circle, he brought a world view to the psychoanalytic movement. His psychology and therapeutic method were precursors of the third force or humanistic psychology.

VIII. **Karen Horney (1885–1952)**

A. The social and emotional environment

Unlike Freud and Jung, Horney felt that conflict is an outgrowth of social conditions and not part of human nature. She focused on the dynamics of social and environmental factors in personality development.

B. Sexuality
   1. Horney did not accept the Freudian theory of the libido and his emphasis on infantile sexuality.
   2. She discounted the theory of penis envy.
C. Anxiety
   Horney stressed the principle of basic anxiety.
   1. The child's apprehension and insecurity result from relationships with parents who are overindulgent, dominating, erratic, or indifferent.
   2. As a consequence, the child is left without a feeling of belonging.
   3. Hostility and conflict derive from this basic anxiety.
D. Personality
   1. She delineated three main directions a child could take in coping with the environment:
      a) *Moving toward people* (i.e., accepting one's helplessness and attempting to win the affection of others);
      b) *Moving against people* (fighting the surrounding hostility); or
      c) *Moving away from people* (remaining apart and neither belonging or fighting).
   2. Three types of persons would typify these three basic attitudes.
      a) Compliant
      b) Aggressive
      c) Detached
E. Self
   Central to Horney's theory is the concept of *self*, which could be viewed in three ways.
   1. The *actual self* (the sum total of an individual's experiences)
   2. The *real self* (the unique total force and sense of integration found in each person)
   3. The *idealized self* (a glorified self-image, closely related to the current concept of narcissism), and a sign of neurosis
F. Therapy
   In therapy, she emphasized the self and the environment, concentrating on:
   1. Self-realization
   2. Self-actualization
   3. Dealing with the here-and-now.
G. Although her emphasis on the influence of culture and the importance of the here-and-now are commonly accepted today, they were unacceptable to the larger psychoanalytic community in her time. A very important contribution to our present day understanding of women was her belief that much of their behavior was the result of cultural enforcement.

H. Both Horney and Harry Stack Sullivan emphasized the environmental and social aspects of personality and disease.

I. They emphasized the importance of security, trust, and warmth in avoiding and resolving conflicts.

IX. Harry Stack Sullivan (1892–1949)

A. Interpersonal theory of psychiatry
1. Harry Stack Sullivan espoused an *interpersonal theory of personality,* that is, interpersonal relationships provide the experiences that are crucial in personality formation, both normal and abnormal.
2. Interpersonal relations mediate the basic human needs that Sullivan believed are tenderness, security, intimacy, and peers.
3. Social psychiatry has developed from Sullivan's principles.

B. Anxiety
1. Sullivan emphasized the need for security, which he felt could be satisfied only through interpersonal relationships.
2. He conceived of anxiety in the infant as stemming from a disturbance in the relationship between the child and the mothering one.
3. He regarded anxiety as the major factor in personality development as well as in the development of all emotional illnesses and psychopathology.

C. Parataxic distortions
This was a term coined and used by Sullivan to describe attitudes toward other persons that are based on distorted evaluations of them or on an identification of such persons with figures from one's past life. As a consequence, one develops certain manners of coping with the significant people in his or her life and uses these in later interpersonal relationships.

D. Personality
1. Sullivan believed that personality evolves from the action of personal and social forces in the individual from the time of birth onward.
2. He believed that the *power motive* underlies all other impulses and operates from birth onward to overcome an inner sense of helplessness.
3. He regarded intrapsychic conflicts (from within the personality) as being derived from interpersonal conflicts, that is, they are internalized interpersonal conflicts.

E. Therapy
Sullivan believed that treatment must include management of the patient in his or her milieu (environment).

F. Both Sullivan and Horney were greatly influenced by concepts of learning theory (simply stated: behavior is modified as a function of learning).

X. Erich Fromm (1900–1980)

A. Fromm was a Marxist who rejected Freud's emphasis on the biological nature of man, especially disputing Freud's inclusion of aggression as a basic part of human nature.

B. Alienation

Fromm believed that individuals are a product of their culture and that, in an industrialized society, they have become estranged from their culture and themselves.

C. Personality

1. Fromm emphasized that character is shaped by social and cultural influences and not by internal determinants.
2. He described five character patterns:
   a) *Receptive* (depends on others for support).
   b) *Exploitive* (exercises power over others or takes things by guile).
   c) *Marketing* (defines worth in terms of success; regards people as commodities to be bought and sold).
   d) *Hoarding* (possessive; bases security on saving and keeping).
   e) *Productive* (achieves his or her own capacity for love and creative work; has developed fully).

D. Therapy

The cultural environment must be considered in the treatment approach.

XI. Erik Erikson (1902–   )

A. Theory

His psychosocial theory of personality extends beyond the nuclear Freudian model to the social world. He views development as extending beyond the infantile sexuality of Freud. (Thus, he rejects the notion that the childhood experiences are the sole determinants of development.) He introduced the term *epigenesis* to refer to the stages of ego and social development.

B. Identity

1. Erikson emphasizes the concepts of *identity* (an inner sense of sameness that perseveres, despite external changes), *identity crisis,* and *identity confusion.*
2. His contributions are built upon basic Freudian tenets (in this regard he differs from Jung, Adler, and Horney, who rejected Freud's theories and substituted their own).
3. Like Adler, he minimizes the role of sexuality in personality dynamics.

C. Psychosocial stages

Erikson identifies eight *psychosocial stages* in personal development (the human life cycle or ego development).

1. Sensory-oral

   The *sensory-oral stage* is characterized by trust vs. mistrust (corresponds to Freud's oral stage and usually extends through the first year of life).

2. Muscular-anal

   The *muscular-anal stage* is characterized by autonomy vs. doubt (corresponds to the anal stage; spans the second and third years of life).

3. Genital

   The *genital stage* takes place during ages four and five; this is the play age.

4. Latency

   Latency involves industry vs. inferiority (ages six to eleven; the school age).

5. Puberty and adolescence

   a) *Puberty and adolescence* involve ego identity vs. role confusion (roughly, ages twelve to eighteen, when the adolescent is developing a personal identity).

   b) *Identity crisis* is a term used by Erikson to describe the inability of the adolescent to accept a role he or she believes to be expected by society.

6. Young adulthood

   Young adulthood is characterized by intimacy vs. isolation (roughly, the period of courtship and early family, extending from late adolescence until middle age).

7. Adulthood

   Adulthood is characterized by generativity vs. stagnation or self-absorption (middle age).

8. Maturity

   Maturity is characterized by ego integrity vs. despair (the individual's major efforts are nearing completion and there is time for reflection and the enjoyment of any grandchildren).

D. At each stage of development, basic psychosocial crises must be resolved.

XII. Adolf Meyer (1866–1950)

A. Psychobiology

1. Adolf Meyer founded *psychobiology* ("psychobiology studies not only the person as a whole, as a unit, but also the whole man").

2. His therapy theory was characterized as distributive analysis and synthesis.
   a) Patients, under the guidance of the therapist, critically evaluate the situations with which they are confronted and their responses to them.
   b) Through discussion and reasoning, the patients try to formulate a way of dealing with their problems more constructively.
3. His was a comprehensive or pluralistic approach to the understanding of mental illness. Thus, he emphasized the need to consider all pertinent information about the life of an individual as a biological, psychological, and social organism.
4. This is sometimes called *holism,* or the holistic approach (the understanding of the individual personality is based on the interplay of his inherited structure, his uniqueness, and the cultural pattern in which he lives).
5. Despite his holistic approach, he did not focus at all on the family.
6. American psychiatry has been greatly influenced by Meyerian thinking.
7. His approach has relevance to the community mental health movement.

B. Ego development
1. He did not systematize his thinking and never outlined developmental stages and their critical tasks.
2. He spoke of reactions rather than diseases.

C. Therapy
1. He introduced the concept of *commonsense* psychiatry, which refers to understanding the patient in the simplest terms possible.
2. He believed that treatment began with the first patient contact, and that one of the first steps in the evaluation of the patient was an assessment of the patient's assets and liabilities.
3. The essential goal of therapy was to help the patient modify his unhealthy adaptations ("habit training"). The emphasis was always on the current life situation.

XIII. Ego-psychologists
A. Heinz Hartmann, Ernst Kris, Rudolph Lowenstein.
B. *Ego psychology* shifted the emphasis from depth psychology to increased emphasis on autonomous or independent functions of the ego (reality testing, control of movement, perception, thinking, etc.).

C. Ego psychology complements but does not replace the older id psychology. It is the part of the personality that is most attuned to the outer world and has the task of maintaining a relationship through reality. This new interest in the ego included but was not limited to those aspects of the ego functioning that are more or less conscious or preconscious.

D. Described an undifferentiated phase from which both the id and the ego are gradually formed.

XIV. **Existential psychoanalysis**

A. Existential psychoanalysis is based on the philosophy of Sartre, Kierkegaard, and others.

B. This theoretical approach stresses the here and now rather than the past in the evaluation of personality disorder.

    1. It primarily focuses on three themes: (1) the person and himself or herself; (2) the person and other persons; and (3) the person and the world he or she lives in.

    2. Anxiety is seen as resulting from the fear of not being—the fear of death.

    3. Therapy emphasizes the use of the therapist's own inner feelings as a therapeutic tool. Emphasis is on expression of feelings by both the patient and the therapist and on the uniqueness of each individual and his or her "way-of-being-in-the-world." In contrast to behavior therapy, existential therapy calls for the therapist to share his or her feelings, values, and existence. The therapeutic process is highly subjective.

    4. Like psychodynamic psychotherapy, existential therapy is not for everyone but rather is directed primarily toward the intelligent and verbal individual who appears to be having an existential crisis.

    5. *Logo therapy* is an existential psychoanalytic method used by Victor Frankl. It is a type of psychotherapy based on a system of spiritual values. It stresses the search for the meaning of human existence.

    6. This theoretical approach has had little influence on present-day psychiatry.

C. Rollo May (1909–   )
Rollo May's special contributions to self-theory come from the European influence of existentialism.

XV. **Margaret Mahler (1897–   )**

A. She described the separation-individuation process—the child's sense of separateness from the world about him.

B. This process begins in the fourth or fifth month of life and is completed by age three.

C. She described four phases.
  1. Differentiation—the ability to distinguish between self and others.
  2. Practicing period—the infant's discovering the ability to separate by crawling and climbing, and later by upright ambulation (from seven to ten months until fifteen to sixteen months).
  3. Rapprochement—the need and desire for the mother to share the infant's newly found experiences and skills (sixteen months to twenty-five months of age).
  4. Consolidation—achievement of individuality and attainment of a certain degree of object constancy (twenty-five to thirty-six months of age).[1]

XVI. **Heinz Kohut (1913–1981)**
  A. Kohut is considered the founder of modern self-psychology.
  B. Kohut focused attention on "holistic" matters, dealing with the problems of the whole man. His ultimate concern was the future of man as a complete being and the primacy of "self-transmission" throughout succeeding generations: the "Odysseus complex."
  C. He viewed man as composed of the confluence of psychic forces (versus Freud's perceptual bias: envisioning a man constituted of isolated mental fragments).
  D. Only through persistent empathy and comprehension of the narcissistic super structure of modern man was it possible to assess this "tragic man" and aid him through the trials and tribulations of his mechanized jungle (insane society).
  E. He defined empathy as "vicarious introspection": the mode of cognition attuned to the affective and cognitive states of another.
  F. Kohutian psychotherapy (self-psychological psychotherapy) is identical to classical psychoanalysis and its basic tenets: free association and transference analysis. However, it involves the analysis of the whole personality as opposed to drive derivatives and formulates this interpretation with that bias.

XVII. **Humanistic perspectives on personality**
  The ascendance of humanistic psychology as a "third force" in psychology (in addition to psychoanalysis and behaviorism) is attributed particularly to the influence of Abraham Maslow and Carl Rogers.
  A. General characteristics of humanistic psychology
    1. It is defined as the study of the experiencing person.
    2. It is concerned primarily with choice, creativity, and self-realization.

1. H. I. Kaplan, and B. J. Sadock, *Modern Synopsis of Comprehensive Textbook of Psychiatry/ III,* 3rd ed. (Baltimore: Williams & Wilkins, 1981), pp. 19, 20.

3. Personally and socially significant problems are taken as a special focus of interest.
4. The goal of study is the enhancement of the lives and dignity of human beings.
B. Maslow's motivational theory
   1. A distinction is made between higher needs and lower needs in which higher needs emerge later in evolutionary and individual development, are less directly related to survival, and have more environmental preconditions to their satisfaction.
   2. Needs for a hierarchy (from lowest to highest levels)
     a) Physiological needs (e.g., food, water, sex, sleep)
     b) Safety (e.g., structure, security, predictability)
     c) Belongingness and love
     d) Esteem (e.g., recognition, acceptance, confidence)
     e) Self-actualization (e.g., full knowledge, acceptance of one's personal trend toward integrity, and expression of human potential)
   3. Relative satisfaction of needs more basic in the hierarchy is necessary for the next level of needs to emerge.
   4. Self-actualization is a level of need that is reached by few people, according to Maslow. (The concept of self-actualization was first expounded by Kurt Goldstein in 1939.)
   5. Maslow objected to personality theories developed from the study of abnormal people and developed his approach to personality from the study of healthy, creative people. He informally collected information about a group he considered to be self-actualized—among these were historical figures such as Abraham Lincoln, Henry David Thoreau, Eleanor Roosevelt, Albert Einstein, and some of Maslow's friends.
C. Rogers' phenomenological theory
   1. The major motivating influence in personality development is the *actualizing tendency,* the striving to maintain and enhance the experiencing person.
   2. The actualizing tendency motivates the person toward greater complexity, greater independence, and greater social responsibility.
   3. It is *phenomenological reality,* the subjective, personal interpretation of experience rather than physical reality, that determines behavior.
   4. The best conditions for development are those that encourage a positive self-regard and feeling of worth.
   5. Distortions of self-regard may occur when a person is confronted with an *incongruency* between perceived experience and self-concept.

6. Under conditions of incongruency a person is vulnerable to anxiety and may respond with defensive denial or distortion to such a degree that psychotherapy is required to reduce the incongruency.

D. Humanistic therapy

1. Humanistic therapy is oriented toward releasing the individual's potential by encouraging self-acceptance "as is" with both strengths and weaknesses.

2. The therapy is viewed as an "authentic" encounter between two individuals, and the client plays a major role in directing the course of treatment. The assumption is that people have within themselves the resources to understand and alter their view of the self and direct their own behavior.

3. The role of the therapist is largely a demonstration of empathetic understanding and unconditional positive regards.

References

Blum, G. S. *Psychodynamics: The Science of Unconscious Mental Forces*. Belmont, Calif.: Brooks/Cole, 1966.

Bromberg, W. *The Mind of Man*. New York: Harper & Brothers, 1959.

Ewalt, J. R., and D. L. Farnsworth. *Textbook of Psychiatry*. New York: McGraw-Hill, 1963.

Freinhar, J. P. "Oedipus or Odysseus: Developmental Lines of Narcissism. *Psychiatric Annals* 16 (August 1986): 476–85.

Goldman, H. H., ed. *Review of General Psychiatry*. Los Altos, Calif.: Lange Medical Publications, 1984.

Kaplan, H. I., and B.J. Sadock. *Modern Synopsis of Comprehensive Textbook of Psychiatry/III*. 3d ed. Baltimore: Williams & Wilkins, 1981.

Kolb, L. C., and H. K. H. Brodie. *Modern Clinical Psychiatry*. 10th ed. Philadelphia: W. B. Saunders, 1982.

Millon, T. *Theories of Psychopathology*. Philadelphia: W. B. Saunders Co., 1967.

Nicholi, A. M., Jr., ed. *The Harvard Guide of Modern Psychiatry*. Cambridge: Belknap Press of Harvard University, 1978.

Rolo, C. *Psychiatry and American Life*. New York: Delta (Dell Publishing), 1963.

Wyss, D. *Psychoanalytic Schools, From the Beginning to the Present*. New York: Jason Aronson, 1973.

The ideas of goblins and sprights have really no more to do with darkness than light; yet let but a foolish maid inculcate these often on the mlnd of a child . . . possibly he shall never be able to separate them again so long as he lives but darkness shall forever afterward bring with it those frightful ideas. . . . Many children imputing the pain they endured at school to their books . . . so join those ideas together that a book becomes their aversion . . . and thus reading becomes a torment to them, which otherwise possibly they might have made the greatest pleasure of their lives.
John Locke

by Walter D. Mink, Ph.D., and the late Shirley H. Mink, Ph.D.

BEHAVIORAL AND COGNITIVE CONCEPTS

I. Introduction

A. The experimental psychology of behavior change has been the source of many concepts and techniques that have been useful in the explanation and treatment of psychiatric disorders.

B. In the first half of this century psychologists tended to emphasize the control of behavior by environmental stimuli and the alteration of behavior by the manipulation of environmental stimuli.

C. In the second half of the century there has been a shift in emphasis to a view of behavior as the outcome of the processing of environmental information in relation to the accumulated knowledge of the individual.

D. The current emphasis is more on understanding behavior in terms of cognitive process than just in terms of the acquisition of responses.

II. Interpretation

A. Those who view learning as the basis of psychiatric disorders interpret such disorders as the outcome of experiences in which inappropriate or maladaptive learning, particularly emotional learning, has occurred.

B. A major assumption is that the same principles of learning that account for the development of disordered behavior can be applied to its correction.

C. Cognitive approaches to psychiatric disorders stress the distortions that may occur in a person's belief system and the effect these distortions may have on the way expectations and judgments are expressed in behavior.

D. Cognitively based corrective approaches are directed toward altering false or unwarranted thoughts and beliefs.

III. Learning

Modern experiments in learning began in Russia with Ivan Pavlov and continue, primarily in the United States, as a fundamental research area in psychology.

A. Ivan Pavlov (1849–1936)

Pavlov was a Russian physiologist who discovered classical conditioning during his studies of digestion. He was awarded the Nobel Prize in 1903 for his achievements.

1. The conditioned reflex

Pavlov showed that a reflexive response can, with proper training, be linked to a stimulus that does not normally elicit it.

a) His famous experiments demonstrated that salivation, which occurs reflexively when food is put in the mouth, can also be caused to occur predictably in the presence of a neutral stimulus such as a bell or light.

b) His training procedure involved the presentation of a neutral stimulus (e.g., a bell) slightly before putting food in a dog's mouth. The food caused the dog to salivate. Repeated pairings of the two, bell and food, eventually resulted in salivation when the bell alone was presented.

   c) In the standard terminology of classical conditioning, a conditioned stimulus (CS), such as a bell, is repeatedly presented slightly before an unconditioned stimulus (US), such as a piece of food that elicits salivation, an unconditioned reflex or response (UR). The CS will eventually elicit the response, which is then referred to as a conditioned reflex or response (CR).

   d) Schematically:

US $\rightarrow$ UR

(food) (salivation)

CS $\rightarrow$ CR

(bell) (salivation)

2. Other phenomena in the conditioning of reflexes

   a) Extinction

When the CS is repeatedly presented without the US, the CR will decrease and eventually disappear. This phenomenon is called *extinction*.

   b) Generalization

When a subject has been trained to make a CR in the presence of a CS, the CR tends to occur as a response to stimuli that resemble the original CS. This is known as *generalization*.

   c) Discrimination

When a subject is trained to respond to the original CS and, during the same training, to ignore stimuli similar to the CS, the subject is said to exhibit *discrimination*.

3. Experimental neurosis

   a) Pavlov noted a disorganization in the behavior of animals that were required to make extremely difficult conditioned discriminations; he called this phenomenon *experimental neurosis*.

   b) Pavlov applied his analysis to the study of hysteria and obsessional neurosis and, during the late part of his career, to schizophrenia. His ideas have had a major influence on contemporary Russian psychiatry.

4. Conditioning of emotional behavior

Classical conditioning may occur particularly in learned reactions that are mediated by the autonomic nervous system, as is the case with emotional reactions.

5. Some food aversions reflect the powerful one-trial conditioning of food characteristics, such as taste or odor, to experiences of nausea or disgust.

B. Behaviorism
John B. Watson (1878–1958), an American psychologist, formulated the methodological position in psychology known as *behaviorism.*
1. Definition
   a) Watson believed that psychology should be the study of observable behavior and should avoid references to unobservable mental functions such as consciousness.
   b) Watson insisted that the experimental study of animal behavior could contribute to the understanding of human behavior and used Pavlov's principles of conditioning to explain human behavior.
2. Watson demonstrated, in 1920, that fears could be induced by classical conditioning.
   a) A one-year-old boy named Albert became fearful of a white rat, which had not frightened him previously, when a loud noise was made behind him while playing with the rat.
   b) After a few trials, Albert became fearful of any white rat *without* the noise, and his fear became *generalized* to other furry animals and objects.
   c) A few years later, Mary Jones replicated Watson's findings and also demonstrated that a conditioned response (fear) could be *eliminated* by conditioning procedures.
C. Operant conditioning (experimental analysis of behavior)
B. F. Skinner (b. 1904), an American psychologist, refined Watson's methodology and explored what he called *operant conditioning.* (An operant is an action that "operates" on the environment; this kind of response is also called "instrumental.")
1. Operant behavior
   Skinner developed experimental procedures for demonstrating how the consequences of an act influence the subject's tendency to repeat the act. Operant conditioning consists in reinforcing or not reinforcing the consequences of an act so that it tends to be repeated or extinguished. There are several notable features of operant conditioning.
   a) Contingency
      Skinner has shown that the temporal relation of an act to an outcome, such as food or escape from an annoying situation, influences the likelihood that the act will be repeated. The occurrence together of the response and the consequence is called a *contingency.*
   b) Reinforcement
      In the terminology of operant conditioning, the consequence of a response is called *reinforcement.* The experiment procedure allows the subject (e.g., a rat) to perform a random act (e.g., pressing a lever). If the act results in the delivery

of food (a reinforcer), it is said to be reinforced. Repeated pairings of the response and the reinforcement will increase the subject's tendency to press the lever.

(1) *Positive reinforcement* is the presentation of a reward.

(2) *Negative reinforcement* is the removal of a noxious or aversive stimulus.

(3) In either case, the response that produces the changed situation for the subject is the one that is reinforced.

(4) *Stimulus control* of a response can also be established by reinforcing the response only in the presence of a particular stimulus, such as a light.

(5) Schematically:

S————————R ————————→ S

light   press lever   reinforcement (food)

c) Some other phenomena of operant conditioning

(1) *Extinction* means that repeated performance of a response in the absence of reinforcement will lead to a decreased occurrence of the response.

(2) *Discrimination* results when a response to one stimulus, but not to another stimulus, is reinforced. The stimulus that signals the reward becomes a *discriminative stimulus*.

(3) *Schedules of reinforcement* involve varying the amount of time between reinforcements (*interval schedule*) or the required number of responses between reinforcement (*ratio schedule*). These schedules influence the rate of the response and the resistance to its extinction.

d) Aversive learning

(1) Sometimes the consequences of a response are unpleasant or aversive and these consequences also have an effect on learning.

(2) *Punishment* occurs when an aversive or noxious stimulus follows a response. Punishment will suppress a response that produces the punishment but will not necessarily extinguish it.

(3) *Escape learning* occurs when a response is learned that terminates or allows withdrawal from the source of discomfort.

(4) *Avoidance learning* occurs when the onset of aversive stimulation is signaled by another stimulus and a response is made to the signal that prevents the onset of discomfort.

2. Application of operant conditioning

a) The principles of operant conditioning have been used to analyze social learning, aggressive behavior, classroom learning, and many other complex forms of behavior.

b) Many students and collaborators of Skinner have interpreted disordered behavior in operant terms and have developed training procedures for use in hospitals and other institutional settings.

c) *Autonomic responses*
Within limits, operant conditioning also affects autonomic responses, as in the self-regulation, through training in biofeedback, of heart rate, blood pressure, and skin temperature.

D. Social learning
1. Social learning approaches pay special attention to the ways in which people learn life skills, cultural rules, and values through interactions with others.
2. Albert Bandura emphasizes the importance of learning observationally from the models of behavior of other persons.
   a) Imitation depends on attention to the model, retention of what has been observed, reproduction of the model's behavior, and the consequences (reward, punishment) that follow the model's action.
   b) Observational learning is assumed to be particularly important in childhood and may account for the expectations that are developed about what will happen if particular actions are engaged in.
   c) Television programs, motion pictures, and literature also provide opportunities for observational learning to occur.

IV. Behavioral psychology and psychiatry
Many examples of behavioral interpretations of psychiatric concepts can be provided, but those that follow may be sufficient to illustrate the style of behavioral analysis.

A. Conflict
1. A behavioral interpretation of conflict stresses the existence of incompatible responses of equal or nearly equal probability.
2. The most compelling kind of conflict occurs when an *approach response* is elicited by the same situation in which an *avoidance response* is elicited.
3. An example of an approach-avoidance conflict might be provided by a child who enjoys playing at a neighborhood playground but has been teased there by a bully.

B. Anxiety
1. Anxiety may be interpreted as an autonomic nervous system reaction that occurs in fearsome or threatening situations but becomes conditioned to irrelevant, coincidental, or unlabeled aspects of the situation (e.g., Albert's fear of the white rat).
2. Insofar as situations that produce anxiety are aversive, learned ways to escape or avoid the situations may be reinforced.

C. Symptoms
 1. Symptoms are viewed as learned reactions that are the result of previous reinforcement (e.g., avoiding anxiety-producing situations or obtaining sympathetic support from another person).
 2. If a symptom persists in a situation, then something in the situation is reinforcing it.
 3. Symptoms, just like any other learned response, can be altered by changing the conditions of reinforcement.

V. **Behavioral research and clinical application**
 A. Laboratory studies of animal learning have sometimes produced findings of direct relevance to the interpretation of psychiatric disorders.
 B. Two examples of laboratory investigation that have influenced clinical thinking are the demonstrations of the operant conditioning of autonomic nervous system responses in rats and the investigations of learned helplessness in dogs and rats.
  1. Voluntary control of involuntary responses (Neal Miller and associates).
   a) Within limits, laboratory studies have shown operant conditioning to affect such autonomic responses as heart rate, blood pressure, skin temperature, and gastric secretion.
   b) Through biofeedback training, in which subjects receive information about alterations in autonomic indicators, humans have been able to achieve a degree of self-regulation of some autonomic processes.
   c) Biofeedback procedures directed toward altering both autonomic and muscular responses are an important component in the practice of the new field of behavioral medicine.
  2. Learned helplessness (Martin Seligman and associates)
   a) Animals given unpredictable electric shocks in a situation in which they can neither escape nor avoid the shock show a deficit in behavior in later situations where escape or avoidance is possible.
   b) When placed in situations where shock can be escaped or avoided by making appropriate responses, the animals given "helplessness" training remain in the location, receive the shock, and make no attempt to deal with the circumstances.
   c) Some human subjects show similar tendencies in learning situations that resemble those used in the studies with animals.
   d) The *learned helplessness* syndrome of loss of coping skills, failure to detect opportunities to change situations, and passive capitulation to circumstances has characteristics similar to clinical depression.

VI. Cognitive interpretations of learning

The learning approaches described in the preceding sections emphasize behavioral responses and the primarily environmental influences on them, such as stimulus conditions and reinforcing operations. The current cognitive reformulation in psychology emphasizes behavioral expressions mediated by processes that are traditionally called "mental" but are inferred from behavior.

A. Cognitive interpretations of behavior emphasize the way in which information about the environment is received, identified, and incorporated into new or existing systems of knowledge (memory).

B. Behavior in a given situation is a product of the current perceptual interpretation of the situation and relevant knowledge based on memory of previous experiences and skills.

C. Cognitive activities and processes include the following:

1. *Sensation and perception,* which are concerned with the registration and interpretation of the physical and social environment.

2. *Memory,* which is concerned with the acquisition and later utilization of knowledge about the world and individual experience in it.

3. *Thinking and problem solving,* which involve the transformation and manipulation of knowledge in order to make decisions or reassess experience.

4. *Language,* in which we encode most of our knowledge and communicate it to others.

D. Images, thoughts, memories, and other subjective mental phenomena figure prominently in the theorizing and research of cognitive psychologists in ways that strict behavioral approaches would not utilize.

E. In clinical applications, a compromise between cognitive and behavioral approaches has emerged recently, in which both external environmental stimuli and internal thought processes are viewed as controlling influences on behavior.

References

Bower, G. H., and E. R. Hilgard. *Theories of Learning.* 5th ed. Englewood Cliffs, N.J.: Prentice-Hall, 1981.

Bower, G. H., R. R. Bootzin, and R. B. Zajonc. *Principles of Psychology Today.* Part 2. New York: Random House, 1987.

Kaplan, H. I., and B. J. Sadock. *Comprehensive Textbook of Psychiatry/IV.* 4th ed. Baltimore: Williams & Wilkins, 1985.

The symptoms of disease are marked by purpose, and the purpose is beneficent. The processes of disease aim not at the destruction of life, but at the saving of it.

Frederick Treves: Address to the Edinburgh Philosophical Institution, October 31, 1905

Symptomatology of Mental Disorders

I. Introduction

A. Symptoms of mental disorders are expressions of the whole organism, not just the psyche or soma alone.

B. The manifestations of mental disorders are the result of multiple forces, some of which are extrapsychic (i.e., from the environment) and some of which are intrapsychic (i.e., from within the personality).

C. Thus, although symptoms may seem perplexing and unusual, they have cause and meaning.

   1. Symptoms represent the patient's effort to maintain his or her emotional equilibrium.

   2. In order to understand their meaning, one must know the patient's life history, including the psychological, sociocultural, and biological needs and the forces that have been of importance in the person's development.

D. Symptoms of mental disorders are really psychobiological reactions.

II. Somatic symptoms

Physical symptoms of mental disorders are of three types.

A. Physiological reflections of anxiety

Such symptoms are either

   1. The predominant manifestation of the disturbance as in panic disorders and generalized anxiety disorders, or

   2. Experienced if the person attempts to control symptoms, as in resisting obsessions or compulsions in an obsessive-compulsive disorder or in confronting the feared situation or object in a phobic disorder.

B. Physical symptoms

These symptoms are found in most somatoform disorders in which physical symptoms suggest physical disorder without demonstrable organic findings, without known physiological mechanisms, and for which there is positive evidence or a strong presumption that the symptoms are linked to psychological factors or conflicts (*DSM*-III). Such symptoms are not under voluntary control. Included among these are somatization disorder (Briquet's syndrome), somatoform pain disorder, hypochondriasis, and undifferentiated somatoform disorder.

C. Symbolic expressions of underlying conflicts

   1. Found in the conversion disorders (symbolic somatization).

   2. Examples are

      a) Hysterical deafness as a defense against hearing something feared or forbidden.

      b) Hysterical paralysis as a defense against taking action.

III. Psychological symptoms

Psychological symptoms may be manifested in many ways. They are discussed in each of the sections describing the kinds of mental disorders. However, they are presented here for ready reference.

A. Disturbances of affect (mood, feeling, or emotion)

1. Anxiety

   Anxiety may be defined as a diffuse, unpleasant uneasiness, apprehension, or fearfulness stemming from anticipated danger, the source of which is unidentifiable. It can be divided into degrees

   a) *Free-floating anxiety* is severe, persistent, generalized, and unattached anxiety. It is typically found in anxiety disorders and is often a precursor of panic.

   b) *Agitation* is a state of restlessness and uneasiness often characterized by such muscular manifestations as motor restlessness; mental perturbation. (Anxiety overflows into the muscular system.)

   c) *Tension* is tautness, motor and emotional restlessness, dread.

   d) *Panic* is an acute anxiety attack of overwhelming severity that leads to disorganization of ego functions. It produces physiological changes and terror. (The word is derived from Pan, the Greek god, who suddenly appeared to unsuspecting travelers in the woods, causing them to "panic.")

   e) *Normal anxiety (stress)*. The source of the anxiety is actual and realistic.

2. Depression

   Depression is a feeling of sadness, loneliness, dejection, or hopelessness, typically found in major depressive disorder and bipolar depressive disorder. It must be differentiated from grief, which is a state of sadness proportionate to a loss. It is extremely common in psychiatric patients.

3. Euphoria

   Euphoria is an exaggerated sense of well-being not consistent with reality. Most commonly found in manic disorders and in certain organic mental disorders, including disorders resulting from the use of toxic substances. It may be divided into degrees.

   a) *Elation* is marked euphoria accompanied by increased motor activity.

   b) *Exaltation* is intense elation accompanied by grandiose feelings.

   c) *Ecstasy* is the feeling of intense but tranquil rapture. Religious feelings are often an integral part of this feeling. It is found in dissociative states, depersonalization, convulsive disorders, and schizophrenic disorders.

4. Apathy

Apathy is the lack of feeling, emotion, interest, or concern; impassiveness or unfeelingness.

5. Inappropriateness

Inappropriateness is an affect opposite to what would be expected. Observed in schizophrenic disorders, for example, laughter when a sad message is being expressed.

6. Ambivalence

Ambivalence is the coexistence of two opposing feelings toward the same individual or object; these feeling may be conscious, unconscious, or both. It is characteristic of the unconscious of children. It is found in many emotional disorders, but especially in depressive and obsessive-compulsive disorders, and is one of the fundamental symptoms of the schizophrenic disorders.

7. Hostility

Hostility is anger, antagonism, opposition, or resistance in thought or behavior. It is the affective counterpart of aggression, to which it is closely allied. It is found in an extreme degree in antisocial personalities and in certain other personality disorders. Unexpressed and internalized hostility is important in the psychodynamics of some depressive disorders. (Violence is a behavioral expression of extreme hostility.)

8. Depersonalization

Depersonalization is the pervasive feeling of unreality, strangeness, or altered identity. Found in depersonalization disorder, schizophrenic disorder, and bipolar affective illness. It may occur in normal persons who have suffered exhaustion or shock.

9. Derealization

Derealization is the feeling that the environment has changed. Found in depersonalization disorders and characterized by alternating periods of euphoria or anxiety and depression. Found in cyclothymic disorder (cyclothymic personality).

B. Disturbances of memory

1. Definition

Memory is composed of three processes.

a). Registration

The ability to establish a record of an experience in the central nervous system.

b) Retention

The persistence or permanence of a registered experience.

c) Recall

The ability to recount a registered experience.[1]

2. All of these processes may be disturbed in various ways.

---

1. Adapted from *Modern Synopsis of Comprehensive Textbook of Psychiatry,* vol. 2. Edited by A. M. Freedman, H. I. Kaplan, and B. J. Sadock (Baltimore: Williams & Wilkins, 1976), p. 392.

3. Amnesia

   Amnesia is a pathological loss of memory. It may be of organic etiology (e.g., head injury) or psychogenic, as in certain dissociative disorders (e.g., psychogenic amnesia).

   a) *Anterograde amnesia* is loss of memory of events that occur after a particular time.

   b) *Retrograde amnesia* is loss of memory of events that occurred before a particular time.

4. Fugue state

   A *fugue state* is dissociation, a flight from the immediate environment, characterized by an inability to remember what is happening. The individual escapes from the environment and, during this state, apparently acts purposefully. However, when the person regains consciousness, he or she cannot recall the episode, or fugue. Found in psychomotor equivalents of convulsive disorders and also in the dissociative disorder, psychogenic fugue.

5. Hypermnesia

   Hypermnesia is abnormally vivid or complete memory, or the reawakening of impressions long seemingly forgotten. Found both in normal persons and in certain manic and paranoid disorders.

6. Paramnesia

   Paramnesia is a distortion or falsification of memory in which the individual confuses reality and fantasy. It includes the illusion of remembering scenes and events not experienced before.

   a) *Confabulation* is a falsification of memory in which gaps in memory are filled in by imaginary (fabricated) experiences that seem plausible and are recounted in detail. Found in certain organic mental disorders, especially alcohol amnestic disorder (Korsakoff's syndrome).

   b) *Retrospective falsification* is the unconscious distortion of past experiences to conform to present emotional needs. Found in certain paranoid disorders.

   c) *Fausse reconnaissance* is a false recognition of the unfamiliar.

   d) *Déjà vu* is the sensation that an experience that is really happening for the first time has occurred previously. Occurs in normal people and is found in many mental disorders.

   e) *Jamais vu* is a false feeling of unfamiliarity with a real situation that one has experienced before.

C. Disturbances of consciousness

   1. Definition

      a) *Consciousness* is synonymous with awareness, "clear mindedness."

      b) It also means *apperception,* a mental act in which the mind becomes aware or has knowledge of itself as it perceives.

   2. Both of these aspects of consciousness may be distorted.

3. Confusion

   Confusion is disorientation in respect to time, place, or person and is accompanied by perplexity. Sometimes accompanied by disturbances of consciousness and commonly associated with organic mental disorders.

4. Clouding of consciousness

   Clouding of consciousness is impairment of retention, perception, and orientation. Commonly associated with organic mental disorders, both acute and chronic.

5. Dream state

   Dream state is also known as twilight state. It is a transient clouding of consciousness of intrapsychic origin during which the person is unaware of reality and behaves violently or opposite to his or her usual pattern. Found in dissociative disorders, convulsive disorders, and in association with the use of certain drugs (e.g., scopolamine or atropinelike drugs).

6. Delirium

   Delirium is characterized by disturbance in affect, orientation, memory, and consciousness. There are obvious changes in mood, there are illusions, and there are hallucinations. Delirium may be caused by any agent that produces temporary and reversible cerebral metabolic insufficiency, such as alcohol or drugs. Also seen in delirious disorders from acute infectious diseases.

7. Coma

   Coma is stupor, a state of unawareness, nonreactiveness, profound unconsciousness. Found in certain organic mental disorders and in the stuporous form of catatonic schizophrenia.

8. Deterioration

   Deterioration, or dementia, is the progressive loss of intellectual and emotional functions. Found in degenerative diseases of the brain such as Alzheimer's disease, and in primary degenerative dementia. Reversible deterioration is found in schizophrenic disorders.

D. Disturbances of orientation

1. Definition

   Orientation is awareness of one's relationship to time, surroundings, and other persons.

2. Disorientation

   Disorientation is loss of awareness of one's relationship to time, surroundings, or other persons. Usually reversible in certain substance-induced disorders (toxic deliria) and irrevisible in chronic mental disorders such as senile and presenile dementia.

3. Disorientation in respect to time is the most common, followed by place and person.

E. Disturbances of perception
  1. Definition
  Perception is the awareness and intended integration of sensory impressions of the environment and their interpretation in light of experience.
  2. Perception may be disturbed or heightened in several ways.
  3. Illusions
  Illusions are misinterpretations of sensory experiences, usually optical or auditory. They are frequently normal.
     a) *Optical illusions* are sometimes called mirages as, for example, when heat rays shimmering on a road look like pools of water. Common in acute but reversible substance-induced disorders such as the withdrawal delirium from alcohol, also known as delirium tremens.
     b) *Auditory illusions* are mistaken interpretations of sounds as, for example, the roaring of the wind heard as the moaning of a human voice.
  4. Hallucinations
  Hallucinations are false sensory perceptions that are not caused by external stimuli.
     a) They may be auditory, visual, olfactory, gustatory, tactile (haptic), or kinesthetic (phantom limb is a kinesthetic hallucination).
     b) Hallucinations occur in substance use disorders (caused by alcohol, cocaine, or hallucinogenic drugs such as LSD, peyote, or mescaline). May also be found in certain other psychotic conditions such as schizophrenic and manic disorders. Different types of disorders tend to produce different types of hallucinations.
        (1) Colorful or vivid *visual hallucinations* are most typically found in the deliria from acute infectious diseases or in the substance-induced delirious disorders.
        (2) *Auditory hallucinations* are commonly found in schizophrenic disorders.
        (3) *Olfactory hallucinations* occur in schizophrenic disorders and in lesions of the temporal lobe of the brain.
        (4) *Tactile hallucinations* (hallucinations of touch) are found in cocaine intoxication and alcohol withdrawal delirium (delirium tremens).
        (5) *Kinesthetic hallucinations* are found in phantom limb syndrome.
     c) An exception to these generalizations about hallucinations is amphetamine-induced organic mental disorder, which commonly produces auditory hallucinations, and sometimes tactile and olfactory ones as well.

d) *Hypnagogic hallucinations* (hypnagogic imagery) are mental images that sometimes occur just before sleep. Images seen in dreams that persist after awakening are called *hypno-pompic*. Both types are normal and are familiar to healthy individuals. Hypnagogic states, in particular, are sometimes experienced by persons who are very tired but unable to find the time or place to sleep. Some believe that hypnagogic and hypnopompic hallucinations are found more frequently in persons who ultimately develop hypersomnolence or narcolepsy.

In *Oliver Twist*, Charles Dickens writes: "There is a drowsy state between sleeping and waking when you dream more in five minutes with your eyes half-open and yourself half-conscious of everything that is passing around you, than you would in five nights with your eyes fast closed, and your senses wrapped in perfect consciousness. At such times, a mortal knows just enough of what his mind is doing to form some glimmering conceptions of its mighty powers, its bounding from earth and spurning time and space, when freed from the restraint of its corporeal associate."

Edgar Allan Poe was concerned with such sleepless dreams. In *Marginalia* he writes: ". . . these 'fancies' have in them a pleasurable ecstasy as far beyond the most pleasurable of the world of wakefulness or of dreams, as the Heaven of the Northman theology is beyond its Hell. I regard the visions, even as they arise, with an awe which in some measure moderates or tranquilizes the ecstasy."

e) Both hallucinations and illusions may occur in normal people during prolonged periods of isolation.

f) Pseudohallucinations are transient visual perceptual distortions that may be associated with anxiety or fear.

g) Night terrors (pavor nocturnus) are nightmares occurring in children in which they awaken screaming with fright, the alarm persisting for a time during a state of semiconsciousness. They remain in a twilight state and cannot be awakened. They then fall into a deep, peaceful sleep. There is complete amnesia for the attack as well as the dream content (Campbell).

5. Eidetic imagery
Eidetic imagery consists of vivid, accurate, and detailed visual afterimages sometimes called photographic memory. Such experiences are normal and are to be distinguished from hallucinations. "Perhaps the artists have a greater eidetic power than most adults," wrote Franz Boaz. It is found frequently in young children, much less frequently in adults.

6. Misperceptions
Misperceptions are associated with conversion disorders (hysterical misperceptions).

a) Perceptual distortions may occur in any of the sensory areas.

b) Sensation may be exaggerated or, more commonly, reduced. For example, *hyperesthesia* and *hyperalgesia* or, conversely, *hypesthesia* and *hypalgesia* may occur in conversion disorder.

c) *Macropsia* is visualization of objects as larger than they really are, conversely, *micropsia* is visualization of objects as smaller than they really are.

F. Disturbances of thinking

1. Definition

   Thinking is the exercise of powers of judgment, conception, or inference, as distinguished from simple sensory perception. It is prey to many disorders.

2. Fantasy

   Fantasy, or phantasy, is a fabricated series of mental pictures or sequences of events; daydreaming.

   a) Fantasy may express unconscious conflict, gratify otherwise unobtainable wishes, or provide an escape from reality.

   b) It may serve as the springboard for creative activities.

   c) It may lead to a harmful distortion of reality.

3. Phobias

   Phobias are persistent, irrational fears of specific objects, activities, or situations. Examples include fear of height, closed spaces, open spaces, strangers, animals, dirt, or school. Certain fears, as of harmless bugs and snakes, are extremely common and not considered pathological, but phobias are typically found in phobic disorders.

4. Obsessions

   Obsessions, also called ruminations, are recurrent persistent, ideas, thoughts, images, or impulses that remain conscious despite their irrationality. Typically found in obsessive-compulsive disorders.

5. Preoccupations

   Preoccupations are excessive concerns with one's own thoughts; engrossment.

6. Delusions

   Delusions are fixed, false beliefs that are not in keeping with the individual's cultural or intellectual level. Found in various types of psychotic disorders—organic mental disorders, schizophrenic disorders, and certain of the affective disorders. They may be

   a) *Persecutory,* a belief that one is singled out for oppression, attack, or harassment.

   b) *Grandiose,* an exaggerated belief in one's own importance.

   c) *Somatic,* a deluded interpretation of physical symptoms.

   d) *Referential,* a belief that the irrelevant remarks or acts of others refers to oneself.

    e) *Influential*, a belief that one can control or be controlled by another's behavior or thoughts, most commonly observed in paranoid or schizophrenic disorders.
        (1) Ideas of *active influence,* the psychotic belief that one controls others.
        (2) Ideas of *passive influence,* the psychotic belief that one is being controlled by others.
    f) *Nihilistic,* the belief that oneself, the environment, or the world does not exist.
    g) *Self-accusatory,* the belief that one is responsible for harm.
    h) Other types of delusions include sin, guilt, impoverishment, illness, and infidelity.

7. Blocking
Blocking is difficulty in recalling or interpreting a stream of speech or thought because of emotional forces that are usually conscious. Most often found in schizophrenics who, for example, may stop talking, or block, while listening to an imaginary voice or because of conflicting reactions to the message.

8. Magical thinking
Magical thinking is the imputation of reality to a thought. "Wishing will make it so" is a primitive, prelogical idea believed by small children, encountered in dreams, and found in the thinking of obsessive-compulsive patients.

9. Incoherence
Incoherence is disorderly, illogical thought, sometimes manifested as garbled speech. Found in schizophrenic disorders, manic disorders, and certain organic mental disorders.

10. Irrelevance
Irrelevance is thinking that is erroneous or irrelevant to the subject at hand.

11. Circumstantiality
Circumstantiality is incidental or adventitious thinking. The individual cannot distinguish essentials from nonessentials, although the goal of the thinking is ultimately reached. Commonly found in manic disorder, in some organic mental disorders, and in the mentally retarded.

12. Tangentiality
Tangentiality is inability to reach the goal of the thinking.

13. Perseveration
Perseveration is a persistent, repetitive expression of a single idea in response to various questions. Found in some organic mental disorders, aphasia, and in certain types of catatonia.

14. Condensation
Condensation is the coalition of several concepts into one.

15. Psychomotor retardation
   Psychomotor retardation is the slowing down of mental and physical activity. Most commonly observed in depressive disorders, but also in some schizophrenic disorders.
16. Psychomotor excitement
   Psychomotor excitement is a mentally and physically hyperactive response to internal or external stimuli. Found in manic disorders and in some catatonic schizophrenic disorders.
17. Flight of ideas
   The *flight of ideas* is skipping from one idea to another in quick succession, without reaching the goal of the thinking. Most commonly observed in the manic disorders.
18. Autism
   Autism, or dereism, is a persistent overindulgence in fantasy. Found in child schizophrenics (pervasive developmental disorders).
19. Misidentification
   Misidentification is the incorrect identification of other people. Found in certain psychotic disorders.
20. Intellectualization
   Intellectualization is the overuse of intellectual concepts and words to avoid feeling or expressing of emotion. Found in adolescents who want to escape their sexual impulses, borderline personalities, obsessive-compulsive patients, and some schizophrenics.
21. Clang association
   Clang association is a disturbance in thinking in which the sound of a word, rather than its meaning, sets off a new train of thought. Occurs most often in manic disorders. May lead to senseless rhyming.
G. Disturbances of speech and verbal behavior
   1. Blocking (see "Disturbances of thinking")
   2. Flight of ideas (see "Disturbances of thinking")
   3. Logorrhea
      Logorrhea, or volubility, is uncontrollable, rapid, excessive talking. Most commonly observed in manic disorders.
   4. Pressure of speech
      Pressure of speech is rapid, accelerated, voluble speech that is difficult to interrupt. Sometimes found in manic disorders.
   5. Neologism
      A *neologism* is a coined word or a condensation of several words to express a complex idea. Often known simply as jargon, it is also found in certain schizophrenic disorders.
   6. Wordsalad
      Wordsalad is an incomprehensible and incoherent mixture of words and phrases. Found in some schizophrenic disorders.

7. Echolalia

Echolalia is the pathological repetition of the phrases or words of another person. Found in some schizophrenic disorders, certain organic mental disorders, and in mental retardation.

8. Echopraxia

Echopraxia is the pathological repetition or imitation of movements the subject is observing. Found in catatonic disorders.

9. Verbigeration

Verbigeration is the meaningless repetition of incoherent words or sentences. Observed in certain psychotic reactions and in certain organic mental disorders.

10. Condensation (see also, number 14 on p. 50)

Condensation is the contraction of several different ideas into one phrase, forming a collage of thought.

H. Disturbances of motor behavior, or conation

1. Definition

Conation is the basic striving of an individual as expressed in his or her behavior.

2. Psychomotor retardation (see "Disturbances of thinking")

3. Psychomotor excitement (see "Disturbances of thinking")

4. Agitation (see "Disturbances of affect")

5. Echopraxia (see "Disturbances of verbal behavior")

6. Catalepsy

Catalepsy is a generalized diminished responsiveness or immobility characterized by trancelike states. Found in organic mental disorders and certain psychogenic disorders.

7. Waxy flexibility

Waxy flexibility, or cerea flexibilitas, is a condition in which a patient passively retains the position into which he or she has been placed. Often present in catatonia.

8. Stereotypy

Stereotypy is the persistent repetition of a motor activity. Sometimes found in schizophrenic disorders.

9. Posturizing

Posturizing is the assumption and maintenance of an unusual posture, often an uncomfortable one. Most commonly observed in catatonics.

10. Mannerisms

Mannerisms are stereotyped movements such as blinking, grimacing, and gesturing. Found in schizophrenic disorders.

11. Negativism

Negativism is opposition, resistance, or refusal to accept reasonable suggestions or advice; a tendency to be in opposition. It may be passive or active. Its most extreme form is found in catatonic schizophrenic disorders.

12. Mutism

    Mutism is a form of negativism characterized by refusal to speak, either for conscious or unconscious reasons. Observed in catatonic schizophrenic disorders, profound depressive disorders, and stupors of organic or psychogenic origin.

13. Automatism

    Automatism is unconsciously directed automatic, repetitious, and symbolic behavior observed in schizophrenic, convulsive, and dissociative disorders.

14. Compulsion

    Compulsions are repetitive, compelling acts that develop in an attempt to relieve obsessions or fears. Most commonly found in obsessive-compulsive disorders and include handwashing rituals and self-mutilation.

I. Disturbances of attention

1. Definition

   Attention is the maintenance of focused consciousness to the salient characteristics of the environment.

2. Decreased attention

   Decreased attention may result from a lack of interest in or a deliberate shutting out of impinging stimulation.

3. Preoccupation

   Preoccupation is concentration on one's own problems, which may diminish attention.

4. Fluctuation

   Fluctuation of attention is a greater than normal variation, sometimes to the point of inability to attend in spite of the attempt to do so.

5. Blunting of attention

   Blunting of attention is extreme inattention, so that even noxious stimulation may not elicit a response.

6. Increased attention

   Increased attention, or hyperprosexia, is unusual attention, usually to details of personal significance.

7. Distractibility

   Distractibility is a heightened rapid fluctuation of attention, so that every new stimulus, regardless of its significance, is responded to by rapid shifts.

IV. **Usefulness of symptomatology**

A. Knowledge of the preceding symptoms is of importance in examining the mental status of the psychiatric patient.

B. The symptomatology helps to establish a working diagnosis and a treatment program.

References

Campbell, R. J. *Psychiatric Dictionary.* 5th ed. New York: Oxford University Press, 1981.

Henderson, D., and R. D. Gillespie. *Textbook of Psychiatry.* 8th ed. London: Oxford University Press, 1956.

Kaplan, H. I., and B. J. Sadock. *Modern Synopsis of Comprehensive Textbook of Psychiatry/III.* Baltimore: Williams & Wilkins, 1981.

Kolb, L. C. and H. K. H. Brodie. *Modern Clinical Psychiatry.* 10th ed. Philadelphia: W. B. Saunders Co., 1982.

Soloman, P., and V. D. Patch. *Handbook of Psychiatry.* Los Altos, Calif.: Lange Medical Publications, 1971.

Anxiety and Stress

Joy, interrupted now and again by pain and terminated ultimately by death, seems the normal course of life in nature. Anxiety and distress, interrupted occasionally by pleasure, is the normal course of man's existence.

**Joseph Wood Krutch:
"May,"** *The Twelve Seasons*
(1949)

I. Introduction

Anxiety has played a key role in psychodynamics and psychopathology. Earlier in this century, anxiety was the central concept in the theory of neurosis and was considered to be a major factor to be understood in other psychiatric disorders as well. During the past twenty-five years, anxiety has come to be less of a primary theoretical concept but is still a useful term for identifying both a subjective state and a pattern of response that are common in normal experience as well as in psychiatric practice. During the same time, "stress" has become a prominent concept in psychiatry and is a common term in popular usage. Although the terms are not interchangeable, it is appropriate to discuss them together.

II. Definition

A. *Anxiety,* in psychiatric usage, can be defined as a diffuse unpleasant uneasiness, apprehension, or fearfulness stemming from anticipated danger, the source of which is uncertain or unidentifiable.

B. *Stress* refers to conditions that are extremely unpleasant, noxious, or demanding that produce both the experience of stress (often characterized as anxiety) and effects on the behavior and physiological state of the individual.

III. Character of anxiety

A. Anxiety is really an alerting process, warning the individual of impending danger and stimulating him or her to deal with the threat.

B. It is a highly distressing psychic state, and for this reason one is usually unable to tolerate the symptoms for any sustained period. To deal with it, or manage it, an individual usually enlists one of the coping mechanisms or one of the defense mechanisms.

C. Anxiety is similar to fear.
1. Both are felt responses to danger and have similar physiologic reactions.
2. The distinction between anxiety and fear, the fortuitous result of an error in translating the word *angst* from Freud's original work into English, has been overdrawn. Apparently Freud himself did not distinguish appreciably between the two.
3. Nevertheless, anxiety, in the psychiatric sense, differs from fear. Anxiety is (a) intrapsychic, from within the personality, in origin; (b) a response to an unknown or unrecognized threat; (c) conflictual; and (d) often chronic.

D. Anxiety produces physiological changes during which the body is alerting itself and preparing for vigorous bodily activity (fight or flight).
1. Certain bodily processes are stimulated and others are inhibited.
   a) The cardiovascular system is stimulated. The heart beats faster and blood pressure is maintained or elevated to force more blood to the muscles. The liver secretes sugar and the adrenal glands produce epinephrine.

b) The gastrointestinal system is inhibited. Its secretions and peristaltic activity are reduced.

2. These bodily adjustments prepare the organism for activity. The blood that is temporarily removed from the gastrointestinal tract is made available to the muscular system.

3. These adjustments are under the control of the sympathetic division of the autonomic nervous system.

4. Biological and psychological defenses are mobilized by anxiety to ensure survival.

IV. **Role of anxiety**

A. Anxiety occupies a focal position in the dynamics of all human adjustment.

1. It is a normal response to threat.

2. It is the driving force for most of our adjustments. For example, anxiety resulting from concern about financial security may drive one individual to accumulate excessive wealth, stimulate another to plan a realistic investment, insurance, and retirement program, and cause still a third individual to become completely dependent.

3. The pattern for developing anxiety is inborn and always available. Evidence of this has been noted by child psychiatrists, who have described the underlying *universal* anxieties that are normally associated with the infant's anaclitic dependency on the mother.

a) *Separation anxiety* is the apprehension noted in infants when they are removed from their mothers or mother surrogates. It is most marked from the sixth to the tenth month.

b) *Stranger anxiety* is the apprehension noted in infants when they are approached by strangers.

c) *Nocturnal anxiety* is the infant's fear of the dark.

B. The mechanisms for coping with anxiety and the defenses against it form the basis of psychodynamics and psychopathology. These are discussed in the following chapter, "Adaptations to Anxiety."

C. The consistent utilization of certain defenses leads to the development of personality characteristics or character traits (see chapter, "Personality Disorders").

V. **Components of anxiety**

A. The manifestations of anxiety occur at three levels.

1. Neuroendocrine

Neuroendocrine refers to the chief hormone adrenaline, or epinephrine, secreted by the medulla of the adrenal glands. It is related to norepinephrine, which, in turn, is related to mood disturbance and depression. It accounts for the physiological responses listed below.

2. Psychic

The *psychic* manifestation of anxiety is the sensation of apprehension and the cortical perception of discomfort. It thus includes the appreciation of the physical responses as well as the awareness of the apprehension.

a) Although the individual consciously perceives and realizes the apprehensiveness, the cause of the anxiety usually escapes awareness.

b) There are degrees of anxiety (see "Disturbances of affect" in the previous chapter).

3. Somatic

The *somatic,* or motor-visceral, manifestations of anxiety are the result of the physiological responses of the various bodily systems to the increased secretion of epinephrine.

a) *Dermatological response.* The skin becomes pale, sweat is secreted, the skin hairs become erect, and there is a shivering of the superficial musculature.

b) The *cardiovascular response* usually includes tachycardia or palpitations, an increase in systolic blood pressure, and premature contractions. Occasionally, the cardiovascular response is one of decreased activity, with resulting faintness.

c) *Gastrointestinal response.* The salivary glands are inhibited, with resultant dryness of the mouth. In addition, the individual may experience a foul taste in the mouth, anorexia, nausea, vomiting, cramps, distension, "butterflies in the stomach," diarrhea, or constipation.

d) The *respiratory response* may include rapid breathing, sighing, or hyperventilation.

e. The *genitoruinary response* may include urinary urgency, urinary frequency, dysmenorrhea, dyspareunia, frigidity, impotence, or pelvic pain.

f) The *vasomotor response* may be sweating or flushing.

g) The *musculoskeletal response* may be manifested as trembling muscles (often first seen in the lips), dilation of the nostrils, tension headache, constriction in the back of the neck (cervical muscle tension), quavering voice, complaints of arthritis or arthralgia, or various other symptoms in muscles or joints.

h) The *pupillary response* is dilation (mydriasis).

VI. **Reactions to anxiety**

There is wide variance in individual patterns of response to anxiety.

A. Behavioral

Some individuals evince only behavioral reactions, such as hyperalertness, irritability, fidgetiness, overdependency, preoccupation, or constriction of activity or concentration.

B. Somatic
   1. Some have primarily *visceral* reactions in one or more of a number of systems, for example, the cardiovascular system, the gastrointestinal tract, the genitourinary system, the respiratory system.
   2. Others have symptoms primarily of *muscular tension,* for example, backache, pain in the joints, or headache due to cervical muscle spasm.
   3. Others have *combinations* of visceral and muscular responses.
   4. Why different organ systems are involved in different patients remains incompletely understood.

VII. Interpretations of anxiety

A. Anxiety is essential to survival. It is emotional pain that serves as a warning or an alerting process, like physical pain.

B. Anxiety is often a protective symptom. One could view an emotional world without anxiety as very similar to a physical world without friction.

C. During personality development, various adjustive mechanisms evolve to protect the individual from anxiety.

D. Cultural factors—including religion, education, one's value system, and one's degree of sociocultural integration—influence the production of anxiety.

VIII. The character of stress

Stress is defined and discussed in a variety of ways but commonly the description of stress includes the following:

A. The external events or *stressors* that affect the individual.

B. The individual differences in the interpretation and recognition of stressors and their impact.

C. The effects on the individual of stress.
   1. Subjective experience of stress
   2. Physiological and behavioral effects of stress
   3. Much of what has been presented above about components of anxiety applies equally to the effects of stress.

D. The coping strategies used by the individual to adjust to the situation.

IX. The general adaptation syndrome

Hans Selye has described a sequence of stages that the body passes through when stress is particularly intense or prolonged.

A. The *alarm reaction* is the first response to stress, the "emergency" reaction that prepares the body for activity as described in III. D. above.

B. The *stage of resistance* is the adaptation to persisting stress, which reduces the excesses of the alarm reaction, but may also introduce some potentially maladaptive features.

C. The *stage of exhaustion* follows prolonged stress in which the adaptation of the stage of resistance leaves the individual vulnerable to and unable to respond appropriately to additional stress.

D. Selye's general adaptation syndrome has been applied particularly to the interpretation of stress-related diseases but it also provides a useful way to think about psychological adaptation and defense.

X. **Stresses that create anxiety**

Theoretically, anxiety can result from all sorts of stimuli (psychosocial stressors) without any awareness on the part of the individual.

A. Anxiety can occur from conflict between
   1. The external world and the ego (extrapsychic).
   2. The instinctual drives and the censoring forces (intrapsychic).

B. Cultural factors can play an important role in the production of anxiety.

C. Psychosocial stressors are often highly individual. They depend upon the following:
   1. The individual's vulnerability
   2. The nature of the stress
   3. The individual's ego resources, including capacity to cope and available defenses

D. *DSM*-III-R provides a scale for Axis IV. Severity of Psychosocial Stressors.
   1. The scale ranges from mild to catastrophic.
   2. Stressors are specified as either *acute* (duration less than six months) or *enduring* (duration greater than six months).

E. Types of psychosocial stressors considered in *DSM*-III-R
   1. Conjugal (marital and nonmarital)—for example, discord, separation
   2. Parenting—for example, illness of a child
   3. Other interpersonal relations—for example, problems with a neighbor
   4. Occupational—for example, retirement
   5. Living circumstances—for example, moving to another city
   6. Financial—for example, stock market crash
   7. Legal—for example, arrest
   8. Developmental—for example, "reaching 50"
   9. Physical illness or injury

XI. **Managing stress**

A. Because *stress* is a highly distressing state, individuals usually act to reduce it or be rid of it, by conscious or unconscious mechanisms.
   1. Conscious attempts to *manage stress* are often called *coping mechanisms*.
   2. Unconscious ways of handling stress effects are called *defenses*.

B. Coping techniques

In his book, *Work Stress,* Alan A. McLean lists a number of ways to improve one's ability to cope with stress (or anxiety) and, hence, to reduce to some degree one's vulnerability. Among these are the following:

1. Personal planning

   This can be done at two levels

   a) The concrete level—consideration is given to education, career, geography, monetary needs, family needs, and lifetime goals and objectives.

   b) Assessments of one's assets and limitations.

2. Life-changing philosophies

   In a world of increasing change, all aspects of society are reevaluated and challenged. Alternatives to traditional values appear at a rapid rate.

   a) Some of these are therapeutic (transactional analysis, behavior modification, reality therapy, logo therapy, psychodrama).

   b) Others are aimed at increasing self-awareness and self-actualization (the human potential movement, est, mind control).

   c) Others are concerned with alternative life-styles (marriage encounter groups, Synanon, gay liberation).

   d) Many focus on largely physical experience (jogging, massage, bioenergetics, the martial arts).

3. The use of physical and mental exercises for the essentially healthy person, to aid in more successful adaptation (meditation, transcendental meditation, exercise, progressive relaxation, biofeedback).

C. Since much of the symptomatology of the common clinical psychiatric syndromes is based on the various defense mechanisms, they will be reviewed briefly in the next chapter before discussion of the individual psychiatric disorders.

References

American Psychiatric Association. *Diagnostic and Statistical Manual of Mental Disorders.* 3d ed., rev. Washington, D.C., 1987.

Blum, G. S. *Psychodynamics: The Science of Unconscious Mental Forces.* Belmont, Calif.: Brooks/Cole, 1966.

Eaton, M. T., Jr., M. H. Peterson, and J. A. Davis. *Psychiatry.* 4th ed. Garden City, N.Y.: Medical Examination Publishing Co., 1981.

Goldberger, L., and S. Breznitz, eds. *Handbook of Stress.* New York: The Free Press, 1982.

Kolb, L. C., and H. K. H. Brodie. *Modern Clinical Psychiatry.* 10th ed. Philadelphia: W. B. Saunders Co., 1982.

McLean, A. A. *Work Stress.* Reading, Mass.: Addision-Wesley, 1979.

I shall cut my coat after my cloth.

John Haywood: (1497–1580)
Proverbs, Part 1, Chapter VIII

Adaptations to Anxiety: Coping and Defense Mechanisms

I. Introduction
A. Individuals usually comport themselves in a fairly predictable, consistent fashion. Although there may be some variation in their behavior, their psychological adaptation is generally in a state of equilibrium. Such a state of emotional poise usually results from their having accumulated a store of problem-solving mechanisms during periods of growth and development. Thus, when they are confronted with the usual stresses of life, called *psychosocial stressors,* they have a variety of effective ways in which to adapt to conflict and frustration.

B. Conscious efforts are regarded as *coping mechanisms. Defense mechanisms* are outside the boundaries of awareness. We are unaware of them as long as they are working well.

C. Most of one's daily frustrations and conflicts can be resolved by conscious and deliberate coping mechanisms. More complex frustrations and conflicts are largely dealt with through unconscious defense mechanisms.

D. We all use defense mechanisms continually. They are not in themselves pathological unless they are so overused that they distort reality or limit the flexibility of our adpative behavior. As a matter of fact, defense mechanisms often result in gains; the sublimation of aggressiveness, for example, may result in a successful career in a competitive sport.

II. Definition of defense mechanisms
A. *Defense mechanisms* are specific, unconscious, intrapsychic adjustments that come into play to resolve emotional conflict and reduce the individual's anxiety.

B. They are also called *mental mechanisms, mental dynamisms, ego defense mechanisms, and adjustive techniques.*

III. Character of defense mechanisms
A. They are automatic, not planned; and economical, not wasted.

B. They have a purpose.
   1. They keep us from becoming anxious or they reduce our anxiety.
   2. They protect the ego.
   3. They maintain repression.

C. They are part of both normal and abnormal adjustments and can be regarded as protective devices.

D. Behavioral theorists would stress the effectiveness of defense mechanisms as avoidance or escape reactions, the learning of which is reinforced by the reduction or termination of aversive stimulation, such as anxiety.

E. Pragmatically, defenses are of two types.
   1. Successful
      Successful defenses are those that eliminate the need for immediate gratification or provide substitute, socially acceptable gratification. Some authorities use the term *sublimation* for successful defenses.

2. Unsuccessful

Unsuccessful defenses do not do what is described in 1, and hence do not resolve the conflict and the continuing need for the defense. Thus, there is a repetition of the defense. They also may not reduce the anxiety sufficiently.

IV. Specific defenses

A. Repression

Repression is the involuntary, automatic banishment of unacceptable ideas, impulses, or feelings into the unconscious (motivated unconscious forgetting).

1. It is best known of all the ego defenses and one of the most commonly employed.

2. It retains the central position in psychodynamic theory that was allotted to it by Freud in relation to ego defenses and symptom formation.

3. It is sometimes used as a generic term for all defense mechanisms. It is a primary defense against anxiety and as such is considered the cornerstone of psychodynamics. If it is unsuccessful in preventing anxiety, it may then be coupled with other defense mechanisms to permit the emergence of repressed material in disguised form. Two such combinations follow.

   a) *Repression plus displacement,* also termed *focalization,* produces phobic responses that veil the repressed wish. For example, a thirty-six year-old mother developed the fear that her two-year-old daughter would contract a serious illness. The phobia was a defense against her repressed hostility toward, and rejection of, the girl.

   b) *Repression plus conversion,* also termed *symbolic somatization,* produces a hysterical response. For example, a twenty-year-old soldier developed paralysis of his right hand when firing on the rifle range. His paralysis was a defense against his repressed hostility toward his father, who had abandoned the family.

4. In psychodynamic theory, conflicts that remain repressed are unchanged in quality and intensity. Because they retain their dynamic drive, they constantly seek expression. This is usually called *cathexis.* This requires a constant expenditure of emotional energy, *countercathexis,* to prevent the conflictual material from appearing in awareness. Often such repressed material reemerges in other ways: in our dreams, for example, in slips of the tongue, or in other aspects of everyday behavior. Freud referred to these as *the psychopathology of everyday life.*

5. Not all repressed conflicts cause psychopathology in the individual. Repression is a universally used defense mechanism. For example, we all sometimes forget the name of a well-known person or a frequently called telephone number. Only if abnormal behavior results is repression considered pathological.

B. Suppression

Suppression is the voluntary, intentional relegation of unacceptable ideas or impulses to the foreconscious (volitional exclusion, or conscious forgetting).

1. Technically, since suppression is a conscious process, it is not considered a true defense mechanism by many authorities.
2. The conflict can be readily recalled because it remains in the foreconscious.
3 It is a commonly employed coping mechanism of normal personalities and, thus, is considered a mature defense.
4. Conscious control requires a strong ego.
5. Examples of suppression
   a) A person who behaved foolishly under the influence of alcohol the previous evening may consciously try to forget the behavior the following day.
   b) A student who wishes to study for an examination may consciously set aside distracting fanstasies.

C. Regression

Regression is the unconscious return to an earlier level of emotional adjustment at which gratification was assured.

1. The retreat may be partial, total, or symbolic.
2. Many symptoms of emotional disorder have a regressive aspect, since mature modes of adjustment are replaced by behavior that represents a reversion to an earlier level of adjustment. It is not a desirable adaptation because, in the process, some developmental maturity is lost.
3. Regression may occur normally, as in the following examples:
   a) It occurs normally in play and sleep.
   b) A toilet-trained, firstborn child may temporarily lose bladder and bowel control in response to the arrival of a second child in the family.
   c) A person promoted to a more responsible position may experience the rearousal of underlying uncertainty, insecurity, and indecision, and hence ask to be returned to the old job.
   d) A person hospitalized for any kind of illness may experience the rearousal of underlying, unmet dependency, and hence make unnecessary requests and demands for attention and care.
4. Regression may be a symptom of pathology.
   a) Excessive dependence on oral gratification can represent a return to the breast. This is seen, for example, in alcoholics.
   b) It is a primary defense in the production of obsessive-compulsive disorders.
   c) Schizophrenia is profound regression, in the psychological sense. In the more severe forms, regression is seen in many aspects of the individual's personality.

D. Fixation

Fixation is the arrest of maturation at an immature level of psychosexual development.

1. Fixation may occur when there is excessive gratification or excessive frustration at a particular developmental level.
2. Examples of fixation
    a) An overly dependent attachment to a parent that remains the same over a long period.
    b) Persistence of enuresis into adolescence.
    c) The continued attachment to a nursing bottle beyond infancy.
    d) The infantile behavior sometimes seen in psychosis may be interpreted as fixation or regression.

E. Identification

Identification is the unconscious, wishful adoption, or internalization, of the personality characteristics or identity of another individual, generally one possessing attributes that the subject envies or admires.

1. Normal identification
    a) Identification plays a decisive role in normal personality development, especially the development of the superego (including the conscience), and occurs within the family setting. It requires the continuing presence and emotional support of the parenting ones.
    b) Normally, a boy identifies principally with his father, a girl, with her mother.
    c) Children often emulate other important parent figures, for example, teachers, scout leaders, athletes, or television and movie personalities.
    d) A person's adult identification, or adult individuation, evolves from the success of identification with all of these important figures.
    e) Identification is to be distinguished from imitation, which is a conscious mimicking of the behavior of others.
    f) *Empathy* is the capacity for participating in, or vicariously experiencing, another's feelings, volitions, or ideas. This ability to feel with another is a form of identification found in mature, well-integrated personalities.
    g) The transference occurring in the therapist-patient relationship in psychotherapy may be based on identification with important figures in one's early life. (See Treatment in Psychiatry: Psychotherapy.)
2. Identification may be distorted.
    a) A person may internalize certain undesirable personality traits of parent or authority figures. This is sometimes called *hostile identification*.

      b) Identification with the aggressor is the unconscious internalization of the characteristics of a frustrating or feared person.

      c) A severely pathological kind of identification is seen in the psychotic person who believes he or she is God or some other important personage.

      d) This mechanism operates in shared paranoid disorder, or folie a deux (see the chapter, "Delusional (paranoid) Disorders").

F. Incorporation

Incorporation is a primitive defense mechanism in which the psychic image of another person is wholly or partially assimilated into an individual's personality. Incorporation is a psychoanalytic term.

1. It is a special type of introjection (see the following).
2. It is the primary mechanism in identification.
3. It is assumed to begin during the oral phase of personality development and to be related to the nursing experience. An example is the infantile fantasy that the mother's breast has been ingested and has become a part of oneself.

G. Introjection

Introjection is the symbolic internalization or assimilation (taking into oneself) of a loved or hated person or external object.

1. This mechanism is the converse of projection (see the following).
2. It is sometimes regarded as a form of identification. It is also closely related to incorporation.
3. It plays a fundamental role in the early development of the ego (it antedates identification).
4. It also plays an important role in the development of the superego; that is, the child internalizes parental values and ideals.
5. It operates in the process of mourning, sadness appropriate to a loss.
6. It tends to obliterate the distinction between the loved object and the person.
7. Instead of expressing anger or aggression toward others, people sometimes turn these unacceptable tendencies into self-criticism, self-depreciation, and self-accusation. This is also referred to as turning against the self.
8. In depressive disorders, individuals direct unacceptable aggressive and hostile impulses toward themselves—that is, toward the introjected objects or persons within themselves.

H. Projection

Projection is the attributing, to another person or object, the thoughts, feelings, motives, or desires that are really one's own disavowed and unacceptable traits.

1. Normal projection
   a) Mild forms of projection are normal, everyday activities. We call them alibiing: the "blind" referee, the unfair supervisor, the scapegoat, and various prejudices and other types of suspiciousness and hypervigilance to external danger.
   b) In mythology, human qualities are often attributed to non-human things or events. This is also called anthropomorphism. In the novel *Main Street,* by Sinclair Lewis, Carol Kennicott takes a walk in Gopher Prairie shortly after her arrival. Looking up the street, "oozing out from every drab wall, she felt a forbidding spirit which she could never conquer."
   c) Many of us are often critical of our own shortcomings in other people and, as a consequence, tend to hold others responsible for our own difficulties.
2. Projection as a symptom
   a) To some extent, projection, like rationalization (see the following), is a misinterpretation or distortion of reality, and hence is potentially dangerous.
   b) It is associated with immaturity and vulnerability.
   c) It is a form of displacement and closely associated with denial (see the discussion of denial on page 72).
   d) In a pathological sense, this is the mechanism operating in paranoid disorders of all types (paranoia, shared paranoid disorder, acute paranoid disorder, and paranoid schizophrenia). If the ego becomes disorganized, it leads to
      (1) Delusions or *projected ideation.* The ego loses the capacity to distinguish inner fantasies from external reality.
      (2) Hallucinations, or projections of perception.
      (3) Ideas of reference, also a projection of ideation.

I. Rationalization

Rationalization is the ascribing of acceptable or worthwhile motives to one's own thoughts, feelings, or behavior that really have unrecognized motives. One does something and invents a reason for the action. It can also be thought of as unconscious, retrospective justification.

1. Rationalization, which is an unconscious mechanism, is not to be confused with pretending or lying, both of which are conscious processes because the individual recognizes that the "reasons" for his or her behavior are fictitious.
2. It is a very common defense. Much of our behavior has multiple determinations; that is, several motives are involved. When we "explain" our behavior by the most acceptable of these motives, we are rationalizing.

3. It helps one preserve self-respect and avoid accountability and guilt.
4. It can even be positive in that it enhances self-esteem.
5. A minor element of truth is often involved.
6. Although rationalizing is self-protective, it is also self-deceiving and hence potentially dangerous. As J. B. S. Haldane has written, "let him beware of him in whom reason has become the greatest and most terrible of passions."
7. Examples of rationalization
   a) Punishing someone else, personally or legally, may be a rationalization.
   b) Imbibing extra cocktails may involve rationalization.
   c) The teenager who does not know how to dance, but really wants to, may say that he prefers to stay home.
   d) The "sour grapes" response is a rationalization. In Aesop's fable, *The Fox and the Grapes,* the fox, who was very hungry, strove to obtain some "charming ripe grapes." He failed, then said "let him who will take them! . . . they are green and sour."

J. Intellectualization

Intellectualization is the overuse of intellectual concepts and words to avoid affective experience or expressions of feelings.
1. It is closely related to rationalization.
2. It is a way of controlling affects and feelings by thinking about them instead of experiencing them.
3. Examples of intellectualization
   a) The adolescent who wants to avoid acknowledging his or her sexual impulses.
   b) Borderline personalities.
   c) Patients suffering from obsessive-compulsive disorders.

K. Compensation

Compensation is a conscious or unconscious attempt to overcome real or fancied inferiorities.
1. Status seems to be an important need in all of us, thus compensatory behavior is universal.
2. Compensation may be
   a) Socially acceptable. For example, the blind person who becomes proficient in music, the paraplegic who becomes successful in politics.
   b) Socially unacceptable. For example, the physically handicapped person who becomes a bully or a boor; the physically small person who becomes aggressive and domineering ("the small man syndrome" or "the banty rooster syndrome").

3. Compensation may also be
    a) Direct, that is, an attempt to achieve in an area in which one has failed.
    b) Indirect, that is, an attempt to achieve in a different field than the field in which one has failed.
4. *Overcompensation* is an exaggerated attempt to overcome inferiorities. (The term was made popular by Alfred Adler.)
5. William Wordsworth (1770–1850), in *Character of the Happy Warrior,* describes compensation:
    "who, doomed to go in company with
    pain
    and Fear, and Bloodshed, miserable
    train!
    Turns his necessity to glorious gain!"

L. Reaction formation
Reaction formation is the direction of overt behavior or attitudes in precisely the opposite direction of the individual's underlying, unacceptable conscious or unconscious impulses.
1. It is a two-step defense.
    a) An unacceptable desire is repressed.
    b) The repression is followed by the conscious expression of its antithesis (thus, employing countercathexis).
2. The conscious intent of reaction formation is often altruistic.
3. The use of this adaptive pattern often leads to the production of lasting changes in an individual's behavior. For example:
    a) Uriah Heep, the hypocritical clerk in Charles Dickens' *David Copperfield,* insists that he is a very "humble" person, but his underlying nature is detestable, sly, and conniving.
    b) "Don Juans" may be masking underlying doubts about their masculinity.
    c) Excessive politeness or courtesy may disguise underlying hostility.
    d) Overt oversolicitousness and overprotectiveness toward a child may hide a parent's hostile and rejecting feelings.
    e) Submissiveness, excessive amiability, or excessive concern may be reaction formations against underlying hostility or aggressiveness.
    f) Compulsive meticulousness may cover up strong impulses to soil.

M. Sublimation
Sublimation is the diversion of unacceptable, instinctual drives into socially sanctioned channels.
1. This is socialization of emotion.
2. It is a term often reserved for successful defense mechanisms because, while the underlying impulse is gratified and the goal is retained, they are redirected from socially unacceptable to socially acceptable paths.

3. Unlike other defenses, there is no countercathexis. The emotional energy from an unacceptable impulse is transferred to a new goal-directed activity that is decided upon by the ego and approved by the superego.
4. Since sublimation offers some gratification of the underlying instinctual drive, it is usually considered healthy and often regarded as the most desirable of the mental mechanisms.
5. Examples of sublimation
   a) Sports and games may be sublimations of hostile and aggressive impulses.
   b) Various types of creative activity may be sublimations of sexual drives.
   c) Vocational choices may be sublimations of underlying unacceptable impulses.

N. Denial

Denial is the unconscious disavowal of a thought, feeling, wish, need, or reality that is consciously unacceptable. One behaves as if the problem does not exist. Denial is to be distinguished from lying, which is a conscious process. (It is also known as negation.)
1. Dynamically, denial is the simplest form of ego defense, closely related to rationalization.
2. It is a very primitive defense mechanism, much used by young children. The shutting of the infant's eyes, to avoid seeing a threatening situation, is the prototype of this defense.
3. Denial is also sometimes used to defend oneself against catastrophes.
4. It is also much used by deteriorated psychotics, who may replace the rejected reality with a more satisfying fantasy.
5. Examples of denial
   a) The small child who disclaims pain when a finger has been smashed in the door.
   b) The deaf individual who refuses to admit a hearing loss.
   c) The alcoholic who refuses to admit that he or she cannot handle liquor.
   d) The dissatisifed employee who believes that a change in jobs will solve all of his or her vocational problems.

O. Substitution

Substitution is an unconscious replacement of a highly valued but unattainable or unacceptable emotional goal or object by one that is attainable or acceptable.
1. It is comparable to displacement.
2. To be satisfactory, the substitutive activity must have certain similarities to the original forbidden one. For example, murderous or intensely hostile impulses may be replaced by some impersonal destructive act, such as striking a punching bag or shooting a target rifle.

P. Restitution

Restitution is the supplanting of a highly valued object that has been lost through rejection by, or death or departure of, another object.

Q. Displacement

Displacement is the redirection of an emotion from the original object to a more acceptable substitute.

1. It is closely allied to symbolization (see symbolization on page 74).
2. It is normal, as when hostile feelings are transferred from an employer to some member of the family or some other object or when various feelings are displaced onto political figures or certain minority groups.
3. Feelings of hostility toward parents are also often transferred to parent surrogates or other authority figures.
4. It also occurs in the transference-countertransference relationship in psychiatric treatment.
5. It is found in phobic disorders, where there is transference of anxiety from an unconscious conflict to an external focus.
6. It is frequently found in obsessive-compulsive disorders. For example, handwashing may result from feelings of moral uncleanness. These feelings are displaced onto dirt, which must be continually cleansed away.

R. Isolation

Isolation is the separation of an unacceptable impulse, act, or idea from its memory origin, thereby removing the emotional charge associated with the original memory.

1. The idea is set apart from its attached original affect, by countercathexis.
2. Isolation differs from repression proper, in which the idea as well as the feeling tone is kept out of awareness.
3. Although the individual consciously retains, or can recall, the painful memory of a traumatic incident, the feeling that originally accompanied it has become detached.
4. This mechanism is commonly seen in obsessive-compulsive disorder. Characteristically, the obsessive-compulsive person remains emotionally aloof from loaded situations. For example,
   a) An obsessed person feels he or she might hurt or kill someone but not have the accompanying hostile or aggressive feelings.
   b) It is the basis of many compulsive rituals.
5. It is found in the compartmentalization of two ideas that are antithetical as, for example, in the devoutly religious person who shows racial prejudice.

S. Undoing

Undoing is a primitive defense mechanism in which some unacceptable past behavior is symbolically acted out in reverse, usually repetitiously. It is also called *symbolic atonement*.

1. It is nullification by counteraction.
2. It is treating an experience as if it had never occurred.
3. It is closely related to reaction formation (magical expiation).
4. Examples of undoing
   a) An executive who has recommended that an employee not be promoted later makes complimentary remarks to the person.
   b) A person with an obsessive-compulsive disorder may undo the hostility shown at the beginning of an interview by being ingratiating at the end of the interview.
   c) Handwashing may represent expiation for antisocial or asocial activities. Repetition compulsion represents an attempt to reenact earlier unacceptable emotional experiences in order to be freed from their original unconscious meaning.

T. Dissociation

Dissociation is the unconscious detachment of certain behavior from the normal or usual conscious behavior patterns of an individual, which then function alone (compartmentalization). It is seen normally

1. In the executive who keeps his or her business from interfering with family life.
2. In sleepwalking, or somnambulism, sleeptalking, and automatic behavior such as automatic handwriting.
3. In the dissociative disorders, such as psychogenic amnesia, psychogenic fugue, and depersonalization disorder.
4. In multiple personalities, for example, in *Dr. Jekyll and Mr. Hyde* or *The Three Faces of Eve*. Generally, the primary character is proper and moral, whereas the secondary personality is hedonistic and impulse-ridden.
5. In schizophrenia, where there is a splitting of affect from mental content.

U. Symbolization

Symbolization is the unconscius mechanism by which a neutral idea or object is used to represent another idea or object that has a forbidden aspect.

1. There is a displacement of emotion from the object to the symbol.
2. Symbolization is based on similarity and association. The symbols protect the individual from the anxiety attached to the original idea or object.
3. Symbolization is the language of the unconscious.

4. Examples of symbolization
   a) Dreams are the most common examples of symbolization. In dreams, for example,
      (1) Elongated or projecting objects are often phallic symbols.
      (2) Openings or shrubbery may represent female genitalia.
      (3) A ship, ocean, or mothering figure may represent the mother.
   b) Affectations of speech, dress, or gait may be symbolizations.
   c) Certain psychotic symptoms such as hallucinations, muteness, posturizing, and stereotypy may have symbolic meaning.

V. Idealization

Idealization is the overestimation of admired qualities of another person or desired object. It is normally seen in
   1. Young persons who exaggerate the intelligence and attractiveness of their friends or lovers.
   2. Precinct workers who overevaluate the assets and underestimate the limitations of a political candidate.
   3. Freud said it was "the origin of the peculiar state of being in love."

W. Fantasy

Fantasy is a fabricated series of mental pictures or sequence of events; daydreaming.
   1. Fantasy may provide the basis for creative activities.
   2. Daydreams can express unconscious conflict, gratify otherwise unattainable wishes, provide an escape from reality.
   3. A disproportionate preoccupation with fantasy may lead to harmful distortion of reality.

V. Special defense mechanisms

A. Because of the current interest in borderline and narcissistic personalities (see the chapter, "Personality Disorders"), two additional defense mechanisms are of importance. They are primitive or psychotic defenses that support denial much in the way that displacement, introjection, sublimation, and the other defenses support repression. These defenses are
   1. Splitting
      Splitting is the inability to unite and integrate the hating and loving aspect of both one's self-image and one's image of another person. The loving, fantasied relationships and the hating ones are internally "split." When the individual develops positive fantasies, the negative feeling are dissociated or "split off"; when the person is frustrated, the negative fantasies are elaborated.
   2. Projective identification
      Projective identification is the association of uncomfortable aspects of one's own personality with their projection onto another person, resulting in identification with the other person.

3. For further discussion of these concepts see E. R. Shapiro, cited in the references that follow this chapter.

B. *DSM*-III-R also includes the following as defense mechanisms:

    1. *Acting-out:* a mechanism in which a person acts without reflection or apparent regard for negative consequences. For example, adolescents may "act out" expressions of underlying depression through truancy, running away, aggressiveness, and so forth.

    2. *Autistic fantasy:* a mechanism in which a person substitutes excessive daydreaming for pursuits of human relationships, more direct and effective action or problem solving.

    3. *Passive aggression:* a mechanism in which a person indirectly and unassertively expresses aggression toward others.

    4. *Somatization:* a mechanism in which a person becomes preoccupied with physical symptoms disproportionate to any actual physical disturbance.

VI. Summary

The foregoing are not all of the defenses against anxiety that have been described by various authorities, but they do include the principal mechanisms seen in the day-to-day adjustments of normal persons as well as in the major psychiatric syndromes.

References

American Psychiatric Association. *Diagnostic and Statistical Manual of Mental Disorders,* 3d ed., rev. Washington, D.C., 1987.

Blum, G. S. *Psychodynamics: The Science of Unconscious Mental Forces.* Belmont, Calif.: Brooks/Cole, 1966.

Eaton, M. T., Jr., M. H. Peterson, and J. A. Davis. *Psychiatry.* 4th ed. Garden City, N.Y.: Medical Examination Publishing Co., 1981.

Freud, A. *The Ego and the Mechanisms of Defense.* New York: International University Press, 1953.

Kaplan, H. I., and B. J. Sadock. *Modern Synopsis of Comprehensive Textbook of Psychiatry/III.* 3d ed. Baltimore: Williams & Wilkins, 1981.

Kolb, L. C., and H. K. H. Brodie. *Modern Clinical Psychiatry.* 10th ed. Philadelphia: W. B. Saunders Co., 1982.

Shapiro, E. R. "The Psychodynamics and Developmental Psychology of a Borderline Patient: A Review of the Literature." *American Journal of Psychiatry* 135 (November, 1978): 135.

Solomon, P., and V. D. Patch, eds. *Handbook of Psychiatry.* 2d ed. Los Altos, Calif.: Lange Medical Publications, 1971.

It is an irrepressible conflict
between opposing and enduring
forces.

**William H. Seward: Speech at
Rochester, New York, October
25, 1858.**

Neurotic Disorders

I. Definition
A. Neurosis, or neurotic disorders, as a cetegory has been abandoned in both *DSM*-III and *DSM*-III-R, which take an atheoretical position about mental disorders.
B. In *DSM*-III (1980) a position was taken that there was no consensus among psychiatrists as how to define "neurosis." In the introduction to *DSM*-III (1980) the term neurotic disorder ". . . refers to a mental disorder in which the predominant disturbance is a symptom or group of symptoms that is distressing to the individual and is recognized by him or her as unacceptable and alien (ego-dystonic); reality testing is grossly intact; behavior does not actively violate gross social norms (although functioning may be markedly impaired); the disturbance is relatively enduring or recurrent without treatment and is not limited to a transitory reaction to stressors; and there is no demonstrable organic etiology or factor."
C. *DSM*-III (1980) continues,
"Freud originally used the term 'psycho-neurosis' to refer to four subtypes only: anxiety neurosis, anxiety hysteria (phobia), obsessive-compulsive neurosis, and hysteria. He used the term both *descriptively* (to indicate a painful symptom in an individual with intact reality testing) and to indicate the *etiological process* (unconscious conflict arousing anxiety and leading to the maladaptive use of defensive mechanisms that result in symptom formation)."
D. Thus, *DSM*-III (1980) takes the position that the term nuerotic disorder should be used only descriptively, and the term neurotic process should be used when one wishes to indicate the concept of a specific etiological process involving this sequence: unconscious conflicts between opposing wishes or between wishes and prohibitions cause unconscious perception of anticipated danger or dysphoria, which leads to use of defense mechanisms that result in either symptoms, personality disturbances, or both.
E. *DSM*-III-R (1987) does not mention the term neurosis, neurotic disorder, or neurotic process at all. However, many physicians still accept the psychodynamic positions of neurosis and find them useful in evaluating and treating patients with certain disorders.

II. Etiology
A. There are different theories of causality, including:
1. Social learning
2. Cognitive theory
3. Behavioral theory
4. Biological models
B. However, biologic and genetic factors are not thought to be of major significance.

C. Social factors are felt by many to play some role. Cultural forces and family interactions seem to play a part in many of these disorders. Some psychiatrists feel that the family unit, rather than the individual, is the proper focus of treatment.
D. Psychogenic factors, both predisposing and precipitating, are regarded by most dynamically oriented clinicians as the basic etiological factors.
  1. Predisposing factors
     Predisposing factors operating during the early development years seem to be most significant. These include parental attitudes toward the child and the child's feelings about whether or not he or she was accepted and loved.
     a) The infant's long period of dependency on the mother seems to be a crucial factor.
     b) Disturbances of the child-parent relationship in the earliest years seem particularly significant; for example, a parent who is harsh, overprotective, or inconsistent.
     c) Thus, the therapist tries to connect the current symptomatology with some unresolved childhood conflict.
  2. Precipitating factors
     Precipitating factors, that is, immediate causes that trigger or initiate the disorders, are often evident in the development of the symptoms, which are frequently hostile, sexual, or dependent feelings.
     a) Reality may be a precipitant rather than a cause.
     b) The dehumanizing aspects or modern-day society may be a psychological threat.
  3. Therapists usually regard the etiology as a constellation of factors rather than a single cause. A more general outline of the etiology of neurosis follows the chapter, "Etiology of Mental Disorders," and is also given in the sections of the chapters describing the various types of anxiety disorders, somatoform disorders, dissociative disorders, sexual disorders, mood disorders, and so forth.
     Generally, the dynamic position of most psychiatrists has been largely psychoanalytic in orientation. For elaboration on this position, see the chapter, "Psychodynamic Concepts."

III. **Character of neurotic disorders**
  A. Repression is incomplete in the neurotic disorders.
  B. The relationship between the symptoms and underlying conflicts are usually unrecognized by the individual.
  C. The choice of defenses is in part a product of the individual's character structure, and thus, according to psychoanalytic theory, is determined by the developmental stage in which fixation occurred or from which the person's most prominent character traits were derived. Refer to the chapter, "Adaptations to Anxiety."

D. In some of these disorders, the "neurotic" compromise is never completely satisfactory because the defenses employed produce symptoms (e.g., phobias, obsessions, or compulsions) that are distressful and from which the individual seeks relief.

IV. **Types**

Neurotic disorders are manifest in diverse ways and are now classified among the following disorders in *DSM*-III-R:

A. Anxiety disorders

B. Somatoform disorders

C. Dissociative disorders

D. Sexual disorders

E. Mood (Affective) disorders

F. Some authorities also consider factitious disorders to belong to this group.

References

American Psychiatric Association. *Diagnostic and Statistical Manual of Mental Disorders.* 3d ed., rev. Washington, D.C., 1987.

Cooper, A. M., A. J. Frances, and M. H. Sacks. *The Personality Disorders and Neurosis.* Vol. 1 New York: Basic Books, Inc.; J. B. Lippincott, 1986

Kolb, L. C., and H. K. H. Brodie. *Modern Clinical Psychiatry.* 10th ed. Philadelphia: W. B. Saunders Co., 1982.

Eaton, M. T., Jr., M. H. Peterson, and J. A. Davis. *Psychiatry.* 4th ed. Garden City, N.Y.: Medical Examination Publishing Co. 1981.

My apprehensions come in crowds;
I dread the rustling of the grass;
The very shadows of the clouds
Have power to shake me as they
pass;
I question things and do not find
One that will answer to my mind;
And all the world appears unkind.

William Wordsworth: *The*
Affliction of Margaret (1804)

Anxiety Disorders

I. Definition

A. The characteristic features of this group of disorders are symptoms of anxiety and avoidance behavior.

1. In panic disorder and generalized anxiety disorder, anxiety is usually the predominant symptom and avoidance behavior is almost always present in panic disorder with agoraphobia.
2. In phobic disorders, anxiety is experienced if the person confronts the dreaded object or situation.
3. In obsessive-compulsive disorders, anxiety is experienced if the person attempts to resist the obsessions or compulsions.
4. Avoidance behavior is almost always present in phobic disorders and frequently present in obsessive-compulsive disorders.
5. The classification of post-traumatic stress disorders is controversial because the predominant symptom is the reexperiencing of the trauma, not anxiety or avoidance behavior. However, anxiety symptoms in avoidance behavior are extremely common, and symptoms of increased arousal are invariably present (*DSM*-III-R, p. 235).

B. Psychiatrically, anxiety as a symptom can be defined as a diffuse, unpleasant uneasiness, apprehension, or fearfulness stemming from anticipated danger, the source of which is unidentifiable.

II. Prevalence

A. Recent studies suggest that anxiety disorders are those most frequently found in the general population, simple phobia being the most common anxiety disorder in the general population, but panic disorder the most common in people seeking treatment (*DSM*-III-R, p. 235).

B. It is also a common symptom in general medical practice, and the physiological reflections of it are what often cause people to seek medical help.

III. Etiology

A. See chapters on anxiety and neurotic disorders.

B. Additional factors that are of importance in certain of these disorders are discussed under separate headings.

IV. Types

The anxiety disorders include the following.

A. Panic disorder with agoraphobia and Panic disorder without agoraphobia

B. Agoraphobia without history of panic disorder

C. Social phobia

D. Simple phobia

E. Obsessive-compulsive disorder (or obsessive-compulsive neurosis)

F. Post-traumatic stress disorder

G. Generalized anxiety disorder

V. Panic disorder with agoraphobia
Panic disorder without agoraphobia
  A. Definition
      1. The essential features of these disorders are recurrent panic
         attacks, that is, discrete periods of intense fear or discomfort,
         with at least four characteristic associated symptoms (short-
         ness of breath or smothering sensations; dizziness, unsteady
         feelings, or faintness; palpitations or accelerated heart rate;
         trembling or shaking; sweating; choking; nausea or abdominal
         distress; depersonalization or derealization; numbness or tin-
         gling sensations; flushes or chills; chest pain or discomfort; fear
         of dying; fear of going crazy or of doing something uncon-
         trolled). The diagnosis is made only when it cannot be estab-
         lished that an organic factor initiated and maintained the
         disturbance (e.g., amphetamine or caffeine intoxication, hy-
         perthyroidism) (*DSM*-III-R).
      2. Panic attacks typically begin with the sudden onset of intense
         apprehension, fear, or terror. Often there is a feeling of im-
         pending doom.
      3. In most cases seen in clinical settings, the person has developed
         some symptoms of agoraphobia.
  B. Definition of agoraphobia
     Agoraphobia is the fear of being in places or situations from which
     escape might be difficult (or embarrassing) or in which help might
     not be available in the event of a panic attack (as a result of this
     fear there's either travel restrictions or a need for a companion,
     "phobic partner" or "obligatory companion," when away from home,
     or there is endurance of agoraphobic situations despite intense anx-
     iety) (*DSM*-III-R).
      1. Common agoraphobic situations include being outside the home
         alone, being in a crowd or standing in a line, being on a bridge,
         and traveling in a bus, train, or car. (*DSM*-III-R).
      2. The person often develops varying degrees of nervousness and
         apprehension between attacks, usually focused on the fear of
         having another attack. Depressive disorder is often present.
  C. Age at onset
     Usually in the late twenties.
  D. Course
     Typically, recurrent panic attacks several times a week or even daily.
      1. It may be limited to a single episode, be recurrent, or become
         chronic.
      2. Usually occurs as attacks; between attacks the individual may
         be comfortable, although more commonly he or she is some-
         what tense.

3. If the conflict is not resolved, the individual may utilize one or more of the defense mechanisms and thus develop the picture of one of the other clinical reaction types.
4. Ordinarily, the prognosis is for recurrent episodes.
5. Some cases become chronic.
6. A panic attack may be the precursor of other mental disorders, such as schizophrenia, major depressive disorder, or somatization disorder.

E. Impairment

Panic disorder without agoraphobia may be associated with no, or only limited, impairment in social and occupational functioning. Panic disorder with agoraphobia, by definition, is associated with varying degrees of constriction in life-style.

F. Complications

Psychoactive substance use disorders, particularly alcohol and anxiolytics.

G. Predisposing factors

Separation anxiety disorder in childhood and sudden loss of social supports or disruption of important interpersonal relationships apparently predispose to the development of this disorder.

H. Prevalence

This disorder is common.

I. Differential diagnosis

Disorders that can produce panic symptoms must be ruled out (e.g., hypoglycemia, pheochromocytoma, and hyperthyroidism). Also, panic attacks may be associated with withdrawal from such substances as barbiturates, caffeine, or amphetamines.

J. Etiology and pathogenesis
1. A combination of psychological, social, and biological factors in a complex causal relationship.
   a) Psychological factors include a disturbed childhood or current conflicts.
   b) Biological
      (1) A predisposition to panic and/or depressive disorders may produce hypersensitivities or biochemical and electrophysiologic pathways. Both the noradrenergic and serotoninergic pathway may be involved.
      (2) A person susceptible to panic attacks may develop "psychological" explanations that may lead to phobic response when confronted with similar circumstances (thus, anxiety results when some conflict is aroused or rearoused either by a weakening of the repressive forces or by strengthening—or reinforcement—of the underlying drive or wish). Thus, repressed conflicts press for reemergence. The symptoms are nonspecific and do not offer any clues to the underlying etiology.

However, the precipitating circumstances and the setting in which attacks occur, especially the first attack, usually give some clues to the underlying cause.

K. Treatment
1. Short-term supportive psychotherapy
This is usually indicated and includes:
a) Reassurance and support (not only verbal but attitudinal as well).
b) Clarification and education, including pointing out various dynamic and stress factors and supporting various positions and recommendations about changes. It could also include attempts to provide the patient with an understanding of panic episodes or other related states of mind. Effort should be made to explore the stimuli that trigger the panic attacks.
c) Environmental modification, including changing the environment in some way, modifying whatever stresses may be present, and family therapy.
2. Insight psychotherapy
Although most psychotherapy is aimed at giving some insight, certain cases of this disorder may require long-term interpretative, psychoanalytically oriented psychotherapy.
3. Medications
Reliance is chiefly on benzodiazepines (chlordiazepoxide, diazepam, oxzepam, lorezepam, and so forth. Newer antianxiety medications, such as alprazolam (Xanax) seem to be especially effective). Antidepressant medications such as tricyclics are sometime effective, especially if depressive symptoms occur. Some studies indicate that monoamine oxidase inhibitors are useful in patients with severe protracted panic disorder. Neuroleptic agents such as chlorpromazine or thioridazine are sometimes prescribed.
4. Deconditioning
Since much anxiety is a conditioned response, deconditioning has been tried with some success.

L. Case example

Mrs. J., a thirty-year-old housewife, sought psychiatric treatment because of the following symptoms: irritability, anxiousness, lower abdominal pain, numbness and tingling of her extremities, and fearfulness about her health. Although she had been a "nervous" person most of her life, her presenting symptoms had begun three months earlier and occurred in "attacks."

During a series of interviews, it was learned that the onset of her symptoms occurred the day her sister unexpectedly removed a niece the patient had been caring for in her home while the mother was hospitalized for delivery of a baby. Two factors in her past history were of dynamic significance: she had been the oldest girl in a large family and cared for the other siblings, especially when her mother was in the hospital having babies; and sterility—she had been unable to conceive during ten years of marriage.

Thus, recurrent anxiety attacks were precipitated in a woman desirous of having a family, who in the past had to "give up" children when the mother returned, and who again had been forced to "give up" a child.

From a dynamic viewpoint, the symptoms were manifestations of the patient's conflict between her desire for children and her inability to conceive. The fact that she had to "give up" a child three months earlier reactivated the conflict and precipitated the symptoms.

In this case, the presenting symptoms were panic attacks. The psychodynamic factors seem readily apparent in this case and were the focus of subsequent treatment.

VI. Agoraphobia without history of panic disorder

A. Definition

The essential feature is agoraphobia without a history of panic attacks.

B. Definition of agoraphobia

Agoraphobia is the fear of being in places or situations from which escape might be difficult (or embarrassing) or in which help might not be available in the event of suddenly developing a symptom that could be incapacitating or extremely embarrassing. As a result of this fear, the person either restricts travel or needs a companion ("phobic partner" or "obligatory companion") when away from home or else endures agoraphobic situations despite intense anxiety.

C. Common agoraphobic situations include being outside the home alone, being in a crowd or standing in a line, being on a bridge, and traveling in a bus, train, or car.

D. Usually the person is afraid of having a limited symptom attack (developing a single or small number of symptoms, such as dizziness or falling, depersonalization or derealization, loss of bladder or bowel control, vomiting or having cardiac distress) or in other cases the person may fear that the symptoms "could" develop and incapacitate him or her or be extremely embarrassing (*DSM*-III-R).

E. Associated features

A personality disorder, particularly avoidant personality disorder, may accompany.

F. Age at onset

Usually in the twenties or thirties.

G. Course

Typically chronic (or persistent).

H. Prevalence

Rare in clinical practice.

I. Etiology and pathogenesis
   1. The cause is not known. There may be multiple interacting factors.
   2. Some may be pathologically disposed to developing intense anxiety when threat is anticipated.
   3. Increasing anxiety is often found to have psychological basis (fear of giving way in public to unacceptable wishes). This conflict between impulses and proper social behavior leads to anxiety and thus motivates various psychological defenses such as avoidance, displacement, symbolization, repression and suppression.
   4. The specific train of thought that leads to anxiety once it becomes conscious yields to repression (and thus is out of one's awareness).
   5. Development of avoidance behavior reduces the anxiety, a reward that thus reinforces that behavior.
K. Treatment (See Section V, K.).
J. Case example

Mrs. A. W., the forty-eight-year-old wife of a small-town physician, sought psychiatric treatment because she had a fear of being in church. Actually, as she unfolded her story, she really feared leaving the home and, before she developed the fear of going to church, had become uneasy while shopping and driving the children to school. It became evident, during exploratory interviews, that the onset of this agoraphobic behavior was related to her husband's heart attack two years earlier. Since he was several years her senior, she was fearful that he might have a second heart attack that would prove fatal.

As she became aware of the relationship of her symptom to her concern about her husband's health, she was able to respond to a combined approach of psychotropic medication and a program of gradual desensitization. She began by forcing herself to attend a church of her own denomination in a nearby town and then, by degrees, finally forced herself to attend her own church and sit in the front row.

VII. Social phobia
A. Definition
The essential feature of this disorder is a persistent fear of one or more situations (the social phobic situations) in which the person is exposed to possible scrutiny by others and fears that he or she may do something or act in a way that will be humiliating or embarrassing. The social phobic fear may be circumscribed, such as fears of being unable to continue talking while speaking in public, choking on food when eating in front of others, being unable to urinate in a public lavatory, or having a hand tremble when writing in the presence of others. In other cases the social phobic fears may involve most social situations, such as general fears of saying foolish things or not being able to answer questions in social situations. If

exposed to the specific phobic stimulus, the person develops an immediate anxiety response. Marked anticipatory anxiety occurs if the person is confronted with the necessity of entering into the social phobic situations and such situations are thus usually avoided (*DSM-III-R*).

B. Prevalence

Social phobia involving fear of public speaking and social phobia involving a generalized fear of most social situations are common.

C. Associated features

Panic disorder and simple phobia commonly coexist with social phobia.

D. Course

Usually chronic.

E. Complication

Persons with social phobia are prone to abuse alcohol, barbiturates, and anxiolytics. When social or occupational functioning is severely impaired, a depressive disorder may be a complication.

F. History

1. Shakespeare described phobic behavior in *The Merchant of Venice:*

   "Some men there are love not a gaping pig:
   Some, that are mad if they behold a cat. . . ."

2. In 1872, Westphal published his classic monograph *Agoraphobia (die Agoraphobia).*
3. In 1909, Freud described the case of "Little Hans," a five-year-old who developed a phobia.

G. Symptoms

1. Aside from the phobia itself, the symptoms are ways of avoiding the feared object, activity, or situation. These obviously restrict the individual's freedom of action. The individual has focalized the anxiety and, as long as he or she can avoid the focalized object, activity, or situation, remains relatively comfortable and free of anxiety.
2. The type of fear is in part culturally determined and, as in some conversion disorders, there is a secondary gain factor. For example, fear of airplanes may develop in a person whose job requires air travel.
3. If confronted with the feared object, activity, or situation, the individual develops anxiety that varies in degree from mild uneasiness to panic.
4. The individual recognizes the unreasonableness of the phobia but is unable to control the behavior or explain the fear.
5. There are numerous types of phobias, since they can develop about almost anything.

6. Counterphobic attitude: at times persons with a phobia seek out the very situation of which they are afraid. There is a striving to master excess anxiety through repeated coping with the danger. (Such repetitive behavior makes possible the transformation of passivity to activity.) Some of the involvement in dangerous sports, such as parachute jumping and racing, may be examples of counterphobic behavior.

H. Case example

A twenty-four-year-old single man consulted a psychiatrist because of his fear of speaking before groups of people, particularly in classrooms. He reported that the first episode occurred in the sixth grade, when he was called on to recite in front of his class and that his fearfulness became more evident in high school and worsened during his college days, when he was in smaller classes where more personal participation was demanded. Whenever he had to speak to a group of people, he became shy, nervous, and short of breath.

On examination, he appeared cooperative, pleasant, but unable to look at himself in a psychological way. He did not exhibit any unusual behavior or thinking pattern throughout the interviews and, although somewhat anxious and uneasy to begin with, related later.

Psychological testing revealed that he had superior intelligence and good ego-strengths, but he seemed to view the world about him as a somewhat threatening and conflictual place in which to live. This seemed particularly true of his relationships with men, whom he regarded as competitors. Since his symptoms were not severe and he had good ego-strengths, he was urged to return to school, enroll in a course that required classroom participation, and forcibly confront himself with the situation that might make him fearful.

VIII. Simple phobia

A. Definition

The essential feature of this disorder is a persistent fear of a circumscribed stimulus (object or situation) other than fear of having a panic attack (as in panic disorder) or of humiliation or embarrassment in certain social situations (as in social phobia).

1. Types

The most common simple phobias in the general population involve animals, particularly dogs, snakes, insects, and mice. Others are claustrophobias (fear of closed spaces), acrophobias (fear of heights), and fear of witnessing blood or tissue injury and fear of air travel.

2. Exposure to the simple phobic stimulus provokes an immediate anxiety response. Marked anticipatory anxiety occurs if the person is confronted with the necessity of entering into a simple phobic situation; such situations are thus usually avoided.

3. The diagnosis of simple phobia is made only if the avoidant behavior interferes with the person's normal routine or with usual activities or relationships with others, or if there's marked distress about having the fear.

B. Associated features
Unrelated social phobia and panic disorder with or without agoraphobia are often present.
C. Age at onset
Varies, but animal phobias usually begin in childhood; blood-injury phobias usually begin in adolescence or early adulthood; circumscribed phobias of heights, driving, closed spaces, and air travel appear to begin most frequently in the fourth decade of life.
D. Course
Most simple phobias that start in childhood disappear without treatment or, those that persist into adulthood rarely remit without treatment.
E. Prevalence
Simple phobias are common in the general population but since they rarely result in marked impairment, people with this disorder rarely seek treatment.
F. Etiology and pathogenesis
1. The usual psychodynamic formulation is selected because of special unconscious symbolic significance to the individual. The meaning is repressed and displaced (see chapter, "Adaptations to Anxiety"). Rarely, unknown biological or psychosocial mechanisms cause phobic patients to acquire an ingrained and unconscious stimulus-response association, which generates fear and subsequent exposure to the phobic stimulus.
2. Why certain objects are feared and not others is unknown.
3. Agoraphobia runs in families; most social and simple phobias do not.

IX. **Obsessive-compulsive disorders (or obsessive-compulsive neurosis)**
A. Definition
The essential feature is recurrent obsessions or compulsions that are sufficiently severe to cause marked distress, are time-consuming, or significantly interfere with the person's normal routine, occupational functioning, or usual social activities or relationships.
Obsessions are persistent ideas, thoughts, impulses, or images that are experienced, at least initially, as intrusive and senseless.
Compulsions are repetitive, purposeful, and intentional behaviors that are performed in response to an obsession, according to certain rules, or in a stereotyped fashion (*DSM*-III-R).
B. Prevalence
1. Fleeting obsessions or compulsions are more or less universal.
2. Obsessive-compulsive traits are not uncommon in children and adolescents.
3. Recent community studies indicate the mild forms may be relatively common.

4. The incidence may be somewhat higher because people with this disorder often conceal their symptoms and avoid consulting a physician about them.
5. It is said that a large number of obsessive-compulsive people remain unmarried.
6. Some studies indicate that the disorder is more common among people in the upper socioeconomic class and those of high IQ.
7. Gender is apparently not a factor.

C. Symptoms
1. The symptoms may take many forms. Doubt and vacillation are prominent (folie du doute).
2. Obsessions
These recurring ideas or impulses can be about anything, but the most common themes are about violence, contamination, and doubt. Other themes are sexuality, obscenities, and religion or religious subjects (scrupulosity).
3. Compulsions
These are recurrent, compelling acts that develop in the attempt to relieve obsessions or fears. They are of two types: (1) reactions to or attempts to control the underlying obsession, and (2) direct expressions of the underlying obsessive urges. The second type is rare and similar to counterphobic measures in phobic patients.
   a) The most common compulsions involve handwashing, counting, checking, and touching.
   b) Another common compulsion is self-mutilation, for example, self-inflicted excoriation as a compulsive punishment for guilt about masturbation.
4. As can be seen from the foregoing, the obsessions are mainly asocial in nature and the compulsions are mainly "caricatures of morality." In fully developed cases, there is a 50–50 ratio between the obsessions and compulsions. Such a state of dynamic equilibrium explains the underlying indecision, uncertainty, and ambivalence of these patients.
5. Sometimes the symptoms are less specific, being manifested as a compulsive and ritualistic quality that pervades all of the individual's behavior. Thus, some individuals perform certain rituals on arising in the morning, dress according to a certain pattern, or perform daily tasks and duties in a fixed and exact sequence.
6. Sometimes the compelling idea may be neutral or indifferent, and the term *obsessive-ruminative state* is then used. The central rumination is often of a religious or philosophical nature. The matter is repeatedly meditated upon, consideration is given to the pros, cons, and imponderables, but no resolution of the matter is achieved.

7. The patient is often embarrassed about the compulsions and rituals and may go to great lengths to disguise them from others. If they become more severe or chronic, the person's ability to hide the acts becomes progressively less successful.
8. Depression and anxiety symptoms are common.
9. Frequently there is a phobic avoidance of situations that involve the content of the obsessions. For example, a person with obsessions about dirt may avoid public restrooms; a person with obsessions about contamination may avoid shaking hands with strangers (*DSM*-III-R).

D. Course and prognosis
1. The onset of obsessive-compulsive disorder may occur at any period of life, but commonly begins in adolescence or early adulthood. This is probably because this is a period when there is increased sexual awareness, conflict about dependency and independency, and so forth.
2. Obsessive-compulsive traits found in childhood often clear up or respond promptly to treatment.
3. Some episodes are transitory and relatively circumscribed. Such patients frequently have a good prognosis if they undergo psychotherapy.
4. Unfortunately, some of these reactions tend to become chronic and follow a remitting course. As such, they are often resistant to treatment.
5. In general, the prognosis is more favorable when
   a) The symptoms are of short duration.
   b) Environmental stressors are prominent.
   c) There is a good environment to return to following treatment.
   d) Interpersonal relationships are good.
6. Complications include major depression and the abuse of alcohol and anxiolytics.
7. This disorder is equally common in both males and females.

E. Etiology and pathogenesis
1. Obsessive-compulsive disorder is dynamically much more complicated than any of the other anxiety disorders.
2. Obsessions and compulsions arise in three phases: (a) an internally perceived dangerous impulse, (b) the threat of what would occur if the impulses were acted upon and, (c) the defense to avert the threat. The threat is the danger of actually harming others, fear of punishment, and the pain of guilt.
3. Repression, for some reason, is unsuccessful or only incompletely successful, and the individual makes use of other defenses to reinforce the repression. These subsequent defenses are isolation, reaction formation, undoing, and displacement (see the chapter, "Adaptations to Anxiety").

4. *Ambivalence,* coexistence of two opposing feelings toward the same individual or object, is very prominent in obsessive-compulsive patients. The feelings are usually love and hate. Ambivalence is also evident in undoing.
5. Psychopathology generally and obsessions specifically are found in the families of obsessives.
6. The premorbid personality typically has obsessional characteristics. That is, he or she is rigid, restricted, orderly, meticulous, cautious, deliberate, conscientious, and dependable. The person who possesses such compulsive qualities is also referred to as an *anankastic personality,* or *anal character* (an individual who needs to feel in control of himself or herself and of the environment). The presence of these traits does not constitute abnormality. Most of the people who have obsessive-compulsive traits do not become obsessive-compulsive patients.

   According to psychoanalytic theorists, such anal qualities develop in the infant during the period of toilet training (the anal phase of infantile sexuality). The development of obsessive-compulsive disorder represents fixation at, or regression to, this anal phase of development—a period when the superego is harsh, demanding, and punitive.
7. The function of the compulsive act is to allay (relieve) and bind (tie down or focalize) anxiety.
8. The acts are symbolic and the symbolic nature is often only discovered during psychotherapy.
9. Pathogenesis of the obsessive-compulsive disorder may be clarified by biochemical and neurophysiological studies now underway. (The capacity to regulate anxiety depends in part on the ability to maintain repression as a defense, and impairment of that function interferes with the ability to suppress unacceptable ideas and feelings. Although the mechanism of this impairment is unknown, it could conceivably have a neurobiologic component.)

F. Treatment
1. Only a small number of obsessive-compulsive neurotics enter treatment. Of the treatments available—psychotherapy, behavioral therapy, and pharmacotherapy—none is impressive.
2. Psychotherapy
   a) Intensive psychoanalytically oriented psychotherapy was at one time thought to be the treatment of choice. However, it would appear that only a small number of people with this disorder respond to such treatment. (Even the most optimistic of psychoanalytic writers are unenthusiastic about insight-oriented therapy.)

b) Supportive psychotherapy is often helpful. However, it should be kept in mind that responses to psychotherapy will often last only a matter of hours, and then the individual's doubts recur.

3. Behavioral therapy
   a) Behavioral therapy has been tried recently. In this, the underlying complexities of the disorder are largely ignored, and attempts are made to focus on the person's behavior.
   b) The treatment is similar to behavioral treatment of phobias.

4. Pharmacotherapy
   a) Anxiolygics, neuroleptics, and antidepressants are sometimes useful in relieving some of the symptoms that accompany obsessive-compulsive disorders.
   b) However, with the exception of clonimipramine, an experimental TCA with a specific antiobsessional affect, none of the known psychotropic drugs relieves the underlying stress of compulsive disorder.

5. Somatic therapy
   a) Electroconvulsive therapy has been used in the past, often with disappointing results.
   b) Prefrontal leukotomy had been performed on some patients who had chronic crippling disorders.

G. Case example

Mrs. B., a thirty-three-year-old housewife, consulted a psychiatrist, complaining of fear of germs and dirt, obsessions about religious ideas, and obsessions about the number 3. These symptoms had begun about three months earlier, following the birth of her second child. She had had a similar episode five years earlier, after her first child was born. This had lasted about six months and finally cleared up during counseling with her pastor.

She was a bright person who was always orderly, methodical, conscientious, and dependable. As a child, she was overly concerned with the "normal" compulsions that children have, such as counting the pickets in fences and avoiding the cracks in sidewalk. At ten she became obsessed with the idea that she would die on a certain Tuesday in October.

In her present episode she had developed a number of compulsions in response to her fears and obsessions. For example, she washed her hands repeatedly and relaundered clothes because of her fear of germs and dirt, and she avoided reading automobile license plates and house numbers because she wished to avoid the number 3. After several weeks in the hospital, she improved enough so that she was able to carry on her housework, although she was still troubled somewhat by her symptoms.

In this case, note the previously compulsive personality and the typical obsessions and compulsions. In view of her compulsive personality and incomplete response to hospital treatment, her prognosis was necessarily poor.

X. Post-traumatic stress disorder

A. Definition

1. In *DSM*-III-R, diagnostic criteria for post-traumatic stress disorder are the following:

a) The person has experienced an event that is outside the range of usual human experience and that would be markedly distressing to almost anyone, for example, serious threat to one's life or physical integrity; serious threat or harm to one's children, spouse, or other close relatives and friends; sudden destruction of one's home or community; or seeing another person who has recently been, or is being, seriously injured or killed as the result of an accident or physical violence.

b) The traumatic event is persistently reexperienced in at least one of the following ways:

(1) Recurrent and intrusive distressing recollections of the event (in young children, repetitive play in which themes or aspects of the trauma are expressed)

(2) Recurrent distressing dreams of the event

(3) Sudden acting or feeling as if the traumatic event were recurring (includes a sense of reliving the experience, illusions, hallucinations, and dissociative (flashback) episodes, even those that occur upon awakening or when intoxicated)

(4) Intense psychological distress at exposure to events that symbolize or resemble an aspect of the traumatic event, including anniversaries of the trauma

c) Persistent avoidance of stimuli associated with the trauma or numbing of general responsiveness (not present before the trauma), as indicated by at least three of the following:

(1) Efforts to avoid thoughts or feelings associated with the trauma

(2) Efforts to avoid activities or situations that arouse recollections of the trauma

(3) Inability to recall an important aspect of the trauma (psychogenic amnesia)

(4) Markedly diminished interest in significant activities (in young children, loss of recently acquired developmental skills such as toilet training or language skills)

(5) Feeling of detachment or estrangement from others

(6) Restricted range of affect, for example, unable to have loving feelings

(7) Sense of a foreshortened future, for example, does not expect to have a career, marriage, or children, or a long life

d) Persistent symptoms of increased arousal (not present before the trauma), as indicated by at least two of the following:
   (1) Difficulty falling or staying asleep
   (2) Irritability or outbursts of anger
   (3) Difficulty concentrating
   (4) Hypervigilance
   (5) Exaggerated startle response
   (6) Physiologic reactivity upon exposure to events that symbolize or resemble an aspect of the traumatic event (e.g., a woman who was raped in an elevator breaks out in a sweat when entering any elevator)
   e) Duration of the disturbance (symptoms in b, c, and d) of at least one month.

B. Types
   1. Cases in which the symptoms have their onset within six months after the trauma and do not last more than six months are considered acute, and the prognosis with treatment is good. Those in which the symptoms are delayed more than six months or last longer than six months are considered chronic or delayed, and the treatment is usually more difficult.
   2. Kolb and Brodie (1982) point out that 75 percent of acute war neuroses were anxiety reactions and that the survivors of concentration camps of World War II are the largest group of sufferers of chronic stress reaction. The Vietnam experience is a well-known type of delayed stress disorder.

C. Etiology
   Although a psychologically distressing event is the precipitating stressor in this disorder, individual predisposition may play a role in the development of the disorder.

D. Treatment
   1. Early treatment seems to be essential to help resolve the condition.
   2. The usual treatment is short-term psychotherapy (5–16 weeks) during which the therapist (a) gets a history from the patient, (b) gives the patient a realistic appraisal of the event and the patient's reaction to it, (c) identifies themes that the patient is still resisting, (d) interprets the patient's pathological defenses, (e) encourages active confrontation of feared topics and harsh memories, (f) begins discussing termination, (g) clarifies remaining conflicts and issues, (h) summarizes the gains in therapy, (i) alerts the patient to future concerns, and (j) bids good-bye.[1]

1. Horowitz, "Disasters and Psychological Response to Stress," *Psychiatric Annals* 15(1985):161–67.

XI. Generalized anxiety disorder (GAD)
A. Definition

The essential features of this disorder is unrealistic or excessive anxiety and worry (apprehensive expectation) about two or more life circumstances, for example, worry about possible misfortune to one's child (who is in no danger) and worry about finances (for no good reason), for six months or longer, during which the person has been bothered by these concerns more days than not. In children and adolescents this may take the form of anxiety and worry about academic, athletic, and social performance. When the person is anxious, there are many signs of motor tension, autonomic hyperactivity, and vigilance and scanning. (Symptoms that are present only during panic attacks are not considered in making the diagnosis.) (*DSM*-III-R)

B. Symptoms

In general there are signs of motor tension, autonomic hyperactivity, and vigilance and scanning.

1. Motor tension

   Trembling, twitching, or feeling shaky; muscle tension, aches, or soreness; restlessness; and easy fatigability.

2. Autonomic hyperactivity

   Shortness of breath or smothering sensations; palpitations or accelerated heart rate (tachycardia); sweating, or cold clammy hands; dry mouth; dizziness or lightheadedness; nausea, diarrhea, or other abdominal distress; flushes (hot flashes) or chills; frequent urination; and trouble swallowing or "lump in throat."

3. Vigilance and scanning

   Feeling keyed up or on edge; exaggerated startle response; difficulty concentrating or "mind going blank" because of anxiety; trouble falling or staying asleep; and irritability.

4. Organic factors that might initiate or maintain the disturbance must be ruled out (e.g., caffeine intoxication, hyperthyroidism).

C. Etiology and pathogenesis

1. Neurobiologic factors

   Some persons are biologically predisposed to states of anxiousness.

   a) The physiological reflections of anxiety are produced by discharge of the adrenergic division of the autonomic nervous system.

   b) Noradrenergic pathways originating in the locus caeruleus in the upper pons and projecting to the cortex and limbic system are thought to help regulate anxiety.

c) Central nervous system receptors for the neurotransmitter gamma-aminobuteric acid (GABA) are found to contain a modulating protein that has a binding site for the anxiety-reducing benzodiazepines.

2. Psychological activation of states of anxiousness
Some individuals actually seek anxiety states. People may deliberately pursue excitement such as roller coaster rides, horror movies, sky diving, and so forth, in order to be stimulated, gain a sense of mastery over a fear, escape from some mental state (boredom, apathy, anger), or achieve the sensation that follows fear ("high" relief pleasure and others' admiration and acceptance).

On the other hand, such anxiety states occur because a person unconsciously anticipates the out of control; intolerable and dangerous states of mind may occur if conscious thoughts about threatening ideas are pursued to their conclusion.

Such anxious states of mind may have been experienced or witnessed in the past with results that may have been psychically traumatic so that the person fears the repetition.

D. Associated features
Unrelated panic disorder or depressive disorder are often present.

E. Impairment
Impairment in social or occupational functioning is rarely more than mild.

F. Treatment
Little is known about specific therapy for generalized anxiety disorder, however, the following principles underlining the therapy for anxiety symptoms (from Maxmen) seem appropriate.

1. Pharmacotherapy
Generally, for mild symptoms of anxiety medication should be avoided. However, when symptoms warrant it, benzodiazepines are the preferred drugs (diazepam, alprazolam, etc.)

2. Psychotherapies
Insight-oriented psychotherapy explores the unconscious and symbolic meanings of the patient's anxiety and clarifies its defensive and "signal" functions. It seeks to identify the stressors producing the anxiety and find a better means of handling stress.

Cognitive therapy focuses on particular stress events or circumstances that trigger conscious dysphoric "automatic thoughts" and then rational ways of responding.

3. Behavior therapy
Relaxation, biofeedback, and meditation are frequently helpful, either by themselves or as supplements to other therapies.

References

American Psychiatric Association. *Diagnostic and Statistical Manual of Mental Disorders.* 3d ed. rev. Washington, D.C., 1987.

Goldman, H. H. *Review of General Psychiatry.* Los Altos, Calif.: Lange Medical Publications, 1984.

Kaplan, H. I., and B. J. Sadock. *Comprehensive Textbook of Psychiatry/ IV.* 4th ed. Baltimore: Williams & Wilkins, 1985.

Kolb, L. C., and H. K. H. Brodie. *Modern Clinical Psychiatry.* 10th ed. Philadelphia: W. B. Saunders Co., 1982.

Maxmen, J. S. *Essential Psychopathology.* New York: W. W. Norton Co., 1986.

Nicholi, A. M., Jr., ed. *The Harvard Guide to Modern Psychiatry.* Cambridge: Belknap Press of Harvard University Press, 1978.

The mind has great influence over the body, and maladies often have their origin there.

Moliere: *Love's the Best Doctor* (1665)

Somatoform Disorders

I. Definition

The essential features of this group of disorders are physical symptoms suggesting physical disorder (hence, somatoform), for which there are no demonstrable organic findings or known physiologic mechanisms, and for which there is positive evidence, or a strong presumption, that the symptoms are linked to psychological factors or conflicts. Unlike in factitious disorder or malingering, the symptom production in somatoform disorders is not intentional; that is, the person does not experience the sense of controlling the production of the symptoms. Although the symptoms of somatoform disorders are "physical," the specific pathophysiologic processes involved are not demonstrable or understandable by existing laboratory procedures and are conceptualized most clearly by means of psychological constructs. For that reason, these are classified as mental (not physical) disorders (*DSM*-III-R).

II. Types

The subtypes of somatoform disorders are listed below. Each will be discussed in turn.

A. Body dysmorphic disorder (dysmorphophobia)
B. Conversion disorder (or hysterical neurosis, conversion type)
C. Hypochondriasis (or hypochondriacal neurosis)
D. Somatization disorder (Briquet's syndrome)
E. Somatoform pain disorder
F. Undifferentiated somatoform disorder

III. Prevalence

Many patients seen in general medical practice do not have significant organic disease. Many of these probably have somatoform disorders, but they do not seek psychiatric treatment because they do not perceive themselves as having psychiatric difficulties. General physicians, especially primary care doctors, should be familiar with these disorders so they can be managed properly.

IV. Body dysmorphic disorder (dysmorphophobia)

A. Definition

The essential feature of this disorder is preoccupation with some imagined defect in appearance in a normal-appearing person. The most common complaints involve facial flaws, such as wrinkles, spots on the skin, excessive facial hair, shape of nose, mouth, jaw, or eyebrows, and swelling of the face. More rarely the complaint involves the appearance of the feet, hands, breasts, back, or some other part of the body. In some cases a slight physical anomaly is present, but the person's concern is grossly excessive (*DSM*-III-R).

B. The previous diagnosis as dysmorphophobia seemed to be a misnomer, since the disturbance does not invovle phobic avoidance. The term dysmorphophobia has also been used to include cases in which

the belief in a defect in appearance is of delusional intensity. Associated features include history of repeated visits to plastic surgeons and dermatologists for correction of the imagined defect, obsessive personality traits and depression.
  C. The age at outset is most commonly from adolescence through the third decade of life. (Keep in mind normal adolescence concerns with minor defects such as acne.)

V. Conversion disorder (or hysterical neurosis, conversion type)
  A. Definition
    1. The essential feature of this disorder is an alteration or loss of physical functioning that suggests physical disorder, but that instead is apparently an expression of a psychological conflict or need. The symptoms of the disturbances are not intentionally produced (as in factitious disorder or malingering) and, after appropriate investigation, cannot be explained by any physical disorder or known pathophysiologic mechanism (*DSM-III-R*).
    2. Psychodynamically, it is a disorder in which unconscious conflict is manifested as disguised and symbolic somatic symptoms. That is, the anxiety arising out of some conflictual situation is converted into somatic symptoms in parts of the body innervated by the sensorimotor system (symbolic somatization). Thus, the conflict is reflected as physical symptoms instead of being expressed directly.
  B. The differentiation from factitious disorder and from malingering is sometimes difficult. Conversion disorder must be distinguished from other illness-affirming states:
    1. *Malingering*: signs and symptoms of illness are consciously produced and consciously motivated.
    2. Factitious disorder: the intentional production of symptoms to assume the *patient role*. The presentation may be fabricated or self-inflicted.
    3. The differentiation of conversion disorder from factitious disorder or malingering is sometimes difficult because
      a) Some behavior may be in part consciously determined and in part unconsciously determined.
      b) Many hysterical and factitious patients are so histrionic about their symptoms, and their secondary gain is so obvious, that one sees them as consciulsy feigning or simulating disease.
    4. However, whichever the disorder, psychiatrists must approach it therapeutically.

C. Prevalence
1. Classical conversion disorder is rarely encountered now.
2. Conversion symptoms, however, are fairly common.
3. Conversion elements are commonly seen in compensation cases.
4. Conversion disorder is usually considered to be more common among women, although it is seen in men in the military setting.
5. Classical conversion disorder is rarely seen in ordinary psychiatric practice, but is more commonly seen by neurologists, orthopedic surgeons, and by military physicians, especially in time of war.
D. Predisposing factors
Antecedent physical disorder (which may provide a prototype for the symptoms), exposure to other people with real physical symptoms or conversion symptoms, and extreme psychosocial stress (warfare or the recent death of a significant figure) are predisposing factors (*DSM*-III-R).
E. Persons with histrionic and dependent personality disorders have increased vulnerability for this disorder.
F. Symptoms
1. Somatic symptoms
a) The somatic symptoms can vary widely. Frequently, they simulate organic disease and represent the patient's idea of the disease. The closeness with which the patient's symptoms approximate the symptoms of an organic disease depends in large measure on the patient's medical and psychological sophistication.
b) The somatic symptoms chiefly involve organs that are in contact with the external world.
c) The distribution of the symptoms is unphysiological and nonanatomical.
d) Somatic symptoms can be considered under two headings.
(1) Motor symptoms, such as convulsive states, paralysis, paresis (muscular weakness), or aphonia (inability to produce normal speech)
(2) Sensory disturbances, such as analgesia (diminished sense of pain), anesthesia (absence of feeling), paresthesia ("tingling feeling")
e) The somatic symptoms associated with conversion disorder tend to be singular rather than multiple (as in somatoform disorder).
f) The onset or exacerbation of the symptoms almost always follow a psychologically meaningful environmental stimulus.

2. Psychological symptoms
    a) The mental-status evaluation of the person with conversion disorder reveals no significant abnormalities.
    b) The classical psychological symptom in the conversion disorder is the patient's indifference to the illness (la belle indifference). Though the symptoms are obviously disabling, the patient seems unconcerned and shows no anxiety. However, it should be kept in mind that people with serious medical illnesses may also be indifferent.
    c) Pseudodementia may be a conversion symptom in elderly people. This is characterized by exaggerated indifference to one's surroundings, without actual mental impairment, and reversible decline of mental functioning, which occurs in depression.
    d) Some histories show a preexisting histrionic personality disorder or dependent personality disorder (see chapter, "Personality Disorders").
    e) This disorder is unique in the *DSM*-III-R classification because specific mechanisms are thought to account for it (see primary gain and secondary gain under psychopathology, which follows).
    f) The onset or exacerbation of the symptoms almost always follows a psychologically meaningful environmental stimulus.
G. Historical conceptions of psychopathology
    1. Hippocrates believed that conversion disorder resulted from a wandering uterus.
    2. In the seventeenth century, hysteria was thought to be due to demoniacal possession.
    3. Charcot believed it was a genetic reaction that resulted in degeneration of the nervous system. He demonstrated that the hysterical symptoms could be produced and removed by hypnotic suggestion. (He also believed that normal people could not be hypnotized.)
    4. Janet introduced the concept of dissociated mental processes in the subconscious. He demonstrated that automatisms were of unconscious origin.
    5. Both Babinski and Bernheim believed that the symptoms resulted from suggestion. (Bernheim's extensive work with hypnosis led him to believe that normal people could be hypnotized.)
    6. Breuer and Freud introduced the concept of repressed conflict as the source of conversion. Freud believed that the repressed conflict was the Oedipus complex.
    7. Most authorities now feel that any highly charged instinct or impulse may be involved.

H. Psychopathology
  1. Essentially, the psychopathology is repression of a conflict and conversion of the anxiety into a somatic symptom that is symbolic of the underlying conflict.
  2. It was thought that only sexual conflict produced conversion symptoms. Theorists now believe that all types of instinctual impulses may find expression in this manner.
  3. The premorbid personality is often histrionic. Such individuals are theatrical, shallow, superficial, or insincere. They are often narcissistic and manipulative. They go through the motions of feeling without really experiencing emotion and tend to overreact to minor stimuli.
  4. The precipitating factor may seem trivial but have a special meaning to the person (thus, as in anxiety disorder, it is important to know the setting in which the first hysterical symptoms occurred).
  5. The choice of symptom may be determined in several ways.
     a) Events may tend to focus the conflict in a specific area (e.g., a tonsillectomy or other type of operation on the throat or neck may be a precursor to aphonia that is an expression of some underlying conflict).
     b) The experience of the organ in relation to the conflict may be the determinant (e.g., paralysis of a hand with which the patient has struck someone in anger).
     c) The suitability of the organ to express the conflict symbolically may also dictate the choice (e.g., paralysis of the legs as a defense against meeting a threat by either attack or flight).
  6. In conversion disorder, both primary gain and secondary gain are observed.
     a) The *primary gain* is the relief of anxiety.
     b) The *secondary gain* is the advantage that accrues to the patient by virtue of the illness. Secondary gain is often a factor in illness, both emotional and physical; however, it is most prominent in conversion disorders.
I. Onset, course, and prognosis
  1. A conversion disorder may prolong or exaggerate symptoms that originally resulted from physical illness.
  2. Conversion symptoms may develop following an accident.
  3. In acute cases—in which the onset is abrupt and the duration of symptoms has been short—the prognosis is usually favorable when the patient is treated.

4. When the symptoms have been allowed to endure for a sustained period, the prognosis is less hopeful.
   a) In such cases, the secondary gain operates to decrease the individual's motivation to get well by giving up the symptoms.
   b) However, active treatment of someone who is well motivated is often successful.
5. *DSM*-III states that the course is unknown, but probaby of short duration when the onset is abrupt.
6. Some studies have indicated that, in the long term, some individuals with "conversion symptoms" reveal an underlying neurologic disorder.
7. The relative maturity of the premorbid personality and the intensity of the underlying conflict are factors that must be evaluated in estimating the prognosis.
J. Case example

The twenty-six-year-old soldier previously mentioned in the chapter, "Adaptations to Anxiety," p. 65, developed paralysis of his right hand when firing for the first time on the rifle range. This was a defense against repressed hostility to his father, who had been physically abusive of the soldier's mother many times and who often abandoned the family for long periods. Upon the father's return home, shortly before the young man entered the service, he again threatened his wife. At that point, the young man stepped up to his father and said, "If you ever strike my mother again, I'll kill you." However, he had a very well-developed conscience and obviously would have trouble following through such a threat.

When he first reached the rifle range and saw the target over his gunsights, he recalled the incident and "saw" the face of his father. Because his conscience could not let him "kill" his father, his right hand became paralyzed, thus preventing him from expressing the strong hostile feelings he had for the father.

VI. Hypochondriasis (or hypochondriacal neurosis)
A. Definition
   1. The essential feature of this disorder is preoccupation with the fear of having, or the belief that one has, a serious disease, based on the person's interpretation of physical signs or sensations as evidence of physical illness. A thorough physical evaluation does not support the diagnosis of any physical disorder that can account for the physical signs or sensations or for the person's unwarranted interpretation of them, although a coexisting physical disorder may be present. The unwarranted fear or belief of having a disease persists despite medical reassurance, but is not of delusional intensity, in that the person can acknowledge the possibility that he or she may be exaggerating the extent of the feared disease or that there may be no disease at all (*DSM*-III-R).

2. The term derives from the term for the subcostal abdominal region, the hypochondrium, which at one time was believed to be the seat or the origin of the disorder.
3. It is now presumed to be of psychogenic origin.
4. The hypochondriac is painfully aware of sensations that most people ignore. In general, he or she exaggerates the intensity and importance of the sensations.
5. The hypochondriac's somatic preoccupation precludes any concern with underlying feelings or conflicts.

B. Prevalence

This disorder is much more commonly seen in general medical practice than it is in pyschiatric practice, because the patients are focused on physical symptoms, and are resistant to the interpretation of any of their symptoms being of psychogenic origin.

C. Symptoms
1. Awareness and exaggeration of physical sensations that most others disregard.
2. Sometimes the somatic preoccupation is really an obsessional symptom, representing displacement of anxiety onto the body itself.
3. Anxiety, depression, and compulsive personality traits are commonly associated with hypochondriasis.
4. Sometimes the hypochondriacal symptoms are vague; at other times, they are organ-centered.
5. Physical findings are absent.

D. Psychopathology
1. It should be kept in mind that this diagnosis has had a number of different clinical meanings in the past.
2. Many show obsessive-compulsive traits and/or narcissistic traits. (They are often egocentric and excessively concerned with themselves and their bodies.)
3. In general, hypochondriasis is considered a reaction to any kind of conflictual situation. Thus, it might be considered a reaction to sexual conflict, to repressed hostility, to disappointment, to failure, and so forth.

E. Course and prognosis

The course is usually a chronic one, although it may be intermittent.

F. Treatment
1. No specific treatment has been very effective.
2. Psychotherapy has had only limited value; the best results have been obtained when treatment is begun early.
3. When hypochondriasis is suspected, careful physical and laboratory examinations should be made to rule out any underlying physical disease. It is important to remember that a hypochondriacal person can develop a serious physical disease.

4. Medications of various kinds have been prescribed for symptomatic relief, including antianxiety agents for anxiety symptoms, antidepressants for any depressive features, and so forth. Drugs often have only temporary effects.
5. Perhaps the best treatment program is a generally supportive one, in which a sympathetic physician listens and does not challenge the patient's symptoms. Such a relationship can best be offered by an internist or a general practitioner, with psychiatric consultation and advice available.
6. Environmental modification is occasionally helpful.

G. Examples
1. Dr. Samuel Johnson was a hypochondriac.
2. In Moliére's (1622–1673) play *The Hypochondriac,* Argan is a hypochondriac who gauges his health by the number of purges and clysters he has had the previous month and who enjoys the attention of two physicians and an apothecary. His desire is to have a physician in the family to attend him at all times.

VII. Somatization disorder
A. Definition
The essential features of this disorder are recurrent and multiple somatic complaints, of several years' duration, for which medical attention has been sought, but that apparently are not due to any physical disorder. The disorder begins before the age of thirty and has a chronic but fluctuating course (*DSM*-III-R).

B. Prevalence
From 0.2 percent to 2 percent among females.

C. Symptoms
1. Complaints invariably involve the following organ systems or types of symptoms: conversion or pseudoneurologic symptoms, gastrointestinal discomfort, female reproductive difficulty, psychosexual problems, and cardiopulmonary symptoms.
2. It is a chronic polysymptomatic disorder.
3. A screening list of seven symptoms has been found highly specific for somatization disorder: shortness of breath, dysmenorrhea, burning sensation in the sexual organs or rectum, lump in the throat (difficulty in swallowing), amnesia, vomiting, and painful extremities.
4. Often it is difficult to determine when the illness started or why the patient sought medical examination.
5. The conversion symptoms suggest neurological damage and are sometimes called pseudoneurological or grand hysterical symptoms.

6. Virtually everyone experiences many somatic symptoms, but we do not complain of them and rarely report them to a physician when we are examined because we interpret the physician's questions as referring to "significant" symptoms.

D. Associated features
1. Anxiety and depression are extremely common. It may be the depression for which the individual seeks psychiatric treatment.
2. Hallucinations are also reported, usually hearing one's name called (however, reality testing is intact).
3. Histrionic personality disorder and, more rarely, antisocial personality disorder often are also present (*DSM*-III-R).

E. Onset and course
1. It begins in the teens or twenties (prior to the age of thirty).
2. It is rare in males.
3. The course is chronic but fluctuating.
4. Patients often have many medical examinations, are often admitted to hospitals for evaluation, and are frequently subjected to unnecessary surgery.
5. The patients' lives are often dominated by their symptoms, and they often lead lives as chaotic and complicated as their medical history.
6. They go from physician to physician.
7. They tend to overmedicate or become drug abusers.

F. Etiologic explanations for somatization disorders
The possibilities are nearly endless and include:
1. The specific cause is unknown.
2. The cause is presumed to be psychological and assumptions are based on the usual presumed kinds of psychogenic factors.
3. There is increased incidence among family members but there is not conclusive evidence of a genetic basis.
4. The somatizing person may be alexithymic (that is, he is unable to use emotional words to describe his or her feelings).
5. Social, political, religious, and economic issues place a premium on somatic diagnosis in preference to stigmatizing psychiatric diagnoses.
6. Many patients continue to emphasize their somatic complaints because the physician has made a symptomatic diagnosis such as nervous stomach, insomnia, or spastic colitis, not realizing that such symptoms can be physiological concomitants of psychiatric disorders.

G. Case example

A forty-six-year-old married woman presented herself at a hospital with a twenty-year history of multiple physical complaints, especially abdominal pain, dating back fifteen years. Asked her reason for seeking hospitalization, she immediately recited a long list of physicians, hospitals, and clinics she had visited, underscoring her dissatisfaction with all of them. She was very dramatic in her presentation. Although sexual themes appeared to underlie her symptomatology and behavior, she focused entirely on her physical symptoms, especially those referable to her abdomen. She reported that she had suffered for fifteen years and had continually sought medical care, and she stated, with a sort of glee, that all attempts had failed. Some of her physical symptoms were described in such a way that they seemed self-induced. For example, she said, "I was bleeding from the vagina, but I didn't pick at any specific place." In addition to seeing many internists, gastroenterologists, surgeons, gynecologists, and other specialists, she had seen several psychiatrists, who had attempted psychotherapy and psychotropic medication. A number of neurological examinations by excellent neurologists had been negative. A laparoscopy had been essentially negative. All medication had been unsuccessful.

On psychiatric examination, she was overly dramatic and superficial. She rambled on about her symptoms and tried to control the interview. She focused entirely on her physical symptoms although there was a strong underlying sexual connotation.

After three or four weeks in the hospital, after attempts with various kinds of medication, psychotherapy, and joint therapy with her husband had failed, she left in an angry mood and proceeded to another hospital in a nearby city.

VIII. Somatoform pain disorder
   A. Definition
      1. The essential feature of this disorder is preoccupation with pain in the absence of adequate physical findings to account for the pain or its intensity (*DSM*-III-R).
      2. As in conversion disorder, psychological factors are etiologically involved.
         a) There is a temporal relationship between an environmental stimulus that is apparently related to a psychological conflict or need and the initiation or exacerbation of the pain.
         b) Or the pain permits the individual to avoid some activity that is noxious to him or her, or to get support from the environment that otherwise might not be forthcoming.
         c) Or in some cases, there may be no direct evidence of an etiological role for psychological factors.
      3. Often the pain enables the patient to effect some secondary gain.
   B. Associated features
      1. It may be accompanied by other localized sensory or motor function changes, such as paresthesia and muscle spasm.
      2. The afflicted person frequently visits physicians to obtain relief despite medical reassurance (doctor shopping), uses analgesics to excess without relief of the pain, requests surgery, and assumes an invalid role.
      3. The individual usually refuses to consider the role of psychological factors in the pain.

4. In some cases, the pain has symbolic significance, such as pain mimicking angina in an individual whose father died from heart disease. A past history of conversion symptoms is common.
5. Histrionic personality traits are seldom present, nor is "la belle indifference," though concern about the pain symptom is usually less intense than its stated severity. Symptoms of depression are frequent (*DSM*-III-R).

C. Prevalence

This disorder is probably common in general medical practice, and such patients are probably usually seen by internists or general physicians, rather than psychiatrists because the patient focuses on the somatic aspects of his or her complaint. In addition, such a person is often extremely resistive of accepting even obvious emotional factors, hence refuses psychiatric consultation. Such persons are said to be alexithymic (persons who define their emotions only in terms of somatic sensations or in behavioral reactions rather than relating them to accompanying thoughts).

D. Concept of chronic pain

1. According to Whittington, the present day conception of chronic pain is based on a biopsychosocial model—pain is viewed as a form of abnormal illness behavior influenced by a wide range of biological, psychological, and social factors. This broader conceptualization of chronic pain has emerged from social psychology, neurochemistry, learning theory, and psychophysiology.
2. Some speak of the "sick role" behavior to account for the disparity between the pain/disability and the detectable disease.
3. Since most chronic pain sufferers are emotionally disturbed, it has often been assumed that the emotional disturbance caused the chronic pain. When this emotional disturbance is depression, the pain has been interpreted as a "depressive equivalent." (In part this is supported by the observation that antidepressants sometimes improve chronic pain.)
4. Characteristics of chronic pain patients (according to Whittington 1985)
   a) Generally they have started work at an early age and were dutiful, compliant, subassertive, and industrious in their work career before the injury.
   b) Their world view is essentially moralistic.
   c) They are not psychologically minded or especially insightful.
   d) They frequently feel alienated from the dominant political, social, and economic system.
   e) They do not have good verbal skills (alexithymia). It should be kept in mind, however, that individuals with poor language skills and poor ability to manipulate symbols are most

often relegated to a life of menial labor and because of this are more likely to experience an industrial accident with a consequent injury to cause chronic pain. (The above are all characteristics of the pain patient *before* the pain begins.)

5. After the underlying injury, a very complex social system is brought into play including the patient and his immediate family, his employers, physicians, coworkers, insurers and their agents, attorneys, judges, and workman compensation referees (Whittington 1985, 3).

6. In treatment they are dependent but noncompliant; are passive and have a sense of entitlement, are often very bitter and utilize projection extensively, and many are clinically paranoid by the time they enter a treatment program. Generally they are abusive of medications and of alcohol and show depressed effect. They are self-defeating.

E. The International Association for the study of Pain (IASP) has promulgated a system of five axes as a nontheoretical comprehensive scheme for classifying pain in patients: (1) Region, (2) System, (3) Temporal Characteristics, (4) Intensity and, (5) Etiology.

F. Treatment

1. Treatment of such disorders is extremely difficult.

2. Any psychiatric treatment must necessarily be based on adequate physical, neurological, and laboratory examinations, to rule out the evidence of physical disease. These are also a prerequisite to establishing the patient's trust in the physician's assurances about the patient's physical state.

3. Supportive psychotherapy is probably the most useful approach in the treatment of this condition.

4. The judicious prescription of antianxiety agents and other psychotropic drugs, including tricyclics, for the appropriate symptoms is also often necessary.

5. The physician should be prepared to offer the patient an ongoing treatment plan.

6. Many patients with this disorder are referred to pain programs or pain clinics. These tend to have an eclectic approach and help the patient try to live with his or her difficulty rather than seeking relief through medications or surgery. Pain programs differ considerably in their patient selection and treatment modality. Most of the treatment focuses on rehabilitation rather than on cure, with emphasis on coping rather than curing the pain.

7. However, it should be remembered that there are chronic pain sufferers who have not responded to the usual pain program, and some of these can only be maintained by the judicious prescription of appropriate analgesics and muscle relaxants.

IX. Undifferentiated somatoform disorder

A. Definition

1. In this disorder there is either a single circumscribed symptom, such as difficulty in swallowing (globus hystericus) or more commonly, multiple physical complaints, such as fatigue, loss of appetite, and gastrointestinal problems. These symptoms are not explainable on the basis of demonstrable organic findings or known pathophysiologic mechanisms and are apparently linked to psychological factors (*DSM*-III-R).

2. Disorders in this category do not meet the full symptom picture of somatization disorder.

References

American Psychiatric Association. *Diagnostic and Statistical Manual of Mental Disorders.* 3d ed., rev. Washington, D.C., 1987.

Blackwell, D., J. R. Galbraith, D. S. Dahl. "*Chronic Pain Management.*" *Hospital and Community Psychiatry* 35 (10):99–107 (October 1985).

Goldman, H. H. *Review of General Psychiatry.* Los Altos, Calif.: Lange Medical Publications, 1984.

Portenoy, R. K., and K. M. Foley. "Chronic Use of Opioid Analgesics in Nonmalignant Pain, Report of 38 Cases." *Pain* 25 (1986):171–86.

Whittington, H. G. "The Biopsychosocial Model Applied to Chronic Pain." *Journal of Operational Psychiatry* 16 (2):1–8 (1985).

Not the power to remember,
But its very opposite,
The power to forget,
Is a necessary condition for our
existence.

Shalom Asch: *The Nazarene*
(1939)

Dissociative Disorders (or Hysterical Neuroses, Dissociative Type)

I. Introduction

In previous classifications of mental disorders, psychogenic amnesia and multiple personality were categorized as hysterical neurosis, dissociative type. They are now classified as dissociative disorders, which also include depersonalization disorder (formerly termed depersonalization neurosis), defined as a disorder in which the person has feelings of unreality, altered personality, or altered identity and might deny his or her own existence along with that of his environment.

Thus, the characteristic that is common to all the dissociative disorders is a constellation of recent mental events that is out of the patient's awareness but is capable, under certain conditions, of being brought into consciousness.

II. Definition

A. The essential feature of these disorders is a disturbance or alteration in the normally integrative functions of identity, memory, or consciousness. The disturbance or alteration may be sudden or gradual, and transient or chronic. If it occurs primarily in identity, the person's customary identity is temporarily forgotten, and a new identity may be assumed or imposed (as in multiple personality disorder), or the customary feeling of one's own reality is lost and is replaced by a feeling of unreality (as in depersonalization disorder). If the disturbance occurs primarily in memory, important personal events cannot be recalled (as in psychogenic amnesia and psychogenic fugue) (*DSM*-III-R).

B. Depersonalization disorder has been included in the dissociative disorders because the feeling of one's own reality, an important component of identity, is lost. Some, however, question this inclusion because disturbance in memory is absent (*DSM*-III-R).

C. Although sleepwalking disorder has the essential feature of a dissociative disorder, it is classified as a sleep disorder.

III. Psychopathology

A. Essentially, the disorder reflects the mechanism of dissociation—that is, the unconscious detachment of certain behavior or aspects of personality from the normal or usual patterns of an individual. The detached material then usually functions alone (compartmentalization).

B. It is a more massive type of forgetting than is seen in simple repression.

C. The ego is protecting itself against something that is critically dangerous and defending itself against overwhelming anxiety that develops because of an emotional bind.

D. Although the dissociation is handicapping, it relieves the individual's anxiety.

E. Dissociation is also symbolic and may have more than one meaning to the patient.

F. Primary gain (relief of anxiety) and secondary pain (advantage that accrues to the patient by virtue of the disorder) are evident in this condition (as they are in conversion disorders).

G. The premorbid personality is said to be immature and egocentric and have experienced some type of episodic emotional disturbance early in life. Still others are said to be histrionic, schizoid, or passive.

IV. Types
A. Multiple personality disorder
B. Psychogenic fugue
C. Psychogenic amnesia
D. Depersonalization disorder (or depersonalization neurosis)
E. Dissociative disorder not otherwise specified

V. Multiple personality
A. Definition

The essential feature of this disorder is the existence within the person of two or more distinct personalities or personality states. Personality is here defined as a relatively enduring pattern of perceiving, relating to, and thinking about the environment and one's self, which is exhibited in a wide range of important social and personal contexts. Personality states differ only in that the pattern is not exhibited in as wide a range of contexts. In classic cases, there are at least two fully developed personalities; in other cases, there may be only one distinct personality and one or more personality states. In classic cases, the personalities and personality states each have unique memories, behavior patterns, and social relationships; in other cases, there may be varying degrees of sharing of memories and commonalities in behavior or social relationships. In children and adolescents, classic cases with two or more fully developed personalities are not as common as they are in adults. In adults, the number of personalities or personality states in any one case varies from two to more than one hundred, with occasional cases of extreme complexity. Approximately half of recently reported cases have ten personalities or fewer, and half have more than ten (*DSM-III-R*).

B. The transition from one personality to another is usually sudden.

C. Prevalence

Although at one time considered to be rare, within the last decade, multiple personality disorder has been diagnosed, treated, and studied with increasing frequency. What distinguishes it from all other psychiatric syndromes is the ongoing coexistence of relatively consistent but alternating separate identities plus recurrent episodes of memory distortion, frank amnesia, or both (Kluft 1987).

D. Age at onset

It almost invariably begins in childhood but does not come to clinical attention until much later. Child abuse and incest are very common during childhood (75 to 88 percent experience sexual abuse during childhood).

E. Sex ratio

Has been reported at about 9:1 predominance in females among its victims.

F. Associated feature

Many clinicians working with both multiple personality disorder and post-traumatic stress disorder have remarked on the similarity of the two conditions.

C. While dissociation is the major mechanism operating in this disorder, identification is also evident in the fashioning of the second personality.

VI. Psychogenic fugue

A. Definition

The essential feature of this disorder is sudden, unexpected travel away from home or customary work locale with assumption of a new identity and an inability to recall one's previous identity. Perplexity and disorientation may occur. Following recovery, there is no recollection of events that took place during the fugue. The diagnosis is not made in the presence of an organic mental disorder (*DSM*-III-R).

B. Predisposing factors and course

Heavy alcohol use may predispose an individual to the development of the disorder. The fugue is usually of brief duration. Recovery is usually rapid and recurrences are rare.

C. Prevalence

It is apparently rare but more common in wartime or in the wake of a natural disaster.

D. Somnambulism (sleepwalking)

This is a dissociative state, identical with fugue, except that the episodes begin during sleep. It is common in childhood and is primarily a disorder of males.

E. Case Example

J. R., a twenty-five-year-old soldier, was admitted to the prison ward of a military hospital, accused of desertion. His history revealed that he had served with distinction in combat and was twice wounded. Following his second wound, he was evacuated to the U.S. mainland for further treatment. After a brief period at one hospital, the medical staff decided he could be managed best at another hospital several hundred miles away and placed him on a train for that destination. The man never arrived at the second hospital. Six months later, he was discovered in another section of the country, living the life of a civilian under an assumed name. He was unable to identify himself correctly and could not account for his activities during the entire six-month period. His real identity was established only through his fingerprints.

VII. **Psychogenic amnesia**
  A. The essential feature of this disorder is sudden inability to recall important personal information, an inability not due to an organic mental disorder (*DSM*-III-R). If the person travels to another locale and assumes a new identity, the case is diagnosed as psychogenic fugue.
  B. There are four types of disturbance in recall.
    1. Localized (circumscribed) amnesia
      Localized anmesia is failure to recall all events during a circumscribed period of time, usually the first few hours following a profoundly disturbing event (this is the most common type).
    2. Selective amnesia
      Selective amnesia is failure to recall some, but not all, of the events occurring during a circumscribed period of time (somewhat less common).
    3. Generalized amnesia
      Generalized amnesia is failure to recall the individual's entire life.
    4. Continuous amnesia
      Continuous amnesia is failure to recall events subsequent to a specific time and up to, and including, the present. (Generalized and continuous amnesia are the least common types.)
  C. During an ongoing amnesia episode, perplexity, disorientation, and purposeless wandering may occur (*DSM*-III-R).
  D. Psychogenic amnesia is a pathological loss of memory.
    1. This type of amnesia must be distinguished from the anmesias associated with organic brain damage and alcoholism.
    2. It is more than a mere forgetting. Rather, it is an active "blotting out" of consciousness containing conflictual material.
    3. It is most often a response to intense feelings such as terror, anger, or guilt.
    4. Its onset is usually sudden, and it is of brief duration.
    5. It is apparently rare and is usually seen in wartime or during natural disasters.
    6. The individual is usually indifferent to the loss of memory (a similar indifference is found in conversion disorder).
  E. Case Example

    Mrs. H., a forty-two-year-old housewife, entered the hospital complaining of several brief periods of memory loss. History revealed that the onset of the first episode coincided with her learning that her husband was going out with another woman. Subsequent episodes usually followed some incident in which she was remined of the "other woman."

VIII. Depersonalization disorder (depersonalization neurosis)

A. Definition

1. The essential feature of this disorder is the occurrence of persistent or recurrent episodes of depersonalization sufficiently severe to cause marked distress. The diagnosis is not made when the symptom of depersonalization is secondary to any other disorder, such as panic disorder or agoraphobia without history of panic disorder (*DSM*-III-R).

2. The symptom of depersonalization involves an alteration in the perception or experience of the self in which the usual sense of one's own reality is temporarily lost or changed. This is manifested by a feeling of detachment from and being an outside observer of one's mental processes or body, or of feeling like an automaton, or as if in a dream. Various types of sensory anesthesia and a sensation of not being in complete control of one's actions, including speech, are often present. All of these feelings are ego-dystonic, and the person maintains intact reality testing (*DSM*-III-R).

3. It may be defined as a disorder of affect, in which the person has feelings of unreality, altered personality, or altered identity. Patients may deny their own existence or that of their environment.

4. An essential feature is the frequent occurrence of prolonged episodes.

5. Derealization is frequently present. (This is a feeling that the environment has changed.)

B. Depersonalization

1. Depersonalization disorder is not to be confused with depersonalization, which occurs as a secondary finding in other disorders.

2. Depersonalization as a secondary finding or symptom is not considered an illness or disorder.

3. Brief episodes of depersonalization, without significant impairment, are a common symptom, said to occur in 30 to 70 percent of young adults.

4. Some common examples of depersonalization are hypnagogic hallucinations (the mental images that occur just before sleep) and hypnopompic hallucinations (images seen in dreams that persist on awakening). These are experienced by healthy people.

C. Types

Related to depersonalization disorder, which is described in *DSM*-III as having a chronic, recurrent course with marked exacerbations and remissions, are the following:

1. Trance states and trancelike states

A *trance state* is a psychological stupor characterized by immobility and unresponsiveness to the environment. It usually

has a sudden onset, and amnesia follows. A *trancelike state* is a similar experience, ordinarily induced in normal individuals by prolonged and unusual concentration on a task or object.
  2. Feelings of unreality
     a) *Feelings of unreality* are feelings that one is unreal.
     b) *Feelings of derealization* are feelings that the environment has changed.
     c) *Depersonalization* (see above) is a sense of estrangement from oneself.
  3. Déjà vu
     Déjà vu is a subjective sensation that an experience that is really happening for the first time occurred on a previous occasion. Experienced by normal people, it also occurs in certain disorders, including psychotic disorders and in organic mental disorders.
  4. Feelings of estrangement
     Feelings of estrangement are a sense of detachment from people, the environment, or concepts. The term embraces paramnesia, distortion, or falsification of memory in which the individual confuses reality and fantasy.
  5. Fascination, or fixation
     Fascination, or *fixation,* is a trancelike state induced in individuals (e.g., pilots) who are compelled to focus on a given object for long periods of time.
  6. Cosmic consciousness, or illumination
     Cosmic consciousness, or *illumination,* is a fabulous sense of joy or well-being, sometimes produced by hallucinogenic drugs.
D. Course and prognosis
  1. The course and prognosis depend upon the patient's motivation to get well, his or her ego-strength, the duration of the disorder, and the strength of the secondary gain.
  2. Depersonalization disorder usually begins in adolescence and generally has a chronic course with remissions and exacerbations.
  3. The symptoms of all the dissociative disorders usually increase when the patient is confronted with mounting anxiety.
  4. In general, the immediate prognosis is good when the dissociative episode has an acute onset.
  5. When there is a close relationship between some environmental factor and the onset, the prognosis is good if the person is removed from the threatening environment.
  6. In some cases, the long-term prognosis is only fair.
E. Treatment
  1. The treatment should be dynamic or pschoanalytically oriented psychotherapy.

2. See the treatments listed under conversion disorders in the chapter, "Somatoform Disorders."

IX. **Dissociative disorder not otherwise specified**
  A. Definition
     Disorders in which the predominant feature is a dissociative symptom that does not meet the criteria for a specific dissociative disorder.
  B. Among the examples of this would be Ganser's syndrome: "the syndrome of approximate answers" to questions, commonly associated with other symptoms such as amnesia, disorientation, perceptual disturbances, fugue, and conversion symptoms. This was named for Sigbert J. M. Ganser, German psychiatrist (1853–1931). It is also called the "nonsense syndrome" or prison psychosis because it is often observed in prisoners who, it is believed, hope to be treated leniently by the court in view of their symptoms.

     In *DSM*-III, Ganser's syndrome was listed as a factitious disorder with psychological symptoms.

X. **Course**
  Characteristically, dissociative disorders have sudden onset and sudden termination.

XI. **Treatment**
  A. Most of the dissociative disorders respond to psychotherapeutic intervention.
  B. Often, especially in psychogenic amnesia, the therapist can gain access to the unconscious mental conflict after a few interviews, by permitting the patient to free-associate to dream material or to any incidents that family or other informants may recall about the patient's locale or behavior.
  C. Occasionally it may be necessary to interview the patient under intravenous Amytal to help him or her recount the amnestic material and help him or her to retain these in consciousness after awakening.
  D. The presence of a significant degree of secondary gain may make it difficult to remove the symptoms.

References

American Psychiatric Association. *Diagnostic and Statistical Manual of Mental Disorders.* 3d. ed., rev. Washington, D.C., 1987.

Eaton, M. T., Jr., M. H. Peterson, and J. A. Davis. *Psychiatry.* 4th ed. Garden City, N.Y.: Medical Examination Publishing Co., 1981.

Kaplan, H. I., and B. J. Sadock. *Comprehensive Textbook of Psychiatry/IV.* 4th ed. Baltimore: Williams & Wilkins, 1985.

Kluft, R. P. An Update on Multiple Personality Disorder, *Hospital and Community Psychiatry.* 38 (April, 1987):363–73.

Kolb, L. C. and H. K. H. Brodie. *Modern Clinical Psychiatry.* 10th ed. Philadelphia: W. B. Saunders Co., 1982.

Nemiah, John. "Psychosomatic Disorders." In *The Harvard Guide to Modern Psychiatry,* edited by A. M. Nicholi, chap. 10. Cambridge: Belknap Press of Harvard University Press, 1978.

We are never so easily deceived as when we imagine we are deceiving others.

La Rochefoucauld: *Maxims* **(1665)**

Factitious Disorders

I. Introduction

A. "Factitious" means not real, genuine, or natural. Factitious disorders are, therefore, characterized by physical or psychological symptoms that are intentionally produced or feigned. The sense of intentionally producing a symptom is subjective; it can only be inferred by an outside observer (*DSM*-III-R).

B. Factitious disorders are distinguished from acts of malingering. In malingering, the "patient" also produces the symptoms intentionally, but it is for a goal that is obviously recognizable when the environmental circumstances are known.

C. In contrast, in a factitious disorder there is no apparent goal other than to assume the patient role.

D. Thus, factitious disorders are distinguished from other illness-affirming states, such as malingering and hysterical conversion disorders.

E. Abnormal illness-affirming states

    1. Malingering: signs and symptoms of illness are consciously produced and consciously motivated.

    2. Hysterical conversion disorders (also including somatoform pain, hypochondriasis, and Briquet's syndrome): signs and symptoms are unconsciously produced and unconsciously motivated.

    3. Factitious disorders: signs and symptoms are consciously produced, but unconsciously motivated.

II. Types

Factitious disorders usually present with either

A. Physical symptoms

B. Psychological symptoms

III. Factitious disorder with physical symptoms

A. Definition

The essential feature is the intentional production of physical symptoms. The presentation may be total fabrication, as in complaints of acute abdominal pain in the absence of any such pain; self-inflicted, as in the production of abscesses by injection of saliva into the skin; and exaggeration or exacerbation of a preexisting physical condition, as in the acceptance of a penicillin injection despite a known history of anaphylactic reaction; or any combination or variation of the above (*DSM*-III-R).

The best studied form of this disorder has been called Münchhausen syndrome. In this chronic form of the disorder, the person's plausible presentation of factitious physical symptoms is associated with multiple hospitalizations. The names was suggested by Asher in 1951 (named after Baron Münchhausen, a real character who wandered from city to city and from tavern to tavern telling tall tales during the eighteenth century). He thought this name was appropriate because the patients wandered from hospital to hospital ("hospital hoboes"), feigned acute medical or surgical illness, and gave false and fanciful information. This has also been called "hospital addiction," although it is doubtful that is dynamically similar to addiction, and "peregrinating professional patients." Impostership is common to this disorder. Once hospitalized, the patient is rarely quiet or cooperative. The behavior is frequently described as truculent, evasive, and hostile; when confronted with the evidence of factitiousness, they sign out against advice.

B. Prevalence

The prevalence is unknown. Some believe that it is rare and that those who have the disorder are overreported, whereas others think the disorder is common but rarely recognized.

C. Symptoms

Common clinical pictures include severe right lower quadrant pain associated with nausea and vomiting, dizziness and blacking out, massive hemoptysis (the expectoration of blood from some part of the respiratory tract), generalized rashes and abscesses, fevers of undetermined origin, bleeding secondary to ingestion of anticoagulants, and "lupuslike" syndromes. Any organ system may be involved and the symptoms are reflections of the person's medical sophistication and imagination.

D. Sex ratio

DSM-III-R reports the disorder as "apparently more common in males," but others say that it seems to occur equally in men and women.

E. Etiology

1. From a psychodynamic point of view, the patient seems to be seeking a repetitive relationship with a physician to reenact a maternal type of relationship.

2. The psychodynamic origin seems to lie in early childhood experiences, that is, emotional and/or physical deprivation.

3. Some have noted that their patients often have borderline personality traits (with developmental difficulty during the separation/individuation phase of childhood).

4. The history often includes a period of hospitalization during early childhood. The developmental history may reveal several themes.

   a) A sense of needing to be taken care of

   b) Masochism

   c) Mastery of an early trauma (thus using factitious illness as a means of mastering a relationship with a parental figure)

F. Treatment

1. Treatment is difficult, although gentle nonjudgmental confrontation would seem appropriate. This would include psychiatric consultation as an attempt to develop a supportive relationship with the patient prior to confrontation.

2. Additionally, the staff who have had to deal with the factitiously disordered patient need an opportunity to ventilate their anger at having been deceived.
3. Psychotherapy by an experienced and skilled psychotherapist, with treatment aimed at improving the patients autonomy and self-esteem while reducing the sense of helplessness, vulnerability, and anger.
G. Differential diagnosis
1. The chief consideration is true physical disorder.
2. Somatoform disorder (symptoms are not intentionally produced).
3. Malingering (the goal is usually apparent).
4. Antisocial personality disorder (rarely associated with chronic hospitalization as a way of life).

IV. Factitious disorder with psychological symptoms
A. Definition
1. The essential feature of this disorder is intentional production or feigning of psychological (often psychotic) symptoms suggestive of mental disorder. The person's goal is apparently to assume the "patient" role and is not otherwise understandable in light of the person's environmental circumstances (as is the case in malingering).
2. It is sometimes called "nonsense syndrome" or the syndrome of deviously relevant answers.
B. Associated features
1. Giving the approximate answers or talking past the point (*Vorbeireden*) may be present.
2. This disorder is almost always superimposed on a severe personality disorder. The person surreptitiously uses psychoative substances to product symptoms suggesting a nonorganic mental disorder (e.g., stimulants, hallucinogens, analgesics, hypnotics, etc.).
C. "The conspicuous features of this disorder consist of a childish, ludicrous performance of simple acts, the correct procedure for which is fully known by the patient" (Kolb and Brodie 1982).
D. Sex ratio
Apparently more common in males.
E. Course
May be limited to a single brief episode or may be chronic.
F. differential diagnosis
1. Other mental disorders
2. Dementia

V. Factitious disorder not otherwise specified

A. According to *DSM*-III-R, this is a category for cases that cannot be classified in any other specific categories.

Examples would include disorders with both factitious physical and factitious psychological symptoms.

References

American Psychiatric Association. *Diagnostic and Statistical Manual of Mental Disorders.* 3d ed., rev. Washington, D.C., 1987.

Eisendraft, S. J. "Factitious Illness: A Clarification." *Psychosomatics* (February 1984):110–17.

Goldman, H. H. *Review of General Psychiatry.* Los Altos, Calif.: Lange Medical Publications, 1974.

Kolb, L. C. and H. K. H. Brodie. *Modern Clinical Psychiatry.* 10th ed. Philadelphia: W. B. Saunders Co., 1982.

Livingston, R. "Maternal Somatization Disorder, and Münchhausen Syndrome by Proxie." *Psychosomatics* (April 1987): 213–17.

For so your doctors hold it
very meet,
Seeing too much sadness
hath congealed your blood,
And melancholy is the nurse
of frenzy.

William Shakespeare:
The Taming of the Shrew

Consultation Liaison Issues / Eating Disorders

I. Introduction

A. In neither *DSM*-III (1980) nor *DSM*-III-R (1987) is there a category labeled psychosomatic or psychophysiologic disorders. Instead there is a classification of psychological factors affecting physical condition. This category enables a clinician to note that psychological factors contribute to the initiation or exacerbation of a physical condition to which psychological factors are judged to be contributory. It can be used to describe disorders that in the past have been referred to as either "psychosomatic" or "psychophysiological." Common examples of physical conditions for which this category may be appropriate include, but are not limited to: obesity, tension headache, migraine headache, angina pectoris, painful menstruation, sacroiliac pain, neurodermatitis, acne, rheumatoid arthritis, asthma, tachycardia, arrhythmia, gastric ulcer, duodenal ulcer, cardiospasm, pylorospasm, nausea and vomiting, regional enteritis, ulcerative colitis, and frequency of micturition (*DSM*-III-R).

B. In the past, the term psychosomatic was used in a nosological or classificatory sense to refer to a group of disorders whose etiology, at least in part, was believed to be related to emotional factors. Subsequently, psychiatric nomenclature substituted the term psychophysiological disorders for psychosomatic disorders.

C. Presently, psychosomatic concepts and their application to patient care are viewed more as an approach or a movement rather than a special field of practice or medical inquiry.

D. The psychosomatic approach assumes that psychological and social factors are significant predispositions, onsets, and continuations of any illnesses. As a matter of fact, it can be an approach to all patients rather than to just those, who in the past, had been considered to have traditional psychosomatic illnesses. More specifically, it is a *bio-psycho-social approach.*

E. Modern consultation liason psychiatry is based on the psychosomatic approach. Here, the psychiatrist is part of a medical team and directs attention to the intrapsychic forces within the patient, the ego-defenses (adaptations to anxiety), life-style, and interpersonal relationships with the nurses and phsycians. The psychiatrist directs attention to the special kinds of emotional problems an individual faces in the particular setting (e.g., intensive care unit, coronary care unit, renal dialysis) and also evaluates the family and social roles of the management of the patient.

F. While older theories were somewhat simplistic in their conceptions of psychosomatic approaches, with the advent of more research, we are aware of the complexities of interacting biological, psychological, and social factors.

II. Consultation liaison psychiatry

A. Definition

This is a subspeciality of psychiatry that is concerned with clinical service, teaching, and research at the borderline of psychiatry and medicine (Lipowski 1986).

1. The clinical service includes the provision of formal psychiatric consultation to other physicians and caregivers or liaisons with them to increase their awareness of psychosocial issues of patients.
2. Teaching would include the instruction of medical students and other caregivers in the aspects of psychosocial medicine.
3. Research includes studies by consultation liason psychiatrists about psychosocial issues in relation to various physical illness and physical injury as well as abnormal illness behavior (for example, somatoform and factitious disorders).

B. Historical Background

Among the names of those who have attempted to integrate psychiatry and medicine are the following:

1. Benjamin Rush (1745–1813). He was a physician and a signer of the Declaration of Independence. His *Medical Inquiries and Observations Upon Diseases of the Mind,* published in 1812, was the first American treatise on psychiatry. This is considered the first attempt to integrate psychiatry and medicine in clinical practice into the teaching of medical students. His holistic approach really was a precursor of the modern psychosomatic movement.
2. Adolf Meyer (1866–1950), founder of *Psychobiology,* which was a comprehensive and holistic approach to the understanding of the individual. He became the director of the Henry Phipps Psychiatric Clinic of Johns Hopkins Hospital in the early twentieth century. This helped pave the way for the emergence of the psychosomatic approach and consultation liaison psychiatry.
3. Subsequently, other psychiatrists were engaged in pioneering efforts that would advocate collaboration between psychiatrists and other physicians in teaching clinical work, and research.
4. Edward G. Billings is credited for founding the first formal division of consultation liaison psychiatry at the University of Colorado School of Medicine in 1934 (Lipowski 1986).

III. The psychosomatic movement

A. Historical perspective

1. Specialists in this approach have seen the early origins of this approach in the writings of Hippocrates. Credit is also given to Francis Bacon who spoke of, "the sympathies and concordances between the mind and the body, which being mixed, cannot be properly assigned the sciences of either" (Schwab 1985).

2. Interest in this approach waxed and waned over the centuries, but "faded into obscurity during 1840–1920" (Schwab 1985).
3. Although in the middle of this century, it appeared as if psychosomatic medicine might become a specialty within a short time. The movement, once again, appeared fated for obscurity.
4. Currently, the psychosomatic movement seems to be in a phase of rapid development. "A number of cultural and intellectual processes favor its growth and importance. These include widespread public concern about stress, deleterious life-styles and the diseases of civilization, which many now agree, are psychosomatic" (Schwab 1985).
5. Thus, the psychosomatic concept seems to fit in very well with the current focus on the biopsychosocial model of health and illness.
6. In this chapter, we will discuss eating disorders as the condition that seems to blend itself well into the matters discussed under consultation liaison psychiatry in the psychosomatic movement.

IV. **Eating disorders**
   A. Introduction
      1. Most everyone is aware of the relationship between emotions and the gastrointestinal tract. It is thought by many that food is, very early on, associated with feelings of security, attention, and love. Various types of psychosomatic disturbances are associated with eating, digesting, and eliminating food.
      2. In 1676, Morton described the characteristic triad—loss of appetite, amenorrhea, and extreme wasting without lassitude—in cases of "nervous consumption" or "prodiginous abstinence."
      3. About 200 years later, Gull and Laseque labeled this condition anorexia nervosa.
   B. Classification
      1. Eating disorders are characterized by gross disturbances in eating behavior.
      2. Included in this group are: anorexia nervosa, bulimia nervosa, pica, and rumination disorder of infancy. Pica and rumination disorder are primarily found in young children and very likely not related to the other two. Anorexia nervosa and bulimia nervosa seem to be related and typically begin in adolescence or early adult life.
      3. Obesity, which is probably many disorders, is *not* classified as an eating disorder in *DSM*-III-R.
   C. Anorexia nervosa
      1. Definition
      The essential features are: refusal to maintain body weight over a minimal normal weight for age and height; intense fear of gaining weight or becoming fat, even though underweight; a distorted body image; and amenorrhea in females (*DSM*-III-R).

2. Description
    a) 95 percent are females. The typical anorectic is a white teenage female from a middle- or upper-class family who plans to attend college.
    b) It must be distinguished from other illnesses that are accompanied by weight loss, such as endocrine and other organic illnesses that produce malnutrition, loss of appeitie, and loss of weight.
    c) Clinical picture
        (1) Refusal to maintain body weight over the normal minimum for one's age and height.
        (2) Loss in weight of 25 percent; or, if under eighteen years of age, a 25 percent loss in weight when the gain in weight projected from pediatric growth charts is added.
        (3) Disturbance of body image and inability to perceive body size accurately.
        (4) Intense fear of becoming obese that does not diminish as weight is lost.
        (5) There is no known medical illness to account for the loss of weight.
        (6) Amenorrhea in females.
    d) Anorexia is rare.
    e) Essentially, the behavior of the person with this illness is governed by the desire to lose weight and the intense fear of gaining it. The behavior includes marked dietary limitation; abuse of laxatives or diuretics or both; and, sometimes, self-induced vomiting. (The last is a symptom of bulimia nervosa, which also may be present.)
3. Etiology
    The etiology of this disorder remains unknown.
    a) Many of these patients are described as "model" children, with perfectionistic tendencies and above average achievement in school. (After the onset of the anorexia nervosa, they become terrified of their lack of control and immobilized by their own perceived helplessness.)
    b) Two prominent features of this disorder are:
        (1) Distorted perception of their body image.
        (2) Dread of not being in control.
    c) Theories of etiology
        Early psychoanalytic interpretations regarded this as "fear of oral impregnation." Later psychoanalytic interpretations regarded it as prevention of individuation and separation by a domineering mother. Family theorists point to ineffective

fathers and overbearing mothers but it is difficult to determine whether this is cause or effect. Biological theories include this disorder as a "variant of depression" (41 percent of anorectics have depression).

4. Clinical course

According to *DSM*-III-R, the most common course is a single episode with return to normal weight but it is important to keep in mind that anorexia nervosa can be a lethal disease and the course may be "unremitting until death."

5. Treatment

No specific treatment exists because the etiology of this disorder remains unknown and the needs of patients are far from uniform. Treatment should be pragmatic and designed to improve major areas of dysfunction (Hsu 1986).

a) Hospitalization may be indicated to effectively assess the patient's condition and needs and also to foster the development of a therapeutic alliance. In some instances it may be "life-saving." It might also provide an opportunity to teach the patient how to eat properly. However, many patients can be treated in an outpatient setting.

b) Traditional psychoanalytic interpretative approaches are ineffective. However, psychotherapy has been found useful.

c) Pharmacotherapy

Certain psychotropic medications may enhance weight gain in the short term when used in conjunction with behavior or milieu therapy. (Included in these would be thorazine and tricyclic antidepressants.)

Because of the coexistent depression commonly found in anorexia nervosa, many clinicians have used antidepressants, either tricyclics or MAOI drugs. (However, one must keep in mind the tyramine-free diet in the use of the latter.)

d) Outpatient therapy

The less emaciated, less severely ill patients who are not vomiting, purging, or suicidal may be treated as outpatients, using psychotherapy in an attempt to resolve underlying psychological problems.

e) Relapses

Although *DSM*-III indicates that a single episode is the most common story, some authors feel relapses are common, especially within the first year.

f) Summary

The prevalence of anorexia nervosa has been increasing. Despite this fact, there has been no major breakthrough in treatment in recent years. However, it does seem that use of coercive treatments such as hyperalimentation and tube feeding are rarely necessary anymore.

D. Bulimia nervosa
  1. Introduction
     Although anorexia nervosa was described three hundred years ago, bulimia was not recognized until the 1950s.
  2. Definition
     The essential features are recurrent episodes of binge eating (rapid consumption of a large amount of food in a discrete period of time); a feeling of lack of control over eating behavior during the eating binges; self-induced vomiting, use of laxatives or diuretics, strict dieting or fasting, or vigorous exercise in order to prevent weight gain; and persistent overconcern with body shape and weight (*DSM*-III-R).
     Amenorrhea is uncommon and there usually is no weight loss.
  3. Description
     Bulimics view their binging behavior as pathological and dread their difficulty in controlling their eating. Their self-induced vomiting is usually common. Binging usually stops when the patient is discovered, falls asleep, induces vomiting, or develops abdominal pain. They are preoccupied with their appearance and body image. Some of the people with this disorder also have psychoactive substance abuse or dependence, most frequently involving alcohol, amphetamines, sedatives, or cocaine.
  4. Clinical Course
     This is usually a chronic disorder arising in the teens or twenties.
  5. Etiology
     The cause of bulimia nervosa is largely unknown. Some psychodynamic theories see binging as a gratification of sexual and aggressive wishes and vomiting as a symbolic "purging of the bad self." Descriptive and biological psychiatrists see it as having some relationship to depression.
  6. Treatment
     Medication (tricyclic antidepressants or MAOIs, which reduce binging) and group therapy seem to be helpful. However, there are still many unanswered questions about treatment.

References

Amercian Psychiatric Association. *Diagnostic and Statistical Manual of Mental Disorders*. 3d ed., rev. Washington, D.C. 1987

Hsu, L. K. G. "The Treatment of Anorexia Nervosa" *American Journal of Psychiatry* 143 (May 1986):5.

Lipowsui Z. J. "Consultation-Liaison Psychiatry: The First Half Century." *General Hospital Psychiatry* 8 (1986):305–15.

Maxmen, J. S. *Essential Psychpathology*. New York: W. W. Norton Co., 1986.

Schwab, J. J. "Psychosomatic Medicine: Its Past and Present" *Pyschosomatics* 26, Period #7 (July 1985).

There is something in the character of every man which cannot be altered: It is the skeleton of his character. Trying to change it is like trying to train sheep to pull a car.

G. C. Lichtenberg: *Reflections* (1799)

Personality Disorders

I. Definition

Personality traits are enduring patterns of perceiving, relating to, and thinking about the environment and oneself, and are exhibited in a wide range of important social and personal contexts. It is only when personality traits are inflexible and maladaptive and cause either significant functional impairment or subjective distress that they constitute personality disorders. The manifestations of personality disorders are often recognizable by adolescence or earlier and continue throughout most of adult life, although they often become less obvious in middle or old age (*DSM*-III-R).

II. Personality development

A. Definition: There are very likely as many definitions of personality as there are authorities who have written about it. No single definition of personality exists.

B. Personality is defined by Campbell as follows: character (q.v.); the characteristic, and to some extent predictable, behavior-response patterns that each person evolves, both consciously and unconsciously, as his or her style of life. The personality represents a compromise between inner drives and needs and the controls that limit or regulate their expression. Such controls are both internal (e.g., conscience and superego) and external (reality demands). The personality functions to maintain a stable, reciprocal relationship between the person and the environment; it is thus a composite of the ego defenses, the autoplastic and the alloplastic maneuvers that are automatically and customarily employed to maintain intrapsychic stability.[1]

C. The APA *A Psychiatric Glossary* defines personality as "The characteristic way in which a person thinks, feels, and behaves; the ingrained pattern of behavior that each person evolves, both consciously and unconsciously, as the style of life or way of being in adapting to the environment."[2]

D. More simply stated, personality is the sum total of a person's internal and external patterns of adjustment to life. Although there may be some variation in a person's behavior, the individual's adjustment is generally in a state of equilibrium because he or she has accumulated a repertoire of problem-solving techniques during growth and development.

Personality reflects those coping mechanisms and ego defenses that one uses to maintain emotional equilibrium. (See chapter, "Adaptation to Anxiety: Coping and Defense Mechanisms," page 63.) It also reflects the compromise that one has made among the pressures from instinctual drives, the environment, and the superego.

1. R. J. Campbell, *Psychiatric Dictionary*, 5th ed. (New York: Oxford University Press, 1981).
2. American Psychiatric Association, *A Psychiatric Glossary*, 6th ed. (Washington, D. C., 1988).

Thus, personality usually reflects the individual's techniques of getting along with other people and results from early developmental factors, including the influences of society, culture, and childrearing patterns. Certain well-developed personality traits such as compulsiveness, narcissism, or dependency may be so minimal that they do not interfere with the individual's functioning.

III. **Characteristics of personality disorder**
  A. Individuals with personality disorders do not develop symptoms that bother them. In psychoanalytic terminology, they have a *character neurosis* (in which impulses and ideas are acceptable to the ego as consonant and compatible with its principles) rather than a *symptom neurosis* (in which the stimuli from any source are rejected by the ego or are prevented from reaching ego for consideration).
  B. The personality disorder is characterized by its lifelong nature and the person's repetitive, maladaptive, and often self-defeating behavior (rather than discomfort or physical and psychological symptoms).
  C. The disorders usually begin in childhood or adolescence and persist throughout most of adult life.
  D. People with personality disorders are usually anxiety-free except when they are confronted with environmental stress.
  E. Because problems are expressed in a maladaptive form of living rather than in symptoms, it is rare for character-disordered individuals to seek help at their own initiative. In general, such people tolerate stress poorly. If they are confronted by minor stresses, they are apt to become anxious; if confronted by moderate stresses, they may develop transient psychotic reactions.
  F. It should be remembered that many of the difficulties people have adjusting to the world may be due to social stress or disarrangement rather than to disordered character.
  G. When the occupation or environment accepts or rewards the individual's behavior, such personality patterns may be compatible with success and satisfaction. For example, a narcissistic person might be very successful in the entertainment world.
  H. Some evidence suggests that individuals with personality disorders are at greatest risks for other psychiatric disorders.

IV. **Etiological factors**
  Among the possible causal factors are
  A. Constitutional predisposition
  B. Childhood experiences that have fostered deviant behavior
    1. Being rewarded for "acting-out" behavior (such as temper tantrums or hostile-aggressive behavior).
    2. Being encouraged when overly conforming and being discouraged when creative.

3. Circumstances in which normal behavior is not allowed to develop, for example, having a rigid, unreasonable parent who adamantly refuses to accept any reason for nonconformity.
    C. Identification with parents or other authority figures who have similar deviancies
V. **Types of personality disorders**
    A. The personality disorders have been grouped into three clusters
        1. Cluster A (previously referred to as odd or eccentric). This group includes paranoid, schizoid, and schizotypal personality disorders.
        2. Cluster B (previously described as dramatic, emotional or erratic). This group includes antisocial, borderline, histrionic, and narcissistic personality disorders.
        3. Cluster C (previously described as anxious or fearful). This group includes avoidant, dependent, obsessive-compulsive, and passive-aggressive personality disorders.
    B. Included under this classification are
        1. Paranoid personality disorder
        2. Schizoid personality disorder
        3. Schizotypal personality disorder
        4. Antisocial personality disorder
        5. Borderline personality disorder
        6. Histrionic personality disorder
        7. Narcissistic personality disorder
        8. Avoidant personality disorder
        9. Dependent personality disorder
        10. Obsessive-compulsive personality disorder
        11. Passive-aggressive personality disorder
    C. In the new multiaxial classification of *DSM*-III-R, these disorders are listed under Axis II. This Axis includes specific developmental disorders of children and adolescents. This Axis allows for the inclusion of diagnostic entities that are usually not given consideration when the usually more florid Axis I disorder is under treatment (e.g., major depressive disorder, substance use disorder, etc.). Such a classification assumes that the attention to more than one clinical parameter of the disorder will "provide greater specificity and objectivity and a firmer basis for identifying subtypes."
    D. The definitions of the personality disorders discussed in the rest of this chapter are based on the descriptions in *DSM*-III-R.
VI. **Paranoid personality disorder**
    A. Definition
    The essential feature of this disorder is a pervasive and unwarranted tendency, beginning by early adulthood and present in a variety of contexts, to interpret the actions of people as deliberately demeaning or threatening.

B. Prevalence

People with this disorder rarely come to clinical attention so its prevalence is unknown.

C. Associated features

1. Persons with paranoid personalities rarely seek psychiatric treatment on their own.
2. The disorder is more common in men.
3. Most paranoid people avoid intimacy.
4. Such a person may be "litigious, moralistic, and a collector of injustices" (Kaplan and Sadock).
5. Paranoid patients often "personalize" fortuitous or coincidental events.
6. Impairment tends to be minimal because people with this personality disorder realize that it is wise to keep their unusual ideas to themselves.

D. Case example

J. H., a thirty-eight-year-old married man, was referred to the court's psychiatric consultant for evaluation after he had pleaded guilty to a charge of assault growing out of a complaint filed by his wife, whom he had beaten up one evening in a bar.

He admitted to one previous court appearance for leaving the scene of an accident and also admitted to being jailed overnight once for drunkenness. In an interview, he admitted to having beaten his wife once previously, but said that he only slapped her with his open hand. He admitted to arguing with his wife but claimed the arguments were not too different from those most married couples have.

His wife reported that he carried a chip on his shoulder most of the time and felt that people owed him something. She indicated that he was "very suspicious" of her friends and that he would not talk to them. He constantly suspected that his wife was unfaithful and was unable to place any trust and confidence in physicians even though, by neglecting to do so, he had impaired his health. His Minnesota Multiphasic Personality Inventory profile was consistent with a diagnosis of paranoid personality. He seemed to be the sort of person who could keep his paranoid feelings under control as long as he did not drink. When he drank, his suspicions and projected feelings were enhanced, and he acted on them.

VII. Schizoid personality disorder

A. Definition

1. The essential feature of this disorder is a pervasive pattern of indifference to social relationships and a restricted range of emotional experience and expression, beginning by early adulthood and present in a variety of contexts.

People with this disorder neither desire nor enjoy close relationships, including being part of a family. They prefer to be "loners," and have no close friends or confidants (or only one) other than first-degree relatives. They almost always choose solitary activities and indicate little if any desire to have sexual experiences with another person. Such people are indifferent to the praise and criticism of others. They claim that they rarely experience strong emotions such as anger and joy, and in fact display a constricted affect. They appear cold and aloof (*DSM*-III-R).

2. Also known as *introverted personality.*

B. Prevalence

The prevalence in clinical settings is low.

C. Associated features

People with this disorder are often unable to express their aggressiveness or hostility. They lack social skills.

D. Impairment

Socialization is severely restricted and occupational functioning may be impaired.

E. Case example

C. N., a twenty-five-year-old single woman, was referred to the court's psychiatric consultant for evaluation after she had been arrested in the lobby of a downtown hotel for drunkenness. Aside from her drunken state, no behavioral disturbance had brought her to the attention of the authorities. She had never been arrested previously.

During the interview, she was very quiet. Most of the information obtained from her was through a question-and-answer approach. She responded to direct questions, but volunteered very little about herself. She had a somewhat disheveled appearance and wore an unusual amount of cheap jewelry. Although she was a college graduate, she was working as a cocktail waitress in one of the local country clubs. She readily admitted to having a drinking problem and estimated that about twice a month she drank to the point of blacking out. Most of her drinking was done alone, although some of it was in the company of other waitresses. She did not seem to be very introspective or reflective. When asked to give her opinion of herself, she said that she never thought much about herself. She admitted to being very passive and said that she felt easily led. The probation officer who had investigated her reported that she was a very shy, withdrawn person, sadly lacking in self-confidence.

VIII. **Schizotypal personality disorder**

A. Definition

The essential feature of this disorder is a pervasive pattern of peculiarities of ideation, appearance, and behavior and deficits in interpersonal relatedness, beginning by early adulthood and present in a variety of contexts, that are not severe enough to meet the criteria for schizophrenia.

The disturbance in the content of thought may include paranoid ideation, suspiciousness, ideas of reference, odd beliefs, and magical thinking that is inconsistent with subcultural norms and influences the person's behavior. Examples include superstitiousness, belief in clairvoyance, telepathy, or "sixth sense," or beliefs that "others can feel my feelings" (when it is not a part of a cultural belief system). In children and adolescents, these thoughts may include bizarre fantasies or preoccupations. Unusual perceptual experiences may include illusions and sensing the presence of a force or person not actually present (e.g., "I felt an evil presence in the room"). Often speech shows marked peculiarities, but never to the point of loosening of associations or incoherence. Speech may be impoverished, digressive, vague, or inappropriately abstract. Concepts may be expressed unclearly or oddly, or words may be used in an unusual way. People with this disorder often appear odd and eccentric in behavior and appearance. For example, they are often unkempt, display unusual mannerisms, and talk to themselves.

B. Prevalence

According to *DSM*-III-R, approximately 3 percent of the population has this disorder.

C. Associated features

During periods of extreme stress, such individuals may experience transient psychotic episodes.

D. Impairment

Social or occupational function is commonly impaired.

E. Family

There is some evidence that people with this disorder are more common in the first-degree biologic relatives of schizophrenics.

IX. Antisocial personality disorder

A. Definition

The essential feature of this disorder is a pattern of irresponsible and antisocial behavior beginning in childhood or early adolescence and continuing into adulthood. For this diagnosis to be given, the person must be at least eighteen years of age and have a history of conduct disorder before the age of fifteen.

B. Prevalence

1. Recent estimates indicate a prevalence of about 3 percent of American men and less than 1 percent of American women

2. It is more common in lower socioeconomic groups with backgrounds of rejection, deprivation, neglect, and abuse

3. Predisposing factors are attention deficit hyperactivity disorder and conduct disorder during prepuberty years

4. The fathers of those affected often have the same disorder

C. Symptoms, according to *DSM*-III-R criteria

1. Current age at least eighteen

2. Evidence of conduct disorder before the age of fifteen—at least three of the following: truancy; running away from home overnight; frequent initiation of physical fights; the use of a weapon in more than one fight; forced someone into sexual

activity; physical cruelty to animals; physical cruelty to other people; deliberate destruction of other's property; deliberate engagement in fire-setting; lying; stealing (with and without confrontation of the victim)

3. Irresponsible and antisocial behavior after the age of 15—at least four of the following:

   a) Inability to sustain consistent work behavior (significant unemployment, repeated absences from work unexplained by illness in self and family, abandonment of several jobs without realistic plans for others)

   b) Failure to conform to social norms with respect to lawful behavior

   c) Irritability and aggressiveness as indicated by repeated physical fights or assaults

   d) Repeated failures to honor financial obligations

   e) Failure to plan ahead or impulsivity as indicated by one or both of the following: traveling from place to place without a prearranged job or clear goal and lack of a fixed address for a month or more

   f) No regard for the truth

   g) Reckless regard for his or her own or others' personal safety

   h) If a parent lacks the ability to function as a responsible parent (inattention to a child's basic needs)

   i) Inability to sustain a totally monogamous relationship for more than one year

   j) Lacks remorse

4. Generalizations

   Antisocial personalities persistently violate the laws, customs, and mores of the community in which they live. They show a lifelong pattern of acting-out behavior (disordered behavior) rather than the subjective discomfort.

D. Etiology

   1. The causes of antisocial personality disorder are not clearly understood.

   2. Family history

      a) A history of antisocial personality disorder is often found in the fathers of both males and females with the disorder.

      b) Findings in twin studies and adoption studies support the hypothesis of a genetic component.

   3. Multiple causation

      Recent studies indicate that both genetic and environmental influences are important (*DSM*-III-R).

4. Organic

   At present there is no evidence that organic brain damage contributes to antisocial personality disorder. In the past, some cases of antisocial behavior have been precipitated by brain damage, for example, by severe head trauma or encephalitis. Although the behavior may be classified as antisocial, technically such individuals are not usually considered antisocial personalities, but are more properly diagnosed as having organic mental disorders.

5. Psychosocial

   Some authorities consider psychological and social factors to be chiefly responsible for the development of antisocial personality disorder.

   a) Social factors

      (1) The antisocial personality comes largely from the lower socioeconomic groups. There is a high rate of delinquency in the slum areas of larger urban communities.

      (2) Living according to the pleasure principle without regard for the reality principle is in part determined by social factors as well as by parental relationships.

      (3) The families and environment from which antisocial persons come have high rates of broken homes, alcoholism, and antisocial behavior.

   b) Psychological factors

      (1) Johnson and Szurek (1952) describe the "superego lacunae" that developed in antisocial personalities as a result of unconscious fostering of such behavior by the parents during the developmental years.

      (2) Antisocial personality disorder has been correlated with maternal deprivation in a child's first five years of life.

      (3) Some studies report that the mothers of children who develop this disorder show a lack of consistent discipline, lack of affection, and increased incidence of alcoholism and impulsiveness.

E. Psychopathology

   1. The essential defect in antisocial personalities involves their character structure (hence, this disturbance is sometimes called a *character disorder* or *character neurosis*).

   2. Like infants, antisocial personalities give direct expression to their impulses. They are seemingly incapable of adapting their urges to the demands of society and unable to postpone immediate gratification of their desires.

3. They defy, or come into conflict with, authority, and they lack sensitivity to other people's feelings.
4. Since they are dominated by unsocialized drives, they have difficulty in their relationships with others. Although intellectually they recognize that their acts are illegal or unethical, they seem uninfluenced by such knowledge.
5. They might be considered emotionally deficient. They are egocentric, selfish, make excessive demands, and are unable to view their own behavior objectively. They are usually free of anxiety, remorse, or guilt.
6. From the foregoing, it becomes apparent that the antisocial person has a poorly developed conscience (defective superego).
   a) Conscience is largely dependent upon relationships with parents or parent substitutes. One's value system is usually developed through one's relationships with parents (largely by identification) and is based on affection and trust.
   b) In antisocial persons, the identification process is faulty. Either they are unable to evolve a value system through the normal process of identification or they develop pathological types of identification.
      (1) *Hostile identification* is internalization of undesirable personality traits of parents or authority figures.
      (2) *Identification with the aggressor* is internalization of the characteristics of a frustrated or feared parent or parent substitute.
   c) We often find a history of difficulty with parents or authority figures from the earliest years.
   d) This history seems related to parental attitudes that are commonly unreasonable, neglectful, cruel, hypocritical, or inconsistent (e.g., vacillating or unpredictable). The child has difficulty attaching himself to either parent as an example to follow or as a source of security because there has been a lack of mutual affection, tenderness, or trust.
   e) Because of this detachment from parents and parent-figures, the behavior of antisocial personalities develops no sense of direction (i.e., they are uninfluenced by any concepts of right and wrong).
   f) Some authorities feel that, in a sense, their willful, unsocialized behavior is a seeking for attention, affection, and acceptance.

F. Case report

Bob, the eighteen-year-old son of well-to-do parents, was brought to the hospital for psychiatric examination upon the order of a judge. One night four weeks earlier, the patient had, in the company of three other boys, entered a cemetery, tipped over several gravestones, and mutilated a monument.

When Bob first entered grade school, he had some minor difficulties. He performed below his intellectual capacity and frequently did things that the other children considered "daring," such as letting the air out of automobile tires. At nine, he began to smoke, not just experimentally, like some of the other boys, but often and somewhat defiantly.

He first came into difficulty with the law at the age of eleven when he stole two cigarette lighters and a wristwatch from a jewelry store. Following this, he was sent to a military boarding school upon the advice of the judge and the family physician. Two months after he entered the new school, he broke into the school store, stole candy and cigarettes, and ran away to a nearby city. He was found two days later in a hotel room by himself. He was returned to his home and completed the school year at the local school.

At thirteen, he and two other boys stole a large amount of gasoline from a nearby storage plant. This was used in a "jalopy" purchased for the patient by his father. At first, he denied the theft but, when confronted with irrefutable proof, admitted his guilt; however, he was unable to give any reason for wanting the gasoline. From the age of thirteen until seventeen, he was frequently involved in minor delinquencies but always escaped punishment because of his family's position in the community and because his father always made restitution. At seventeen, he began drinking beer and shortly was getting "high" regularly.

Bob was the older of two brothers but was reared as an only child because his infant brother died when Bob was four. After this, the parents overindulged him. At five, he fell from a horse, following which he had a few convulsions. He was examined at a well-known clinic and placed on anticonvulsants. After a few weeks of this treatment, he quit taking the medications. He says he has never been really close to anyone and has never felt toward his parents as other youngsters do. Although the parents verbally disapproved of his behavior, they encouraged it in subtle ways; for example, increasing his already overly generous allowance after he was caught stealing from a hardware store.

At no time has he ever shown any guilt for his delinquent and antisocial behavior, and he always seems free of anxiety. His case illustrates some of the typical aspects of the antisocial personality disorder.

X. Borderline personality disorder
A. Definition
The essential feature of this disorder is a pervasive pattern of instability of self-image, interpersonal relationships, and mood, beginning by early adulthood and present in a variety of contexts (*DSM*-III-R).

1. A marked identity disturbance is almost invariably present (as manifested by uncertainty about several life issues such as self-image, sexual orientation, career choice, friends, etc.).
2. Unstable and intense interpersonal relationships, including alternation of the extremes of overidealization and devaluation.
3. Affective instability is common (as evidenced by mood shifts from baseline mood to depression, irritability, or anxiety). In addition these people often have inappropriately intense anger or lack of control of their anger. They tend to be impulsive particularly in activities that are potentially self-damaging, such as shopping sprees, psychoactive substance abuse, reckless driving, casual sex, shoplifting and binge eating.
4. Recurrent suicidal threats, gestures, or behavior and other self-mutilating behavior (e.g., wrist scratching) are common in the more severe forms of this disorder. This behavior may serve to manipulate others, may be a result of intense anger or may counteract feelings of "numbness" and depersonalization that arise during periods of extreme stress.
5. Chronic feelings of emptiness and boredom.
6. Frantic efforts to avoid real or imagined abandonment.
7. Previous labels for borderline personality disorder include *ambulatory schizophrenia, latent schizophrenia, preschizophrenia, schizophrenic character, abortive schizophrenia, pseudoneurotic schizophrenia,* and so forth.

B. Prevalence

It is apparently common and more frequently diagnosed in females.

C. Associated features

Features of other personality disorders such as narcissistic, histrionic, schizotypal, and antisocial are commonly present.

D. Etiology and psychopathology
1. Early formulations of borderline psychopathology were based on the ego-psychological model of psychoanalysis, thus the borderlines were viewed as having weak ego structures that remained intact and able to cope with reality when reality was structured and consistent but that could be easily flooded by primary process thinking (largely unconscious psychological expressions of underlying basic drives that follow the pleasure principle) when external structure was lacking or internal pressures had upset the ego's precarious equilibrium (thus such diagnostic terms as: *borderline psychosis, borderline schizophrenia, ambulatory schizophrenia, preschizophrenia*).

More recent formulations have been influenced by object relations theory (the psychoanalytic description of the internalization of interpersonal relations and the organizing effects of internalized human object relationships on the structure of psyche), leading to the concept of borderline disorganization.

2. Most causal theories have been based on cases treated with psychodynamically oriented therapy. Most of the theoretical formulations have been psychoanalytic in orientation.

    a) Masterson (1972) sees the borderline personality in adolescence as characterized by a persistent symbiosis with parental figures. There is a predominance of negative feelings that are shared by parent and child, which persists and yet binds the two together by mutual guilty and bad feelings.

    b) Kernberg (1975) suggests that early pathological object relations are internalized and maintained by the use of primitive defense mechanisms that healthier people give up in normal development. These psychoticlike defensive operations are denial, projection, splitting, and projective identification (see the chapter, "Adaptations to Anxiety"). Further, Kernberg sees the person with borderline personality disorder as categorizing people as all good (nurturant) and all bad (hateful). He relates this to the patient's early stages of psychosexual development, in which the mother figure is experienced in two contradictory ways (good and bad).

    Thus Kernberg hypothesized that the arrest in normal psychological development, with failure to integrate ambivalent feelings, originally arose against the primary caretaker but later occurred in other close relationships as well.

3. Mahler and Masterson (1972) have hypothesized that this disorder results after a disturbance occurring in children between sixteen and twenty-five months of age during the rapprochement phase of separation and individuation. In this phase, the child practices independent behavior and returns to the primary caretaker for approval, admiration, and emotional "refueling." The critical, rejecting parent or the suffocating, smothering parent interferes with optimal progression of attachment-separation sequences.

4. Although most authorities regard etiology as largely psycho-dynamic and hereditary, some feel there is a genetic role, and Kernberg (1975) and Klein have suggested that patients with borderline personality have a "constitutionally based" inability to regulate affects, especially anger. There may also be a relationship between borderline personality and depressive illness.

E. Course and prognosis
   1. In the past, short-term follow-up studies have suggested that borderline patients do not change much.
   2. Recent evidence suggests that the long-term prognosis of this condition is relatively good with gradual improvement (provided the patient does not commit suicide or succumb to alcohol abuse).

F. Treatment
   1. Psychotherapy
      a) Attempts at long-term psychotherapy for borderline personality disorder are fraught with anguish and hostility for both the patient and therapist. Regression is a repeated problem.
      b) In general, there are two viewpoints about treatment approaches:
         (1) A modified psychoanalytic approach is considered helpful and aims at the resolution of the underlying psychopathology. Such treatment may require special ongoing support systems.
         (2) In supportive reality-oriented therapy the patient is offered a limited psychotherapeutic relationship, but the therapist expects to be indefinitely available. The goal in this treatment is gradual social adjustment. (Such an approach may include some behavioral approaches as well.)
   2. Psychotropic medication
      a) Antipsychotic drugs may be useful during brief psychotic periods and lower doses may be indicated for anger, hostility and suspiciousness, paranoid thinking, and so forth.
      b) Carbamazepine may increase impulsivity.
      c) Tricyclic antidepressants may be helpful during periods of depression and monoamine oxidase inhibitors may also be helpful in improving mood (caution: dietary restrictions).
      d) Those who have bipolar traits might benefit from lithium.
   3. Some authorities suggest use of pharmacotherapy together with psychotherapy in the context of an ongoing supportive relationship with the therapist.
   4. Treating borderline patients is a challenge.

G. Case example

A sixteen-year-old white female was admitted to a residential treatment center upon referral of a psychiatrist who had treated her in an acute adolescent hospital for approximately six months. In his referral note, he reported that she was unable to function in her chaotic home situation. In addition to this, she was depressed in the hospital, had made suicidal gestures, specifically, cutting herself with fragments of glass and drinking bottles of cologne. In addition, he reported that she was showing academic underachievement, truancy, poor peer relationships, and had frequent headaches and temper outbursts.

Evaluation at the residential treatment center revealed that her manifest symptoms had begun to surface about a year and a half earlier, following a move from one part of the country to another. About this time, she became truant and engaged in activities that kept her four other siblings in constant turmoil. In addition, her peer relationships at school deteriorated and she showed bellicosity toward her teachers. She even became physically assaultive of others in her school. There was evidence of a great deal of intense ambivalence, on her part, surrounding her mother and her relative degree of separation from and closeness to her mother. (The mother had had a series of men living with her, and about six months before the girl was admitted to the residential treatment center, her stepfather entered into a sexual relationship with her, of which the mother was unaware until just before the girl's hospitalization.) Shortly before her initial hospitalization, she had run away from home for a two-week period and suddenly reappeared in the police station to report that she had been physically abused by her mother and raped by her stepfather. After the parents were cleared of these accusations by an investigation, she was placed in a crisis home and then admitted to the local hospital.

From assessment performed at the residential center, it was learned that she had developed an ever-increasing degree of separation anxiety as a result of her impaired separation-individuation process. The periods of acting out seemed to be correlated with the imminent separation from her mother, and the speculation was that her sexual involvement with her stepfather was perhaps a search for a lost nurturant mother. Her identification seemed confused. She seemed to lack a consistent role model.

Her treatment plan, which included intense individual psychoanalytic therapy, lasted for approximately two and a half years. She made good progress in therapy and was able to surrender unstable relationships that were patterned after her mother; she also was able to express vulnerability instead of covering it up. In treatment, she showed a great deal of splitting and projective identification.

XI. Histrionic personality disorder
A. Definition

The essential feature of this disorder is a pervasive pattern of excessive emotionality and attention-seeking, beginning by early adulthood and present in a variety of contexts. In other classifications this category is termed hysterical personality.

B. People with this disorder constantly seek or demand reassurance, approval, or praise from others and are uncomfortable in situations in which they are not the center of attention. They characteristically display rapidly shifting and shallow expression of emotions. Their behavior is overly reactive and intensely expressed; minor stimuli give rise to emotional excitability. Emotions are often expressed with inappropriate exaggeration; for example, the person may appear much more sad, angry, or delighted than would seem to be warranted. People with this disorder tend to be very self-centered, with little or no tolerance for the frustration of delayed gratification. Their actions are directed to obtaining immediate satisfaction.

C. These people are typically attractive and seductive, often to the point of looking flamboyant and acting inappropriately. They are typically overly concerned with physical attractiveness. In addition, their style of speech tends to be expressionistic and lacking in detail. For example, a person may describe his vacation as "Just fantastic" without being able to be more specific.

D. Prevalence

DSM-III-R notes that the disorder is "apparently common" and diagnosed "much more frequently in females," in part because of the sex class and its description.

E. Associated features

People with this disorder are lively and dramatic and are always drawing attention to themselves. They are prone to exaggeration in their interpersonal relations and often act out a role such as that of "victim" or "princess" without being aware of it. They crave novelty, stimulation, and excitement and quickly become bored with normal routine. Others frequently perceive them as superficially charming and appealing, but lacking genuineness. They are often quick to form friendships, but once a relationship is established, can be egocentric and inconsiderate. They may constantly demand reassurance because of feelings of helplessness and dependency. Their actions are often inconsistent and may be misinterpreted by others.

In relationships they attempt to control the opposite sex or to enter into a dependent relationship. Flights into romantic fantasy are common. The actual quality of their sexual relationships is variable. Some are promiscuous; others, naive and sexually unresponsive; and still others, apparently normal in their sexual adjustment.

Usually these people show little interest in intellectual achievement and careful, analytic thinking, but they are often creative and imaginative.

People with this disorder tend to be impressionable and easily influenced by others or by fads. They are apt to be overly trusting of others and suggestible, and to show an initially positive response to any strong authority figure who, they think, can provide a magical solution for their problems. Though they adopt convictions strongly and readily, their judgment is not firmly rooted, and they often play hunches.

Frequent complaints of poor health, such as weakness or headaches, or subjective feelings of depersonalization may be present. During periods of extreme stress, people with this disorder may experience transient psychotic symptoms, but they are generally of insufficient severity or duration to warrant an additional diagnosis.

F. Symptoms

In addition to the symptoms listed under the definition above, the patient often displays "la belle indifference." Women with this disorder may be coquettish and men with the disorder may play the "Don Juan" role.

G. Case example

Scarlett O'Hara, the heroine of Margaret Mitchell's *Gone with the Wind,* seems to be a histrionic personality type. At the end of the novel, after she is rejected by Rhett Butler, she can't think of letting him go and thinks, "I won't think of it now—I'll go home to Tara tomorrow—I'll think of it all tomorrow at Tara. I can stand it then. Tomorrow, I'll think of some way to get him back. After all, tomorrow is another day."

XII. Narcissistic personality disorder

A. Definition

The essential feature of this disorder is a pervasive pattern of grandiosity (in fantasy or behavior), hypersensitivity to the evaluation of others, and lack of empathy that begins by early adulthood and is present in a variety of contexts (*DSM*-III-R).

1. There is a grandiose sense of self-importance. Sometimes this alternates with feelings of special unworthiness.
2. The fantasies are associated with unlimited success, power, brilliance, beauty, or ideal love and with chronic feelings of envy for those perceived as being more successful.
3. Self-esteem is fragile.
4. Interpersonal relationships are invariably disturbed. Empathy is lacking.
5. Entitlement, an unreasonable expectation of especially favorable treatment, is usually present.
6. Interpersonal exploitativeness is common.
7. Friendships are often made only after the person considers how he or she can profit from them.

B. Prevalence

It seems to be more common recently than in the past, although this may be due to recent clinical interest in this disorder.

C. Associated features

Histrionic, borderline, and antisocial personality characteristics are frequently found in association with this disorder. Depressed mood is common.

D. Clinical notes

1. Although borderline and narcissistic personality disorders were originally regarded as discrete entities, they are now regarded by some as part of a continuum.

2. Much attention has been focused on the subject of narcissism not only in the psychiatric literature but also in the popular press as well. (For example, Tom Wolff has labelled the 1970s the "the 'me' decade.")

3. Renewed interest in narcissism has been fostered by the works of Otto Kernberg and Heinz Kohut.

    a) Kohut believes that the diagnosis of narcissistic personality disorder can be established only by observing a spontaneously developing transference relationship in a trial analysis. He differentiates a narcissistic personality disorder from the borderline states.

    b) Kernberg's description of the narcissistic personality agrees in general with the *DSM*-III-R proposed classification and regards that the defensive organization of narcissistic patients as quite similar to that of borderline patients.

4. Margaret Mahler postulates a sequence of three "phases" of infantile development, directed ultimately toward the child's attainment of a selfness separateness from the mother.

    a) Absolute autism—the period of William James's "blooming, buzzing, confusion"—occupies the first postnatal month and is characterized by the operation of basic life sustaining reflex activities, and responses are essentially devoid of mental representation. During this period the infant's kaleidoscope world is organized around a "primitive good-bad" dichotomy of perceptions in accordance with the pleasure principle, which dictates that whatever reduces it is "good tension" and whatever increases or fails to reduce it is "bad."

    b) Symbiosis, the second through the sixth postnatal month. During this phase the infant's "good-bad" perceptual dichotomy undergoes organization in relation to the figure or person of the mother.

c) The separation-individuation process. The child's sense of separateness from the world about him. This is divided into four phases
    (1) Differentiation
    (2) Practicing
    (3) Rapprochement
    (4) Consolidation
        (See chapter, "Psychodynamic Concepts".)
E. Case example

J. C., a thirty-two-year-old corporate junior executive, was initially seen in consultation, jointly with his wife, because of marital distress. This was his second marriage and the couple had two children in elementary school. His wife complained that he was extremely self-centered and was always cool and distant with her. He was also remote from the children, but expected them to accomplish much to enhance his own name.

At work, he prided himself on his ruthless decisiveness in dealing with subordinates who might show signs of incompetency. About his superiors, he privately acknowledged that he would "play on their sympathy and compassionate feelings" to enhance his corporate position. He also confided that he had numerous brief extramarital affairs, and on a few occasions had homosexual encounters. A handsome man, he prided himself on his sexual technique and his ability to be able to enjoy both sexes.

In discussing his work relationships, it became clear that he had no loyalty to any colleague or company policy and felt that he would leave to establish his own business to "run things my own way." He had had some strong disagreements with some of his superiors about his own practices, which were at odds with the ethics of the company.

It was believed that part of his own motivation for seeking joint consultation was that he felt a divorce would cost him more financially and hinder his business plans. He felt that he could reduce the financial cost by superficially complying with his wife's wishes.

He abruptly announced his plans to terminate the counseling, and did so.

XIII. Avoidant personality disorder
A. Definition

The essential feature of this disorder is a pervasive pattern of social discomfort, fear of negative evaluation, and timidity, beginning by early adulthood and present in a variety of contexts (*DSM*-III-R).

1. Most persons with this disorder are concerned about how others assess them. They are easily hurt by criticism and are devastated by the slightest hint of disapproval. They are generally unwilling to enter into a relationship unless given an unusually strong guarantee of uncritical acceptance; consequently, they often have no close friends or confidants (or only one) other than first-degree relatives.

2. Social or occupational activities that involve significant interpersonal contact tend to be avoided.
3. They fear being embarrassed by blushing, crying, or showing signs of anxiety before other people.
4. Generalized timidity often produces resistance to doing anything that will deviate from the person's normal routine.
5. Unlike people with schizoid personality disorder, who are socially isolated, but have no desire for social relations, those with avoidant personality disorder yearn for affection and acceptance.
6. This is a new term in *DSM*-III-R.
7. Avoidant disorder in childhood or adolescence is a predisposing factor. Disfiguring physical ailments may be predisposed to this disorder.

B. Prevalence

According to *DSM*-III-R, it is currently apparently common.

C. Associated features

Depression, anxiety, and anger at oneself for failing to develop social relations are commonly experienced. Specific phobias may also be present (*DSM*-III-R).

D. Case example

A twenty-nine-year-old single white male consulted a psychiatrist with complaints of loneliness and lack of friends.

He had grown up in a small community in a resort area and attended college for approximately two years, with a goal toward entering forestry. However, he never did complete college and worked in resort areas in the West until he entered the Marines, where he served honorably for four years. He did not feel lonely during his military service because "There always seemed to be people around me." His parents were divorced when the patient was about nine years of age. His father was absent from the home a lot because of his employment. The patient felt that he did not have a close relationship with his mother and had "negative" feelings toward his father. He was not close to his sister, who was two years older, or to his brother who was four years younger.

In discussing his personality, he reported that he felt there was "something wrong with me." He saw himself as self-centered and wanting friends but unable to make them. "I just can't make friends," he said. He was a weekend drinker and at such times went out to bars to play pool or stayed at home to watch television. He did not speak with any of the residents of his apartment building, and although he was able to converse some with fellow employees, he still said, "I'm kind of a stranger to them." He also realized that he did something to "keep people away from me."

Despite the fact that he had an isolated life, he did express an underlying yearning for affection and acceptance and was seeking help in how he might learn to relate to others.

XIV. Dependent personality disorder

A. Definition

The essential feature of this disorder is a pervasive pattern of dependent and submissive behavior beginning by early adulthood and present in a variety of contexts (*DSM*-III-R).

1. Such persons are unable to make everyday decisions without an excessive amount of advice and reassurance from others and will even allow others to make most of their important decisions.

2. Their excessive dependence on others leads to difficulty in initiating projects or doing things on one's own. People with this disorder tend to feel uncomfortable or helpless when alone and will go to great lengths to avoid being alone. They are devastated when close relationships end and tend to be preoccupied with fears of being abandoned.

3. Such individuals are easily hurt by criticism and disapproval and tend to subordinate themselves to others, agreeing with people even when they believe them to be wrong, for fear of being rejected.

B. Associated features

1. Commonly another personality disorder is present (e.g., histrionic, schizotypal, narcissistic, or avoidant personality disorder. Anxiety and depression are common).

2. People with this disorder invariably lack self-confidence.

C. Prevalence and sex ratio

This disorder is apparently common and is diagnosed more frequently in women.

D. Predisposing factors

Chronic physical illness or separation anxiety disorder may predispose to the development of this disorder.

XV. Obsessive-compulsive personality disorder

A. The essential feature of this disorder is a pervasive pattern of perfectionism and inflexibility, beginning by early adulthood and present in a variety of contexts.

1. These people constantly strive for perfection, but this adherence to their own overly strict and often unattainable standards frequently interferes with actual completion of tasks and projects.

2. People with this disorder are always mindful of their relative status in dominance-submission relationships.

3. Work and productivity are prized to the exclusion of pleasure and interpersonal relationships. Often there is preoccupation with logic and intellect and intolerance of affective behavior in others.

4. Decision making is avoided, postponed, or protracted, perhaps because of an inordinate fear of making a mistake.
5. People with this disorder tend to be excessively conscientious, moralistic, scrupulous, and judgmental of self and others.
6. People with this disorder are stingy with their emotions and material possessions (*DSM*-III-R).

B. Prevalence and sex ratio

This disorder seems to be common and is more frequently diagnosed in males.

C. Complications

Obsessive-compulsive disorder, hypochondriasis, major depression, and dysthymia may be complications. Many of the features of obsessive-compulsive personality disorder are apparently present in people who develop myocardial infarction, particularly those with overlapping "Type A" personality traits of time urgency, hostility-aggressiveness, and exaggerated competitiveness (*DSM*-III-R).

D. Etiology

1. The person who possesses such traits is referred to as an *anankastic personality* or *anal character* (such an individual needs to feel in control of himself or herself and the environment).
2. According to psychoanalytic theory, such anal qualities develop in the infant during the period of toilet training (the anal phase of infantile sexuality).
3. According to Erikson, disturbance in this stage of development characterized by the issues of autonomy versus shame and self-doubt predisposes to the development of obsessive-compulsive personality disorder.
4. The compulsive personality probably has encountered excessive discipline during the developmental years.
5. Family life is characterized by constrained emotions and members are often criticized and socially ostracized if they express anger.
6. According to learning theory, obsessions are conditioned responses to anxiety and compulsions are behavioral patterns that reduce the anxiety.

E. Course and prognosis

This is variable and not predictable. As noted above, persons with compulsive personality traits do well in positions demanding accurate, deductive, or detailed work. People such as this are rigid and are usually vulnerable to unexpected changes. Such personalities may also develop frank obsessions and compulsions and are susceptible to major depressive disorders, especially those of late onset.

F. Treatment

Unlike persons with the other personality disorders, compulsive personalities often are aware of their discomfort and are more apt to voluntarily seek treatment. However, treatment of obsessive-compulsive personalities is not easy and may be protracted. Focus should be on feelings rather than thoughts and on clarification of the defenses of intellectualization and displacement of hostility

XVI. **Passive-aggressive personality disorder**

A. Definition

The essential feature of this disorder is a pervasive pattern of passive resistance to demands for adequate social and occupational performance, beginning by early adulthood and present in a variety of contexts. The resistance is expressed indirectly rather than directly, and results in pervasive and persistent social and occupational ineffectiveness even when more self-assertive and effective behavior is possible. The name of this disorder is based on the assumption that such people are passively expressing covert aggression.

1. People with this disorder habitually resent and oppose demands to increase or maintain a given level of functioning. This occurs most clearly in work situations, but is also evident in social functioning. The resistance is expressed indirectly through such maneuvers as procrastination, dawdling, stubbornness, intentional inefficiency, and "forgetfulness." These people obstruct the efforts of others by failing to do their share of the work.

2. These people become sulky, irritable, or argumentative when asked to do something they do not want to do. They often protest to others about how unreasonable the demands being made on them are, and resent useful suggestions from others concerning how to be more productive. As a result of their resentment of demands, they unreasonably criticize or scorn the people in authority who are making the demands (*DSM-III-R*).

B. Prevalence and sex ratio

Unknown. Oppositional defiant disorder in childhood or adolescence apparently predisposes to the development of this disorder.

C. Associated features

Often people with this disorder are dependent and lack self-confidence. Typically, they are pessimistic about the future, but have no realization that their behavior is responsible for their difficulties.

D. Etiology
   1. Prospective studies of this disorder are lacking.
   2. A reasonable hypothesis seems to be that the passive-aggressive personality person is one whose parents were both assertive and aggressive in their relationships with him or her, yet blocked the expression of normal assertiveness-aggressiveness in the child and reluctantly met his dependency needs. As a consequence, the child learns to retroflex his anger and at first glance, appears polite and undemanding, but overtly punishes the oppressor with inefficiency. (He adopts the style of pseudopoliteness, hiding resentment, which then can only be covertly expressed.)
E. Treatment
   1. Insight-oriented psychotherapy, involving examination of the patient's covert expression of hostility, with a goal of gradually converting passive-aggressive behavior to more successful behavior, has been helpful.
   2. Supportive psychotherapy seems to be the more practical approach. The therapist must repeatedly confront such individuals with the consequences of their behavior.
   3. Psychotropic medication is indicated on those rare occasions where severe anxiety or severe depression can bring on symptoms.

XVII. **Personality disorders needing further study**
   DSM-III-R, Appendix A, lists proposed diagnostic categories needing study. Three diagnoses are included. These are late luteal phase dysphoric disorder, sadistic personality disorder, and self-defeating personality disorder.
   A. Late Luteal Phase Dysphoric Disorder
      1. Definition
         a) The essential feature of late luteal phase dysphoric disorder is a pattern of clinically significant emotional and behavioral symptoms that occur during the last week of the luteal phase and remit within a few days after the onset of the follicular phase. In most females these symptoms occur in the week before, and remit within a few days after, the onset of menses.
         b) The diagnosis is given only if the symptoms are sufficiently severe and cause marked impairment in social or occupational functioning and have occurred during the majority of the menstrual cycles of the past year.
         c) The diagnosis should not be made if the person is experiencing only a late luteal phase exacerbation of another disorder such as major depression, panic disorder, dysthymia, or a personality disorder.

2. Symptoms

Among the most commonly experienced symptoms are marked affective lability (sudden episodes of tearfulness, sadness, or irritability); persistent feelings of irritability, anger, or tension (feeling "on edge"); and feelings of depression and self-deprecating thoughts. Also common are decreased interest in usual activities, fatigability and loss of energy, a subjective sense of difficulty in concentrating, changes in appetite, cravings for specific foods (especially carbohydrates), and sleep disturbance. Other physical symptoms, such as breast tenderness or swelling, headaches, joint or muscle pain, a sensation of "bloating," and weight gain, may also be present.

3. Associated features

Some studies suggest that there may be a higher frequency of depressive disorder in females with this disorder.

4. Females seeking treatment generally report that this condition worsens with age.

5. Prevalence

Unknown.

B. Sadistic personality disorder

1. Definition

The essential feature of this disorder is a pervasive pattern of cruel, demeaning, and aggressive behavior directed toward other people, beginning by early adulthood. The sadistic behavior is often evident both in social relationships (particularly with family members) and at work (with subordinates), but seldom is displayed in contacts with people in positions of authority or higher status.

a) Many people with this disorder use physical violence or cruelty to establish dominance in interpersonal relationships. Other people with this disorder are never physically violent, although in many cases they are fascinated by violence, weapons, martial arts, injury, or torture.

b) A variety of behaviors reflect the basic lack of respect or empathy for others (e.g., humiliation or demeaning; such a person often gets others to do what he or she wants by frightening them with tactics ranging from intimidation by hostile glances to terror through threats of violence).

c) Often people with this disorder seem to be amused or enjoy psychological or physical suffering of others (including animals).

2. Associated features

Almost invariably the sadistic behavior is ego-syntonic, and the person rarely comes to clinical attention unless this has been mandated by the courts. Often these people victimize others who suffer from self-defeating personality disorder. Frequently many features of narcissistic and antisocial personality disorder are present.

3. Predisposing factors

People with this disorder have been physically, sexually, or psychologically abused as children or have been reared in a family in which there was abuse of a spouse.

4. Prevalence

It is rarely seen in clinical settings but is not uncommon in forensic settings.

5. Sex ratio

It is far more common in males.

6. Differential diagnosis

Sexual sadism, in this sadistic behavior, is for the purpose of sexual arousal.

C. Self-defeating personality disorder

1. Definition

The essential feature of this disorder is a pervasive pattern of self-defeating behavior, beginning by early adulthood and present in a variety of contexts. The person may often avoid or undermine pleasurable experiences, be drawn to situations or relationships in which he or she will suffer, and prevent others from helping him or her. The diagnosis is not made if the self-defeating behaviors occur only in situations in which the person is responding to or anticipating being physically, sexually, or psychologically abused. Similarly, the diagnosis is not made if the self-defeating behaviors occur only when the person is depressed.

a) The disorder has been called masochistic personality disorder, but the name of the category has been changed to avoid the historic association of the term *masochistic* with older psychoanalytic views of female sexuality and the implication that a person with the disorder derives unconscious pleasure from suffering. A variety of theories—psychoanalytic, cognitive, and social learning—have been offered to explain the origins of this pattern.

b) The person repeatedly enters into relationships with persons or places himself or herself in situations that are self-defeating and have painful consequences even when better options are clearly available.

c) Reasonable offers of assistance from others are rejected.

d) The person's reaction to positive personal events, such as graduation, a job promotion or raise, or any form of praise or encouragement from others may be depression or feelings of guilt.

e) Characteristically, people with this disorder act in such a way as to cause others to be angry or to reject them.

f) Opportunities for pleasure may be repeatedly avoided.

g) The person reports a number of situations in which he or she had the opportunity to accomplish a task crucial to his or her personal success, but despite having the capacity to complete the task, failed to do so.

h) People who consistently treat the person well are often experienced as boring or uninteresting.

i) The person frequently attempts to do things for others that require excessive self-sacrifice, even though these sacrifices are unsolicited by the intended recipients.

2. Associated features
Other personality disorders are common, particularly borderline, dependent, passive-aggressive, obsessive-compulsive, and avoidant personality disorders.

3. Complications
Dysthymia and major depressive episodes are common complications.

4. Predisposing factors
Physical, sexual, or psychological abuse as a child, or having been reared in a family in which there was abuse of a spouse may predispose.

5. Prevalence
Initial studies suggest that this disorder may be one of the more common personality disorders in clinical samples.

6. Sex ratio
3:2 to 2:1 females to males.

XVIII. Treatment of personality disorders

A. Treatment of the personality disorders is very difficult because the patients usually lack any fundamental motivation for change.

B. The positive rewards of their behavior overbalance the socially incurred ill-feeling that may result.

C. When they do seek treatment it is often likely to be
1. Because of anxiety developing secondarily in response to the social repercussions of their behavior.
2. At the insistence of another person (a parent, spouse, or employer).
3. Because of the slowly developing awareness of an unsatisfactory life-style.

D. Intensive psychoanalytically oriented psychotherapy is useful in narcissistic personality disorders and borderline personality disorders.

E. In individual therapy, the therapist may focus on the individual's maladaptive behavior rather than on a discussion of his inner life.

F. The therapist's negative countertransference feelings must be dealt with in many of these disorders; recognizing feelings of resentment is an important cornerstone in developing an appropriate management strategy that will create a favorable therapeutic alliance to help facilitate change.

G. Such persons often need a different model with whom to identify and from whom to obtain reliable information about their emotional impact on others. In general, the therapist must remain flexible and be prepared to take an active role in the treatment process if necessary.

H. In general, the therapist should focus on the behavior rather than trying to deal with the "reasons" for it.

I. Limited setting and structure are also important in treating many disorders.

References

American Psychiatric Association. *Diagnostic and Statistical Manual of Mental Disorders.* 3d ed., rev. Washington, D.C., 1987.

Cleckley, H. *The Mask of Sanity.* 4th ed. St. Louis: C. V. Mosby Co. 1964.

Gunderson, J. G. "Pharmacotherapy for Patients with Personality Disorder." *Archive of General Psychiatry* 43 (July 1986): 698–700.

Jacobsberg, L. B. et al. "Symptoms of the Schizotypal Personality Disorder." *American Journal of Psychiatry* 143(10): 1222–27 (October 1986).

Johnson, A. M., and S. A. Szurek. "The Genesis of Antisocial Acting Out In Children and Adults." *Psychoanalytic Quarterly* 21 (1952): 323–43.

Kaplan, H. I., and B. J. Sadock. *Comprehensive Textbook of Psychiatry.* 4th ed. Baltimore: Williams & Wilkins, 1985.

Kernberg, O. *Borderline Conditions and Pathological Narcissism.* New York: Jason Aronson, 1975.

Kolb, L. C., and H. K. H. Brodie. *Modern Clinical Psychiatry.* 19th ed. Philadelphia: W. B. Saunders Co. 1982.

Masterson, J. *Treatment of the Borderline Adolescent: A Developmental Approach.* New York: Wiley-Interscience, 1972.

Nicholai, A. M., Jr., ed. *The Harvard Guide to Modern Psychiatry.* Cambridge: Belknap Press of Harvard University Press, 1978.

Perry, J. C. et al. "Passive-Aggressive Personality Disorder." *Journal of Nervous and Mental Diseases* 170(3): 164–73 (1982).

Rinsley, D. B. "Developmental Etiology of Borderline and Narcissistic Disorders." *Bulletin of the Menninger Clinic* 44(2): 127–34 (1980).

Wong, N. "Borderline and Narcissistic Disorders, A Selected Overview." *Bulletin of the Menninger Clinic* 44(2): 101–26 (1980).

In order to do certain crazy things, it is necessary to behave like a coachman who has let go of the reins and fallen asleep.

Jules Renard: *Journal,* **November, 1888.**

DISORDERS OF IMPULSE CONTROL

I. Introduction

A. Not all antisocial behavior is identified with persons diagnosed as having *antisocial personality disorders*.

B. Excluded from the antisocial personality disorders are a group called neurotic characters, or acting-out neurotics, whose disturbance is characterized by the irresistible, repetitious expression of a *single* pleasurable impulse.

C. Antisocial behavior may be the expression of any type of impulse, but the specific symptom has a symbolic significance as related to the patient's life history.

D. In these disorders, the superego is usually well developed and is only defective to the extent that it permits acting out of one type of antisocial behavior.

E. In the past, these disorders were called impulse neuroses or impulse-ridden states. In the current nomenclature, they are called *disorders of impulse control.*

II. Definition

The essential features of disorders of impulse control are

A. Failure to resist an impulse, drive, or temptation to perform some act that is harmful to the person or others. There may or may not be conscious resistance to the impulse. The act may or may not be premeditated or planned.

B. An increasing sense of tension or arousal before committing the act.

C. An experience of either pleasure, gratification, or release at the time of committing the act. The act is ego-syntonic (acceptable to the ego) in that it is consonant with the immediate conscious wish of the individual. Immediately following the act there may or may not be genuine regret, self-reproach, or guilt (*DSM*-III-R).

III. General psychodynamic considerations

A. From the psychoanalytic point of view, these disorders could be considered as resulting from the temporary loss of control of the reality principles (thus allowing the individual to express a pleasurable drive).

B. Psychodynamically, the expression of the impulse represents an attempt to relieve underlying anxiety, depression, guilt or other painful affects (and, secondarily, to provide distorted satisfaction of underlying instinctual drives).

C. Some have stressed the oral fixation of such people (in the psychoanalytical model).

D. The impulsive (ego-syntonic) character of the disorders distinguishes it from compulsive (ego-dystonic) and ego-alien drives. (This is not always easy to verify clinically.)

E. Some believe that the tension-relieving aspect of the impulse expression is not goal directed and that the underlying need is for the relief of pain rather than the production of pleasure.

F. Organic factors: cerebral atrophy; alcohol and drugs may permit release of underlying impulses.

IV. Types

A. Intermittent explosive disorder
B. Kleptomania
C. Pathological gambling
D. Pyromania
E. Trichotillomania
F. At one time, substance use disorders (including alcoholism) and paraphilias (see chapter, "Sexual Disorders") were considered disorders of impulse control.

V. Intermittent explosive disorder

A. Definition

The essential features of this disorder are discrete episodes of loss of control of aggressive impulses, resulting in serious assaultive acts or destruction of property. The degree of aggressiveness expressed during the episodes is grossly out of proportion to any precipitating psychosocial stressors. There are no signs of generalized impulsivity or aggressiveness between the episodes.

The person may describe the episodes as "spells" or "attacks." The symptoms are said to appear within minutes or hours and, regardless of duration, remit almost as quickly. Genuine regret or self-reproach about the consequences of the action and the inability to control the aggressive impulse may follow each episode.

Other disorders that are sometimes associated with loss of control of aggressive impulses must be ruled out before the diagnosis can be made. These include psychotic disorders, organic personality syndrome, antisocial or borderline personality disorder, conduct disorder, or intoxication with a psychoactive substance (*DSM*-III-R).

This category has been retained in *DSM*-III-R despite the fact that many doubt the existence of a clinical syndrome characterized by episodic loss of control that is not symptomatic of one of the disorders that must be ruled out before the diagnosis of intermittent explosive disorder can be made.

B. Prevalence

The disorder apparently is very rare.

C. Sex ratio

Apparently more common in males.

D. Differential diagnosis (see paragraph above)

E. Etiology

In addition to the factors listed in III, some authorities suggest that the disorder neurophysiological factors may play a role in the disorder.

F. Case example

A twenty-two-year-old married man was referred to the court psychiatric consultant for evaluation after he had pleaded guilty to a charge of simple assault, growing out of an incident in which he was verbally and physically abusive to his wife. He was on probation at the time of the offense for a similar disorderly conduct offense committed nine months earlier.

At the interview, he was cooperative and pleasant but did not spontaneously volunteer much about himself. He was quiet, nonverbal, and not at all reflective. In discussing his difficulty he said, "Basically it's temper," which had been an issue in his marriage for the preceding three years. He said that the difficulty was that his temper began during the time that he was in the service for two years following his eighteenth birthday. "It just seemed to come on by itself." It had its onset shortly before he was sent overseas to Vietnam where he served as an infantry rifleman and was wounded.

The kind of subsequent anger that included the physical and verbal abuse of his wife occurred about every six months. At such times he usually would awaken angry and, as a consequence, would overreact throughout the entire day.

Mental status evaluation revealed him to be free of anxiety and depression. He didn't think that there was anything wrong with his mind and he denied delusions, hallucinations, and other types of perceptual distortions. He denied any thinking disturbance. He thought that it was sometimes hard for him to trust others.

It was the consultant's opinion that this man had an explosive personality. Since the outbursts seemed to develop chiefly in relationships with his wife, it was suggested that they both be referred for marriage counseling if the wife planned to remain in the marriage.

VI. Kleptomania
A. Definition

1. The essential feature of this disorder is a recurrent failure to resist impulses to steal objects not needed for personal use or their monetary value; the objects taken are either given away, discarded, returned surreptitiously, or kept and hidden. Almost invariably the person has enough money to pay for the stolen objects. The person experiences an increasing sense of tension immediately before committing the act and intense gratification or relief while committing it. Although the theft does not occur when immediate arrest is probable (e.g., in full view of a policeman), it is not preplanned, and the chances of apprehension are not fully taken into account. The stealing is done without long-term planning and without assistance from, or collaboration with, others. Further, there is no association between the stealing and anger or vengeance (*DSM*-III-R).

2. The diagnosis is not made if stealing is due to conduct disorder or antisocial personality disorder.

B. Associated features

The kleptomaniac may exhibit depression, anxiety, and guilt over the possibility of apprehension.

C. Sex ratio

The majority of the individuals apprehended for shoplifting are female, but only a small portion of these have kleptomania.

D. Case example

A twenty-seven-year-old married man, who had just formed his own small business, consulted a psychiatrist about difficulties in his relationship with his wife and the hostile feelings he had toward his hypercritical father. He expressed a great deal of anger and negativism toward both parents, but especially toward the father, who was unreasonable, paranoid, and insensitive.

In discussing his past history, he reported that he had a habit of stealing small items from the shops he visited for business or personal reasons. These items were almost never of any use to him, and usually were inexpensive. He saved all of them and kept them in drawers in his workshop at home. No one knew of his stealing habit—not even his wife, who was irritated by what he described to her as his "impulse buying."

At first he reported no associated feelings with the stealing incidents, but later in therapy, he recalled that he felt anxious before and at the time of the thefts—and remorseful afterward. He could not relate these incidents to any psychological determinant, but he suspected it had something to do with his rebellious feelings toward his father. He terminated therapy a few months later, when he left the city. At that time, he still did not know the reasons for his stealing.

(Note in the above: it was not the impulsive stealing that led to his seeking psychiatric treatment. The history of kleptomania was only incidentally reported in the therapeutic process.)

VII. Pathological gambling

A. Definition

The essential features of this disorder are a chronic and progressive failure to resist impulses to gamble, and gambling behavior that compromises, disrupts, or damages personal, family, or vocational pursuits. The gambling preoccupation, urge, and activity increase during periods of stress. Problems that arise as a result of the gambling lead to an intensification of the gambling behavior. Characteristic problems include extensive indebtedness and consequent default on debts and other financial responsibilities, disrupted family relationships, inattention to work, and financially motivated illegal activities to pay for gambling (*DSM*-III-R).

B. Associated features

1. Generally, people with pathological gambling disorder have the attitude that money causes and is also the solution to all their problems. As the gambling increases, the person is usually forced to lie in order to obtain money and to continue gambling.

There is no serious attempt to budget or save money. When borrowing resources are strained, antisocial behavior in order to obtain money is likely (*DSM*-III-R).

2. The gambler usually appears overconfident, energetic, easily bored and is a "big spender"; but at other times he may show signs of personal stress, anxiety, and depression.

C. Etiology

1. *DSM*-III-R considers the following to be predisposing factors: inappropriate parental discipline (absent, inconsistency, or harshness); exposure to gambling activities as an adolescent; high family value placed on material and financial symbols; and a lack of family emphasis on saving, planning, and budgeting.

2. Some psychoanalysts have regarded it as related to conflicts about masturbation.

3. Others have seen it as an Oedipal conflict.

D. Case example

Mrs. J. P., the fifty-two-year-old wife of a social agency executive, was referred for psychiatric treatment because of her "addiction to bingo." Her gambling had its onset after she learned of the tragic death of her thirty-year-old scientist-son. Her irresistible urge to gamble (and lose) at bingo seemed to represent an equivalent of depression.

Repeated efforts at out-patient psychotherapy and hospital treatment were to little avail. She wrote worthless checks, stole, and went into debt to continue her habit. Ultimately, her husband divorced her. Unfortunately, there was no follow-up beyond that point.

VIII. Pyromania

A. Definition

The essential features of this disorder are deliberate and purposeful (rather than accidental) fire setting on more than one occasion; tension or affective arousal prior to setting the fires; and intense pleasure, gratification, or relief when setting the fires or witnessing or participating in their aftermath. In addition, there is fascination with, interest in, curiosity about, or attraction to fire and its situational context or associated characteristics (e.g., uses, consequences, exposure to fires). The fire setting is not done for monetary gain, as an expression of sociopolitical ideology, to conceal criminal activity, to express anger or vengeance, to improve one's living circumstances, or in response to a delusion or hallucination.

Although the fire setting results from a failure to resist an impulse, there may be considerable advance preparation for starting the fire, and the person may leave obvious clues. People with the disorder are often recognized as regular "watchers" at fires in their neighborhoods, frequently set off false alarms, and show interest in fire-fighting paraphernalia. Their fascination with fire leads some to seek employment or volunteer work in fire fighting. They may be indifferent to the consequences of the fire for life or property, or they may get satisfaction from the resulting destruction (*DSM*-III-R).

B. Age of onset
   Usually in childhood.
C. Etiology
   1. See III.
   2. Lewis and Yarnell wrote a monograph on this disorder in 1951.
D. Case example

An eighteen-year-old married man was arrested for having set a number of fires in the city. In discussing the setting of the fires he indicated that he got a "thrill" or a "feeling of excitement" as he watched the fires. In addition, he experienced some sexual gratification from setting the fires. As a matter of fact, he would set the fires in an area in which he could witness them from his home and he and his wife would become sexually excited and have sexual intercourse while observing the blaze.

Apart from the particular offense that brought him to the attention of the law, there was evidence that he had had adjustment difficulties for many years. Obesity, for example, had been a problem with him for a long time, and he gave a history of an arrest four years earlier for an assault on a two-and-one-half-year-old boy. He felt that he turned to homosexuality at that point because he was not able to date in high school. He denied that he had had any homosexual feelings since he had been married in March of the previous year.

From clinical examination, there was no evidence that he was psychotic. In a general way, he indicated that he probably knew right from wrong and that at the time he set the first fire he knew it was wrong, but after that the rightness or wrongness of his behavior in setting additional fires did not enter his head—"It was just something I needed." There was also evidence that setting the fires relieved sexual, aggressive, and anxious feelings. At the time of psychiatric examination in the county jail, he was still experiencing strong desires to set fires.

E. The pyromaniac must be distinguished from the arsonist.

IX. Trichotillomania
A. Definition
   1. The essential feature of this disorder is recurrent failure to resist impulses to pull out one's own hair. The diagnosis is not made when hair pulling is associated with a preexisting inflammation of the skin or is in response to a delusion or hallucination.
   2. Specific patterns and rituals involving the plucking of the hair and its dispositions are common: trichophagy or mouthing of the hair may follow the plucking.
   3. Unlike in alopecia areata, regrowth of the hair is without pigmentary change, and a scalp biopsy will uncover signs of the traumatic nature of the disorder: catagen hairs, absence of inflammation and scarring, the presence of keratin plugs, and dilated follicular infundibula. Characteristic histopathologic

changes in the hair follicle, known as trichomalacia, are demonstrated by biopsy, and help to distinguish the condition from other causes of alopecia (*DSM*-III-R).

B. Associated features: long-standing denial of the disorder is commonly encountered. Other acts of self-mutilation may be present (head banging, nail biting, scratching, gnawing, excoriation, etc.).

C. Age of onset
Usually begins in childhood.

D. Predisposing factors
   1. Although the disorder is regarded as "multidetermined," onset has been linked to stressful situations in more than one-quarter of the cases.
   2. Disturbances in mother-child relationships, fear of being left alone, and recent object loss are often cited as critical factors in the genesis of the condition. Psychoactive substance abuse may contribute to the development of this disorder.

E. Prevalence
No information. It is more common in people with mental retardation and possibly with schizophrenia or borderline personality disorder.

References

American Psychiatric Association. *Diagnostic and Statistical Manual of Mental Disorders*. 3d ed., rev. Washington, D.C., 1987.

Goldman, H. H. *Review of General Psychiatry*. Los Altos, Calif.: Lange Medical Publications, 1984.

Kaplan, H. I., and B. J. Sadock. *Comprehensive Textbook of Psychiatry/IV*. 4th ed. Baltimore: Williams & Wilkins, 1985.

If venereal delight and the power of propagating the species were permitted only to the virtuous, it would make the world very good.

James Boswell: *London Journal,* March 26, 1763

SEXUAL DISORDERS

I. Introduction

A. Background

1. Sexual deviations have been practiced throughout history and by all races.
2. Some deviant acts may be considered to be within the normal range of sexual expression if indulged in only sporadically or as foreplay to normal coitus.
3. Sexual deviancy includes any sexual behavior that is at variance with more or less culturally accepted norms.
4. To be considered deviant, either the quality or the object of the sexual drive must be deemed abnormal.
5. Our concepts of sexual normalcy and deviancy are related to the values of our society. Since these values change, concepts and definitions of sexual deviance also change.
6. Some authorities speak of "sexual variants" rather than "sexual deviancies."
7. The deviant is usually one who has difficulty achieving normal or satisfactory sexual relations with a mature human partner. Thus, according to Marmor, the deviant practices represent alternative ways of attempting to achieve sexual gratification.

B. Previous classification

In *DSM*-III, published in 1980, the psychosexual disorders were divided into four groups:

1. Gender identity disorders
2. Paraphilias
3. Psychosexual dysfunctions
4. Other psychosexual disorders (which included ego-dystonic homosexuality)

The current classification in *DSM*-III-R is divided into two groups: paraphilias and sexual dysfunctions. There is also a residual class of other sexual disorders for disorders in sexual functioning that are not classifiable in any of the other categories. (This last group includes a place for "persistent and marked distress about one's sexual orientation.")

C. Gender identity disorders including transsexualism are listed in *DSM*-III-R under: Disorders Usually First Evident in Infancy, Childhood, or Adolescence.

II. Definition

The sexual disorders are divided into two groups: the paraphilias, characterized by arousal and response to sexual objects or situations that are not part of normative arousal-activity patterns and that in varying degrees may interfere with the capacity for reciprocal, affectionate sexual activity; and sexual dysfunctions, characterized by inhibitions in sexual desire or the psychophysiologic changes that characterize the sexual response cycle. Other sexual disorders is a residual class for disorders in sexual functioning that are not classifiable in any of the specific categories.

III. **Types**
  A. Paraphilias
    1. Exhibitionism
    2. Fetishism
    3. Frotteurism
    4. Pedophilia
    5. Sexual masochism
    6. Sexual sadism
    7. Transvestic fetishism
    8. Voyeurism
    9. Paraphilia not otherwise specified
  B. Sexual dysfunctions
    The essential feature of this subclass is inhibition in the appetitive or psychophysiologic changes that characterize the complete sexual response cycle. It includes:
    1. Sexual desire disorders
      a) Hypoactive sexual desire disorder
      b) Sexual aversion disorder
    2. Sexual arousal disorders
      a) Female sexual arousal disorder
      b) Male erectile disorder
    3. Orgasm disorders
      a) Inhibited female orgasm
      b) Inhibited male orgasm
      c) Premature ejaculation
    4. Sexual pain disorders
      a) Dyspareunia
      b) Vaginismus
    5. Sexual dysfunction not otherwise specified
  C. Other sexual disorders
    Sexual disorders that are not classifiable in any of the previous categories include nonparaphilic sexual addiction and "persistent and marked distress about one's sexual orientation."

IV. **Gender identity disorders**
  A. Definition
    The essential feature of the disorders included in this subclass is an incongruence between assigned sex (i.e., the sex that is recorded on the birth certificate) and gender identity.
    1. Gender *identity* can be defined as one's sense of femininity or masculinity, or, according to Campbell, it is "the inner conviction that one is either male, female, ambivalent, or neutral."

2. Gender *role* according to Campbell, is "the behavior and appearance that one presents in terms of what the culture considers to be 'masculine' or 'feminine.' " One might also consider this to be the individual's perception of his or her social role as being either masculine or feminine. While gender identity is usually established and fixed early in life, gender role evolves over a period of time.
3. Gender identity is the private experience of gender role, and gender role is the public expression of gender identity. (*DSM*-III).

B. Gender identity disorder of childhood

The essential features of this disorder are persistent and intense distress in a child about his or her assigned sex and the desire to be, or insistence that he or she is, of the other sex (*DSM*-III).

C. Transsexualism

1. Definition

The essential features of this disorder are a persistent discomfort and a sense of inappropriateness about one's assigned sex in a person who has reached puberty. In addition, there is persistent preoccupation, for at least two years, with getting rid of one's primary and secondary sex characteristics and acquiring the sex characteristics of the other sex. Therefore, the diagnosis is not made if the disturbance is limited to brief periods of stress. Invariably there is the wish to live as a member of the other sex. In the rare cases in which physical intersexuality or a genetic abnormality is present, such a condition should be noted on Axis III.

People with this disorder usually complain that they are uncomfortable wearing the clothes of their assigned sex and therefore dress in clothes of the other sex. Often they engage in activities that in our culture tend to be associated with the other sex. These people often find their genitals repugnant, which may lead to persistent requests for sex reassignment by hormonal and surgical means (*DSM*-III-R).

2. Types (Kaplan and Sadock, 1985)

a) Male transsexualism

(1) Male primary transsexualism—so-called because the disorder has its incipiency in the boy's earliest years and remains unchanged throughout life.

(2) Male secondary transsexualism—this refers to a disorder that starts later in life (from childhood upward). Such males appear masculine and have adopted masculine roles.

b) Female transsexualism
   (1) Female transsexuals have seen themselves as masculine since early childhood and have not lived feminine lives.
   (2) Female transsexuals have usually appeared successfully as males, even before "sex change" surgery, and have often found partners (who are not overt homosexuals).
c) *DSM*-III-R types (subdivided according to the history of sexual orientation)
   (1) Asexual—the person denies ever having had strong sexual feelings.
   (2) Homosexual—object choice has been the same anatomic sex.
   (3) Heterosexual—the individual claims to have had an active heterosexual life.
3. Etiology
   a) There is a history of gender identity problems as a child.
   b) Some consider that all types of transsexual disorders stem from unresolved separation anxiety during the early stages of infantile development.
   c) In primary male transsexuals, some believe that the father is distant and passive and the mother is a woman with strong bisexual aspects in her personality.
   d) In female transsexuals, fragmentary evidence suggests that the female child's mother was unavailable for mothering (but not necessarily physically absent). This seems to set up a process in which the female child tries to restore her mother.
   e) No biological factors have been reported in either male or female transsexualism.
4. Course
   Chronic. The long-term prognosis of combined psychiatric, hormonal, and surgical sex-reassignment treatment is not well known (*DSM*-III-R).
5. Treatment
   a) Psychiatric treatment of this disorder has been disappointing.
   b) Psychotherapy has been unsuccessful.
   c) Aversive therapy has also been unsuccessful.
   d) Whether behavior therapy will be of help in the future is unknown.

e) Sex transformation, or reconstructive surgery, has been used for a carefully screened group of patients. Persons with psychotic or borderline behavior, a criminal record, or gross sexual disturbances have been excluded. Although such surgery does not always relieve symptoms (e.g., depression), the patients seem to have done well postoperatively. Some authorities state that in the absence of long-term follow-up studies, the outcome remains controversial.

6. Case example

A twenty-four-year-old, single, genetic male was admitted to the hospital for transsexual surgery. He had been born in a small town in southern Minnesota and had an unusually healthy life.

He stated that from his earliest memories he had regarded himself as a girl and that throughout his life he had never felt differently. Some of his earliest memories were of dressing up in the clothes of his sister, who was two years older. He was interested exclusively in dolls, little girls' games, and playing with girls. He did not like playing with boys or engaging in their games. He was also interested in dolls and cooking and, in high school, baton twirling. He said that he was always accepted "as a girl" by the girls in the small town in which he grew up.

By the end of grade school, he was taunted by boys for his feminine ways. It was during his midteens, while coming across descriptions of a famous case of transsexuality, that it began to dawn upon him that he might be a transsexual.

He denied any overt sexual experiences of any type except for a few anal sexual experiences. He was afraid of having relationships with a male "because he would quickly find out about me." He had never attempted sexual relations with a genetic female—"this would disgust me." He masturbated frequently and in his fantasies played the role of a woman, lying on his back and accepting the penis from his imaginary male lover

About four and one-half years earlier, he had begun to take estrogens and dress and live like a woman. During this time, there was substantial breast development, his male genitalia became "smaller," and he became unable to have erections. He felt disgust for his penis and testicles, never felt them, and kept them constantly tucked between his legs. He also enrolled in a school for beauticians, where he met his first fellow transsexual. About two years before admission to the hospital, he had had his breasts injected with liquid silicone to make them "more solid."

He was a natural blond and had never had much trouble with excessive bodily and facial hair. He had a "peaches-and-cream" complexion, and a depilatory used about every ten days controlled the relatively small amount of facial fuzz. In the hospital, a one-stage transsexual operation was performed.[1]

---

1. Courtesy of the late Donald W. Hastings, M. D., University of Minnesota Hospitals.

D. Gender identity disorder of adolescence or adulthood, nontranssexual type (GIDAANT)
   1. Definition
      The essential features of this disorder are a persistent or re-
      current discomfort and sense of inappropriateness about one's
      assigned sex, and persistent or recurrent cross-dressing in the
      role of the other sex, either in fantasy or in actuality, in a
      person who has reached puberty. This disorder differs from
      transvestic fetishism in that the cross-dressing is not for the
      purpose of sexual excitement; it differs from transsexualism
      in that there is no persistent preoccupation (for at least two
      years) with getting rid of one's primary and secondary sex
      characteristics and acquiring the sex characteristics of the
      other sex (*DSM*-III-R).
   2. Age at onset and course
      Age at onset and course are both variable but in most cases
      before puberty there was a history of some or all of the fea-
      tures of gender identity disorder of childhood.
   3. Sex ratio
      More common in males.

V. Exhibitionism
   A. Definition
      1. The essential feature of this disorder is recurrent, intense
         sexual urges and sexually arousing fantasies, of at least six
         months' duration, involving the exposure of one's genitals to
         a stranger. The person has acted on these urges or is markedly
         distressed by them. Sometimes the person masturbates while
         exposing himself (or fantasizing exposing himself).
            If the person acts on these urges, there is no attempt at
         further sexual activity with the stranger, and therefore people
         with this disorder are usually not physically dangerous to the
         victim (*DSM*-III-R).
      2. The term is sometimes used in the popular sense to describe
         somebody who is "showing off."
   B. Prevalence
      1. Exhibitionistic play among children is common and is not
         considered a deviancy.
      2. It is one of the more common deviations among adults.
      3. It is nearly always a deviation of males. Females usually do
         not derive erotic satisfaction from exhibiting their genitalia,
         but derive more pleasure from displaying other parts of their
         bodies.
      4. The exhibitionist often returns repeatedly to the same scene
         to expose himself. As a consequence, he is frequently ar-
         rested.

5. In senile men, it may be a symptom of impaired judgment and poor impulse control.
C. Etiology
1. Psychodynamically, the exhibitionist seems to be seeking reassurance for this underlying castration anxiety.
2. The exposure may thus be an attempt to seek reassurance by
  a) Having another person react to the sight of his genitalia.
  b) Having other persons show fear of him.
  c) Showing the female what he wishes she could show him, thus reassuring himself that she also has a penis.
3. Some say that exhibitionists suffer from sexual impotence or premature ejaculation and deep-seated feelings of masculine inadequacy.
D. Prognosis
1. The prognosis depends upon the exhibitionist's desire for change.
2. It is also related to the severity of the deviancy.
3. The deviancy usually ceases with aging—at least, few arrests are made in the older age group.
E. Case example

G. J., a thirty-six-year-old married man, was referred to the court's psychiatric consultant for evaluation after he had pleaded guilty to a charge of exposing himself to a woman in the downtown area. His history indicated that he had begun exposing himself several months earlier and, although he could not give any conscious reason for the behavior, it was interesting to note that he had become impotent shortly before he experienced the first urge to expose himself.

Although he indicated that he was worried about his impotence, he had not yet summoned up enough courage to discuss the matter with his personal physician. He seemed to have no understanding that his impotence might be psychogenic and that this might have some relationship to his exhibitionism. Mental-status examination did not reveal any thinking disorder or any major personality disturbance.

VI. Fetishism
A. Definition
1. The essential feature of this disorder is recurrent, intense sexual urges and sexually arousing fantasies, of at least six months' duration, involving the use of nonliving objects (fetishes). The person has acted on these urges or is markedly distressed by them (*DSM*-III-R).
2. Common fetish objects are bras, women's undergarments, stockings, shoes, boots, or other wearing apparel.
3. The person with the fetishism frequently masturbates while holding, rubbing, or smelling the fetish object, or may ask his sexual partner to wear the object during sexual encounters.

4. The fetish is used as the masturbatory object, thus it is clearly a symbolic substitute for the female, rather than the male, genital.
5. Preoccupation with certain parts of the female body (e.g., breasts, buttocks, legs, hips) is called *partialism* (classified as: Paraphilia Not Otherwise Specified in *DSM*-III-R).

B. Prevalence
1. Fetishism seems to be peculiar to men.
2. Kinsey believed that there was a relationship between sadomasochistic behavior and fetishism.
3. No figures are available on its prevalence.
4. Sometimes a fetishist is arrested for stealing an article of female clothing, especially undergarments ("fetish theft").
5. Once established, the disorder tends to be chronic.

C. Etiology
1. Freud attributed fetishism to the castration anxiety originating in early childhood.
   a) The fetish represents a symbolic "female penis" and reassures the male that the female also has a penis, thus allaying castration anxiety.
   b) Such theories are of dubious value because castration anxiety is seen as a cause of many disorders that are not sexual deviations.
2. Like many homosexuals, fetishists do not achieve a healthy identification with their fathers who, according to Marmor, have usually been distant, absent, or rejecting.

D. Treatment
1. As in other sexual deviations, motivation to change is critical.
2. Psychotherapy is focused on the patient's basic feelings of masculine inadequacy and heterosexual inhibition.
3. Group psychotherapy may be helpful.
4. Behavioral therapy has been tried.
5. Marmor believes that a combination of dynamic and behavioral techniques may ultimately prove the most effective therapy.

E. Case example

A twenty-eight-year-old married man was referred to the court's psychiatric consultant after he had been arrested for touching an eighteen-year-old girl on the buttocks on two occasions on a downtown street. He admitted that he had touched between thirty to fifty girls, usually between fourteen and twenty-one-years old, on the buttocks, breasts, or genitalia. He rarely touched the same girl twice. In addition, he admitted that on three or four occasions he had made obscene propositions to the girls. He said the incidents usually occurred on his way to work or on his way home in the evening and were most apt to occur when his wife was menstruating and unavailable for sexual relationships. In all instances he denied having an erection or an orgasm, but he did describe a feeling of "excitement," which he compared to the experience he had in other situations, such as shooting deer. He denied other kinds of sexual problems, claiming that he got along well with his wife.

During the interview, he behaved very much like a schizoid person, showing a rather blunted effect and a lack of verbal spontaneity. He said that on many occasions in the past he had vowed to himself to give up his deviancy but had always found it difficult to stop.

He was recommended for probationary supervision with the stipulation that he attend a psychiatric clinic.

VII. Frotteurism
A. Definition
The essential feature of this disorder is recurrent, intense sexual urges and sexually arousing fantasies, of at least six months' duration, involving touching and rubbing against a nonconsenting person.

The person has acted on these urges or is markedly distressed by them.
B. Prevalence
Usually a male deviation.
C. Is usually committed in crowded places.

VIII. Pedophilia
A. Definition
The essential feature of this disorder is recurrent, intense sexual urges and sexually arousing fantasies, of at least six months' duration, involving sexual activity with a prepubescent child. The person has acted on these urges or is markedly distressed by them.
B. This may be exclusively heterosexual or exclusively homosexual, but heterosexually oriented pedophiles are twice as common as homosexually oriented ones.
C. The person may limit his activities to his own children, stepchildren, relatives, or may victimize children outside his family.
D. Prevalence
1. The disorder usually begins in adolescence.
2. Prevalence is most difficult to estimate, although it is most common in adult males.
3. This is the most common paraphilia that comes to the attention of the law.
4. Heterosexual offenses are more common than homosexual ones.
5. The popular belief that homosexuals tend to be child molesters seems to be a myth.
6. Mostly, the behavior is genital petting. Most pedophiles do not resort to force or aggression.
7. The course is usually chronic, especially in those attracted to boys.

E. Etiology
   1. Most pedophiles are mild-mannered men who have profound feelings of masculine inadequacy and a fear of being castrated by mature women. They are frequently sexually impotent. As a result, they expect rejection and failure in any attempts at adult heterosexual relationships.
   2. On the other hand, the male pedophile is often said to be masochistic.
   3. Many of the men feel that their penis is small, hence children are seen as less threatening or less challenging.
   4. Although no single family constellation is identifiable, a large percentage of pedophiles seem to come from unhappy home situations and to have had a poor relationship with the father.
   5. Incest, although not classified as a perversion, is superficially related to pedophilia because of the frequent selections of an immature sexual child as a sexual object.
F. Types
   Men who approach children sexually can be divided into the following groups:
   1. Occasionally, males who are under the influence of alcohol
   2. Males who are responding to a special situation
   3. Pedophiles
   4. Mentally retarded persons
   5. Sociopathic types
   6. Disorganized schizophrenics
   7. Men with organic brain disease (senile dementia).
G. Case example

Mr. I. H., a thirty-six-year-old single man, was referred to the court's psychiatric consultant after he had pleaded guilty to drunkenness when he was found picking up a three-year-old boy and walking away with him. History revealed that he had been arrested on several occasions and had appeared in court three times. Seven years earlier, he had been picked up by police for questioning after there had been complaints in a neighborhood about his frequent appearances there when there were small children around. He was released. About five years earlier, he had been arrested for drunkenness and held in jail overnight. A few months later, he was arrested for disturbing the peace. On that occasion, he had picked up a three-year-old boy but claimed that he did nothing to him. About four years earlier, he was arrested on a charge of indecent assault after picking up a four-year-old girl. He said that he was so drunk at the time that he could not remember exactly what happened.

During the interview, he was quiet but frank in discussing his problem and his previous court appearances. There were certain schizoid qualities to his behavior. Although he admitted that he had a problem, he was not certain it was sexual. He felt that his basic attraction to children was toward those who were in need of care or attention. Mental-status examination did not reveal any signs of a disturbance in thinking or perception. He was committed to a state hospital under the sexual psychopathic law.

IX. Sexual masochism

A. Definition

The essential feature of this disorder is recurrent, intense sexual urges and sexually arousing fantasies, of at least six months' duration, involving the act (real, not simulated) of being humiliated, beaten, bound, or otherwise made to suffer. The person has acted on these urges or is markedly distressed by them (*DSM*-III-R).

1. *Flagellation* (erotic whipping) is one example of masochism.
2. *Moral masochism* is the seeking of humiliation and failure rather than physical pain.
3. *Hypoxyphilia,* sexual arousal by oxygen deprivation, is a particularly dangerous form of masochism.
4. *Infantilism,* is sometimes used to describe a desire to be treated as a helpless infant and clothed in diapers.
5. Some men with this disorder also have fetishism, transvestic fetishism, or sexual sadism.

B. Prevalence

1. Elements of mild masochism are common.
2. The actual prevalence of this disorder is not known.
3. Masochistic fantasies are likely to begin in childhood, but masochistic activities with partners commonly begin in early adulthood.
4. The disorder is usually chronic.

C. Etiology

1. Again, castration anxiety is the psychoanalytic explanation for both moral and physical masochism.
2. Some think the origins may lie in a child's identification with someone being punished while at the same time experiencing sexual pleasure.

D. Treatment

1. Treatment should be aimed at the underlying feelings of inadequacy.
2. Aversive therapies have been tried.
3. Perhaps a combination of dynamic psychotherapy and some behavioral therapy would offer the best prospect for resolution.

X. Sexual sadism

A. Definition

The essential feature of this disorder is recurrent, intense sexual urges and sexually arousing fantasies, of at least six months' duration, involving acts (real, not simulated) in which the psychological or physical suffering (including humiliation) of the victim is sexually exciting. The person has acted on these urges or is markedly distressed by them.

1. Some people with this disorder are bothered by their sadistic fantasies, which may be invoked during sexual activity but not otherwise acted upon.
2. Others act on their sadistic sexual urges with a consenting partner who willingly suffers pain and humiliation. Still others act on their sadistic sexual urges with nonconsenting victims.
3. In all of these cases it is the suffering of the victim that is sexually arousing (*DSM*-III-R).
4. Rape is an extreme form of sadism.

B. Prevalance
   1. Mildly sadistic trends are common in all males.
   2. The exact prevalance is not known.
   3. Sadism also refers to other acts of excessive cruelty not related to sexuality, such as beating of children.
   4. Extreme sadism is usually a psychotic symptom.
   5. Sadistic fantasies are apt to begin in childhood but the onset of sadistic activities is common in early adulthood.

C. Etiology
   According to psychoanalytic theory, underlying castration anxiety is the cause of this type of behavior, also.

D. Case example

Mr. Creakle, the cruel headmaster of Salem House in *David Copperfield:* "He [Creakle] then showed me the cane, and asked me what I thought of that, for a tooth? Was it a sharp tooth, hey? Was it a double tooth, hey? Had it a deep prong, hey? Did it bite, hey? At every question, he gave me a fleshy cut with it that made me writhe; so I was very soon made free of Salem House—and was very soon in tears also."

XI. Sado-masochism

A. Definition
   1. The occurrence of sadism and masochism in the same person. These two deviancies often occur together, and Freud regarded masochism as sadism turned inward.
   2. The two conditions are sometimes included under the term *algolagnia*. Thus, *active algolagnia* is sadism, and *passive algolagnia* is masochism.
   3. Sadism and masochism often represent the active and passive poles of the subjugation-humiliation axis.

B. Case example

A thirty-seven-year-old man, separated from his wife, was referred for psychiatric consultation by the attorney who was defending him in a suit filed by a woman who accused him of tying her up and beating her.

He reported that he had been aware of sado-masochistic feelings from about the age of eighteen, although he recalled pleasurable responses to being tied up by another boy at the age of eleven, when they played cowboy and Indian. Since his marriage at twenty-one, he had gone out with a number of women. He would derive sexual pleasure from either tying up a woman or being tied up by her. He usually terminated the relationship with sexual intercourse. He said he found that women liked to be treated roughly. For the preceding five years, he had had intermittent sexual impotence.

XII. Transvestic fetishism

A. Definition

The essential feature of this disorder is recurrent, intense sexual urges and sexually arousing fantasies, of at least six months' duration, involving cross-dressing. The person has acted on these urges or is markedly distressed by them. Usually the person keeps a collection of women's clothes that he intermittently uses to cross-dress when alone. While cross-dressed, he usually masturbates and imagines other males' being attracted to him as a woman in his female attire.

1. This disorder has been described only in heterosexual males. The diagnosis is not made in cases in which the disturbance has evolved into gender identity disorder of adolescence or adulthood, nontranssexual type, or transsexualism.
2. Transvestic phenomena range from occasional solitary wearing of female clothes to extensive involvement in a transvestic subculture.
3. Transvestism is to be distinguished from transsexualism. Transvestites, unlike transsexuals, accept their biological gender and get excited by cross-dressing.

B. Prevalence

1. Cross-dressing occurs on a continuum from a single guilt-laden dressing to ego-synotic membership in a transvestite subculture.
2. Children sometimes dress up in the garb of the opposite sex. According to the folklore of people with this condition, "petticoat punishment," the punishment of humiliating a boy by dressing him in the clothes of a girl, is common in the history of those who later develop this disorder (*DSM*-III-R).
3. Transvestism is more frequently found in males. In our culture, dressing in the clothes of the opposite sex is considered less deviant in females.
4. Some authorities say transvestism is frequently associated with other deviations, and some describe a triad of deviancy characterized by transvestism, fetishism, and homosexuality.

C. Etiology

In addition to what has been said previously about the etiology of sexual deviancy:

1. The confusion about sexual identification may date from the earliest years in the lives of such individuals.
2. The parents may have preferred a child of the opposite sex.
3. There may have been envy of the opposite sex role.
4. It is thought that the male transvestite reacts to his castration anxiety by identifying with the phallic woman. The mother of such patients is often reported as being seductive.
5. The female transvestite is regarded as having penis envy.

D. Prognosis

The prognosis is questionable; transvestites are reluctant to surrender their deviancy because the syndrome is pleasurable (egosyntonic). Motivation for change usually results from external pressures.

E. Treatment

Because of the reluctance of transvestites to alter their behavior, treatment has been discouraging. In recent years there have been attempts at aversive behavioral therapy, using electroshocks or emetics.

F. Case example

R. U., a twenty-one-year-old married man, was referred to the court's psychiatric consultant after he had pleaded guilty to a disorderly conduct charge growing out of his arrest in a fitting room of the dress department of a department store, dressed in women's clothing.

Upon examination by the police physician, it was discovered that he was completely dressed in women's clothing, including a padded brassiere and women's hose. He admitted that he had dressed in women's clothing on a previous occasion, about two weeks earlier. He felt his problem was a climax to a rather deep-seated sexual problem and reported that he received a thrill upon entering the women's fitting room in the department store, as he had, previously, when he entered the women's washroom of a downtown theater. Just wearing the clothing stimulated him sexually. He seemed to be immature and naive but did not show other evidences of sociopathic behavior. He was placed under probationary supervision and referred to a psychiatric clinic.

XIII. Voyeurism

A. The essential feature of this disorder is recurrent, intense sexual urges and sexually arousing fantasies, of at least six months' duration, involving the act of observing unsuspecting people, usually strangers, who are either naked, in the process of disrobing, or engaging in sexual activity. The person has acted on these urges or is markedly distressed by them.

The act of looking ("peeping") is for the purpose of achieving sexual excitement, and no sexual activity with the person is sought. Orgasm, usually produced by masturbation, may occur during the voyeuristic activity, or later in response to the memory of what the person has witnessed. Often these people enjoy the fantasy of having a sexual experience with the observed person, but in reality this does not occur. In its severe form, peeping constitutes the exclusive form of sexual activity (*DSM*-III-R).

    1. A voyeur is known as a "peeping Tom."

B. Prevalence
    1. Sexual curiosity is universal, and voyeuristic tendencies are widespread in the male population, as indicated by the extent to which nude or nearly nude women are used in the various communications media.
    2. It is normal to be excited by the sight of a love object.
    3. It is probably a common deviancy, although the extent is not known because voyeurs are quiet and unobtrusive and, hence, rarely caught.
    4. The onset of this disorder is usually in adolescence and the course is usually chronic.

C. Etiology
    1. Voyeuristic urges are universal; it is the inability to keep them within socially accepted limits that poses problems.
    2. The psychoanalytic explanation is centered on feelings of castration anxiety; the deviation provides reassurance.
    3. Some authorities view this deviation as an attempt to re-create exciting and pleasurable childhood experiences with the mother.
    4. Some say a voyeur has been exposed, in an aggressive way, to the nudity of his mother.

D. Prognosis
    1. This depends upon the voyeur's desire for change.
    2. It is also related to the severity of the deviancy.
    3. Although this is usually a harmless paraphilia, there are cases that can proceed from looking to touching, and later to seizing and assault.

E. Treatment
    1. The voyeur rarely seeks help voluntarily.
    2. Treatment is an attempt to help the person deal with underlying feelings of inadequacy.
    3. Some patients say they suffer from impotence and premature ejaculation.

F. Case example

A twenty-three-year-old married man was examined by the court's psychiatric consultant after he had pleaded guilty to a charge of window peeping.

He stated that he began his voyeuristic activities in his first year of college. He estimated that he peeped in windows about once every three or four months. In that period of time he had been picked up by the police on two occasions, but formally charged only once. He was a mild-mannered, frank, and open individual who was basically shy and retiring but could verbalize easily about his problem. He denied any other types of sexually deviant behavior and denied that he had ever been aggressive in any sexual or asocial way. He came from an upper-middle-class family and had an austere father who was emotionally remote from him. He described his mother as a seductive person who had never allowed him to have a warm relationship with his father.

Arrangements were made for him to be seen in a psychiatric clinic.

XIV. Paraphilia not otherwise specified
A. Telephone scatologia
1. *Telephone scatologia (lewdness)* is sexual gratification derived, usually by men who telephone women, make obscene remarks, and suggest that the women meet them and engage in sexual activity.
2. The man is usually apprehended when the woman agrees to meet him where the police can arrest him.
3. Case example

E. L., a twenty-year-old single male, was referred to the court's psychiatric consultant for evaluation after he had been arrested for making obscene phone calls to a sixteen-year-old girl over a six-month period. He would make such comments as, "Do you still have your cherry?" Or, "I want to put my fingers in your hairy cunt." Or, "If you don't let me fuck you, I will force you to fuck me." He admitted that he became sexually excited and on a couple of occasions masturbated when he made these phone calls.

During the interview, he seemed uneasy and defensive and was not very revealing of himself. There was a certain strangeness about his behavior. He was evasive when questioned about his thought processes, although he denied any psychotic mentation, delusions, hallucinations, or other types of perceptual distortions. The MMPI profile suggested depression, passive dependency, and homosexual impulses.

He was recommended for probationary supervision, with the stipulation that he be seen for further evaluation at the local mental health center to see if he could participate in any meaningful kind of treatment.

B. Necrophilia is the deriving of sexual gratification from corpses.
C. Partialism (exclusive focus on part of body)
D. Zoophilia (also called *bestiality*)
 1. Definition: The essential feature is the use of animals as a repeatedly preferred or exclusive method of achieving sexual excitement. The animal may be the object of intercourse or may be trained to sexually excite the human partner by licking or rubbing. Usually the preferred animal is one with which the individual had contact during childhood, such as a household pet or farm animal. The animal is preferred no matter what other forms of sexual outlet are available (*DSM*-III).
 2. Prevalence
  a) It is rare, even though sexual relations with animals are relatively common.
  b) Zoophilia is most commonly found in adolescents and usually involves a household pet or farm animal.
  c) It is said to be more common in people who live in rural areas or are socially isolated.
  d) The disorder is apparently rare in other circumstances.
  e) Such patients are often schizoid, mentally retarded, or psychotic.
 3. Case example
 In the following clinical vignette, the patient does not satisfy the current true criteria for zoophilia but does indicate zoophilic interests.

 Mrs. J. W., a thirty-year-old, married woman, came for psychiatric treatment because of depressive symptoms. These were in part a result of a somewhat estranged relationship with her husband who, although attentive, was not sexually interested in her. During the course of her hospitalization, she became profoundly depressed when her pet dog died. At that point she revealed that on a number of occasions she had engaged in sexual relations with the dog.

E. Coprophilia
 1. *Coprophilia* is a pathological sexual interest in excretions. It includes the desire to defecate on a partner or to be defecated upon.
F. *Klismaphila* is the love of enemas and a dependence on their use for sexual arousal.
G. *Urophilia* is a pathologic love for, or interest in, urine.
XV. **Prognosis for paraphiliacs**
 A. In general, the prognosis for paraphiliacs depends upon the severity and the chronicity of the deviation. When the paraphilia is well developed and firmly fixed, and there is lack of desire for change, the prognosis is extremely poor.

B. The best prognosis seems to exist when there is a relationship between the deviant behavior and some precipitating environmental stress, and for younger deviants (especially adolescents).

C. Since the symptom is pleasurable (ego-syntonic), it is often difficult to treat, especially since deviants seldom seek psychiatric treatment on their own.

XVI. **Treatment of paraphiliacs**

A. There is no ideal treatment.

B. Psychotherapy is a long, drawn-out, tedious process with sometimes doubtful results. For those who are uncomfortable, anxious, or depressed, an indication that they cannot accept their deviance, psychotherapy is more promising. Such treatment is usually psychoanalytically oriented. Such a therapeutic approach affords the opportunity to trace the onset of the disorder and hopefully eliminate it.

C. Behavioral therapy has been tried with some reported success.

D. When the deviance is not well fixed, the patient is more likely to respond to either of the above therapies.

E. Group therapy has shown some promise.

F. Environmental manipulation is sometimes of value.

G. Sometimes confinement of the deviant is necessary for the protection of the community (e.g., the pedophile who repeatedly approaches young children).

H. Psychotropic medications, including antipsychotic drugs, may be helpful in those paraphilias that are acutely or dangerously compulsive.

I. Antiandrogens (e.g., cyproterone acetate, and Depo-Provera) in selected cases have been reported to decrease hypersexual behavior.

XVII. **Sexual dysfunctions**

A. Definition

1. The essential feature of this subclass is inhibition in the appetitive or psychophysiologic changes that characterize the complete sexual response cycle. Ordinarily this diagnostic category will be applied only when the disturbance is a major part of the clinical picture, even though it may not be part of the chief complaint. The diagnosis is not made if the sexual dysfunction is attributed entirely to organic factors, such as a physical disorder or a medication, or if it is due to another Axis I mental disorder (*DSM*-III-R).

2. The complete sexual response cycle can be divided into the following phases (*DSM*-III-R):

a) *Appetitive.* This consists of fantasies about sexual activity and a desire to have sexual activity.

b) *Excitement.* This consists of a subjective sense of sexual pleasure and accompanying physiologic changes. The major changes in the male consist of penile tumescence, leading to erection, and the appearance of Cowper's gland secretion. The major changes in the female consist of vasocongestion in the pelvis, vaginal lubrication, and swelling of the external genitalia. Other changes include development of the orgasmic platform, that is, narrowing of the outer third of the vagina by increased pubococcygeal muscle tension and vasocongestion; vasocongestion of the labia minora; breast tumescence; and lengthening and widening of the inner two-thirds of the vagina.

c) *Orgasm.* This consists of a peaking of sexual pleasure, with release of sexual tension and rhythmic contraction of the perineal muscles and pelvic reproductive organs. In the male there is the sensation of ejaculatory inevitability, which is followed by emission of semen, caused by contractions of the prostate, seminal vesicles, and urethra. In the female there are contractions, not always subjectively experienced as such, of the wall of the outer third of the vagina. In both the male and the female there is often generalized muscular tension or contractions, such as involuntary pelvic thrusting.

d) *Resolution.* This consists of a sense of general relaxation, well-being, and muscular relaxation. During this phase, males are physiologically refractory to further erection and orgasm for a period of time. In contrast, women may be able to respond to additional stimulation almost immediately.

3. Inhibitions may occur during one or more of these four phases of the response cycle.

4. Sexual avoidance (phobic) is not really a psychosexual problem. Many are preoccupied with their sexual performance.

B. Prevalence

This is not really known, but most of these dysfunctions are believed to be common, especially in their milder forms.

C. Types of sexual dysfunctions

1. Sexual desire disorders

a) Hypoactive sexual desire disorder: persistently or recurrently deficient or absent sexual fantasies and desire for sexual activity.

b) Sexual aversion disorder: persistent or recurrent extreme aversion to, and avoidance of, all or almost all, genital sexual contact with a sexual partner.

2. Sexual arousal disorders
   a) Female sexual arousal disorder: (1) persistent or recurrent partial or complete failure to attain or maintain the lubrication-swelling response of sexual excitement until completion of the sexual activity; (2) persistent or recurrent lack of a subjective sense of sexual excitement and pleasure in a female during sexual activity.
   b) Male erectile disorder: persistent or recurrent partial or complete failure in a male to attain or maintain erection until completion of the sexual activity.
3. Orgasm disorders
   a) Inhibited female orgasm: persistent or recurrent delay in, or absence of, orgasm in a female following a normal sexual excitement phase during sexual activity that the clinician judges to be adequate in focus, intensity, and duration.
   b) Inhibited male orgasm: persistent or recurrent delay in, or absence of, orgasm in a male following a normal heterosexual excitement phase during sexual activity that the clinician, taking into account the person's age, judges to be adequate in focus, intensity, and duration.
   c) Premature ejaculation: persistent or recurrent ejaculation with minimal sexual stimulation or before, upon, or shortly after penetration and before the person wishes it.
4. Sexual pain disorders
   a) Dyspareunia: recurrent or persistent genital pain in either a male or female before, during, or after sexual intercourse.
   b) Vaginismus: recurrent or persistent involuntary spasm of the musculature of the outer third of the vagina that interferes with coitus.

D. Course

The course is variable. All of the dysfunctions may be acquired or lifelong. Most commonly have their onset in early adult life.

E. Etiology

It is assumed that physiological factors have been ruled out.

1. Predisposing factors

There is a slight correlation between certain personality traits and the presence of certain psychosexual dysfunctions.
   a) Histrionic characteristics in females are frequently associated with inhibited sexual excitement and inhibited orgasm.
   b) Compulsive traits in males are frequently associated with inhibited sexual desires and inhibited sexual excitement.

      c) Anxiety appears to predispose to the development of premature ejaculation.

      d) Any negative attitude toward sexuality (from internal conflicts, rigid subcultural values, or particular experiences) seem to predispose to psychosexual dysfunction.

2. Psychodynamic theory regards sexual dysfunctions as having their roots in early developmental conflict.

3. Women's sexual responsiveness, more than men's, tends to depend on feelings of tenderness, intimacy, affection, and security. Any factors that interfere with these underlying feelings may also impair the woman's ability to be sexually responsive.

4. A frequent problem in the woman's impaired sexual response is the male's premature ejaculation (some say premature ejaculation in men is disappearing).

5. Perhaps even more common is some disturbance in the total relationship with the partner.

6. Primary male impotence usually indicates serious underlying psychopathology. Such men usually come from backgrounds of sexual repression.

7. Men with secondary impotence are usually responding to some situational factor (e.g., excessive indulgence in alcohol, occupational or economic tensions, depression).

8. Testosterone is the libido hormone in both sexes.

F. Treatment

1. Individual psychotherapy is useful in examining problems with intimacy and dependency (issues often accompanied by sexual dysfunction).

2. Group therapy, whether behaviorally, educationally, or psychodynamically oriented, may be useful adjuncts to other forms of therapy.

3. Dual sex therapy originated with Masters and Johnson. In this therapy the marital dyad is the focus of therapy.

4. In psychoanalytically oriented sex therapy, sex therapy is integrated with psychoanalytically oriented psychotherapy.

5. Focus in hypnotherapy is specifically on the anxiety-producing symptom, that is, the particular sexual dysfunction. Patients are also taught relaxation techniques to use prior to sexual intercourse.

G. Outcome

The most difficult treatment cases involve couples with severe marital discord.

HOMOSEXUALITY

I. Introduction

A. The American Psychiatric Association has officially taken the position that homosexuality does not constitute a psychiatric disorder.

B. However, in *DSM*-III (1980), ego-dystonic homosexuality was listed. The essential features are a desire to acquire or increase heterosexual arousal, so that heterosexual relationships can be initiated or maintained, and a sustained pattern of overt homosexual arousal that the individual explicitly states has been unwanted and a persistent source of distress. Generally, individuals with this disorder have had homosexual relationships, but often the physical satisfaction is accompanied by emotional upset because of strong negative feelings regarding homosexuality. In some cases, the negative feelings are so strong that the homosexual arousal has been confined to fantasy.

II. *DSM*-III-R

A. In *DSM*-III-R, homosexuality is not listed as an actual disorder. However, under sexual disorder not otherwise specified is listed an example of a disorder not classifiable in any other previous categories, "persistent and marked distress about one's sexual orientation."

B. The subject of homosexuality remains controversial and its conceptualization is marked by fundamental lack of consensus.

III. Prevalence

According to Kinsey, about 4 to 6 percent of males consider themselves homosexual and about 2 percent of females. This did not include the ones with occasional or opportunistic same-sex contacts.

IV. Etiology

A. Constitutional factors
   1. There are heterosexual and homosexual components of the libidinal drives of everyone. Sexual behavior is related to sexual identification and, also, the ability to sublimate certain drives.
   2. A surfacing of homosexual drives has been attributed by some to genetic or biologic factors.

B. Psychoanalytic theory
   1. Freud viewed homosexuality as an arrest of psychosexual development. According to his theory, castration anxiety and unresolved Oedipal situations underlie male homosexuality. Unresolved penis envy forms the basis for female homosexuality.
   2. The male homosexual has identified with his mother.
   3. The female homosexual has identified with her father.

C. Environmental theories
   1. Some authorities believe that homosexual men have overly close, intimate, possessive, dominating, overprotective, and "demasculinizing" mothers, and detached, unaffectionate, hostile fathers who treat their sons in a humiliating way.
   2. Similarly, homosexual females are said to have submissive fathers who were distant to their daughters, and mothers who were hostile, competitive, defeminizing, and who favored sons.

3. Confirmed homosexual females give a history of having been exposed to alcoholism and abusiveness.
4. Seduction in early life by a homosexual may, in some cases, play a significant etiological role.

D. Cultural theories
1. Homosexuality has existed in both past and present cultures. It has often been viewed as a normal variant of biological behavior. However, there are cultures in which homosexuality is unknown.
2. Subcultures in which there is an undue restriction on any show of heterosexual interest (e.g., prohibition of dating, dancing, and so forth) may lead to the belief that homosexual behavior is less forbidden than heterosexual behavior.
3. Homosexuality may occur transiently—in adolescents, as an expression of curiosity or experimentation, or in circumstances where heterosexual contacts are unavailable (e.g., American prisons).

E. Treatment
1. Of the basic underlying homosexuality
   a) Most homosexuals do not seek treatment. It is only those who seek surgery or who have incidental psychological symptoms or personality problems that do.
   b) Bieber has reported that with the use of psychoanalytic therapy, approximately one-third of bisexual or homosexually oriented males achieved heterosexual reorientation.
   c) Several behavior modification approaches have been tried. Negative conditioning, in which the showing of homo-erotic pictures has been accompanied by injection of apomorphine (to produce vomiting) or painful electrical stimuli, has had some reported success. Also covert sensitization and anticipatory avoidance have been tried.
   d) Some approach the treatment of the ego-dystonic homosexual to enable him or her to live more comfortably as a homosexual, without change or guilt. (Gay counseling centers are engaged in such treatment programs.)
   e) Few data have been reported on the treatment of women with ego-dystonic homosexuality.
   f) Drug therapy
      (1) Antianxiety agents or antidepressants have been prescribed for coincidental anxiety or depression.
      (2) Male hormones seem contraindicated for homosexual males, since they only increase the sexual drive without changing the aim.
   g) Group therapy has been said to have beneficial results.
   h) Some therapists approach the treatment of homosexuality as if it represents inhibition of sexual desire (inhibited appetitive phase type of psychosexual dysfunction).

2. Of incidental emotional symptoms or personality problems
   In general, treatment follows the same rules that apply to heterosexual people with these problems.

F. Case example

A twenty-seven-year-old single man consulted a psychiatrist after he had been rejected for induction into the army. He said that as far back as the age of ten, he had been troubled with strong homosexual urges. On one occasion in the tenth grade, he developed such a strong attraction for another boy that he became "very ill" for several days and had to remain home in bed.

After graduating from art school, he obtained employment as a commercial artist and had remained successfully employed in that capacity. He had a few casual acquaintances but almost no close friends. Because of his homosexual desires, he purposely avoided forming friendships with other men.

His father was described as a gentle, mild-mannered man. His mother was described as quite the opposite—stern, "unfeminine," and "hot-tempered." She administered the discipline in the family and, though she assumed a rather masculine role, was usually sick in bed one or two days every two weeks. The patient was closer to his mother than to his father.

The patient had been able to control his homosexual desires until about two years earlier when, under the influence of alcohol, he allowed another man to seduce him. Since that time he had had a few homosexual experiences. Because of his great guilt, he has made strenuous efforts to control his urges.

References

American Psychiatric Association. *Diagnostic and Statistical Manual of Mental Disorders*. 3d ed., Rev. Washington, D.C., 1987.

Eaton, M. T., Jr., M. H. Peterson, and J. M. Davis. *Psychiatry*. 4th ed. Garden City, N.Y.: Medical Examination Publishing Co., 1981.

Farnsworth, D. L., and F. J. Braceland, eds. *Psychiatry, the Clergy and Pastoral Counseling*. Collegeville, Minn.: Saint John's University Press, 1969.

Goodwin, D. W., and S. B. Guze. *Psychiatric Diagnosis*. 2d ed. New York: Oxford University Press, 1979.

Hastings, D. W. *Impotence and Frigidity*. Boston: Little, Brown, 1963.

Kaplan, H. I., and B. J. Sadock. *Comprehensive Textbook of Psychiatry/IV*. 4th ed. Baltimore: Williams & Wilkins, 1985.

Kolb, L. C., and H. K. H. Brodie. *Modern Clinical Psychiatry*. 10th ed. Philadelphia: W. B. Saunders Co., 1982.

Marmor, J. "Sexual Deviancy: Part 1." *Journal of Continuing Education in Psychiatry* 39 (7) (July, 1978): 123–34.

———. "Sexual Deviancy: Part 2." *Journal of Continuing Education in Psychiatry*, August, 1978.

Masters, W. H., and V. E. Johnson. *Human Sexual Response*. Boston: Little, Brown, 1966.

———. *Human Sexual Inadequacy*. Boston: Little, Brown, 1970.

Some fell by laudanum, and some by steel
and death ambush lay in every pill.

Sir Samuel Garth: *The Dispensary,* IV 17th Century

PSYCHOACTIVE SUBSTANCE USE DISORDERS

I. Definition

A. According to *DSM*-III-R, this diagnostic class deals with the symptoms and maladaptive behavioral changes associated with more or less regular use of psychoactive substances that affect the central nervous system. Disorders in this section are to be distinguished from psychoactive substance-induced organic mental disorders because psychoactive substance use disorder refers to the maladaptive behavior associated more or less with the regular use of the substances whereas psychoactive substance-induced organic mental disorder describes the direct, acute, or chronic effect of substances on the central nervous system.

B. Classes of psychoactive substances

There are nine classes of psychoactive substances that are associated with both abuse and dependence. These include alcohol; amphetamine or similar acting sympathomimetics; cannabis; cocaine; hallucinogens; inhalants; opioids; phencyclidine (PCP) or similarly acting arylcyclohexylamines; and sedatives, hypnotics, or anxiolytics. A tenth drug, nicotine, shows dependence but not abuse. These ten classes may be grouped into those that share similar features: (1) alcohol and sedatives, anxiolytics or hypnotics; (2) cocaine and amphetamine or similarly acting sympathomimetics; (3) hallucinogens and phencylidine (PCP) or similarly acting arylcyclohexylamines.

C. The psychoactive substance use disorders are subdivided into substance abuse and substance dependence.

   1. Psychoactive substance use dependence

      a) At least three of the following must be present:

         (1) Substance often taken in larger amounts or over a longer period than the person intended.

         (2) Persistent desire or one or more unsuccessful efforts to cut down or control substance use.

         (3) A great deal of time spent in activities necessary to get the substance (e.g., theft), taking the substance (e.g., chain smoking), or recovering from its effects.

         (4) Frequent intoxication or withdrawal symptoms when expected to fulfill major role obligations at work, school, or home (e.g., does not go to work because hung over, goes to school or work "high," intoxicated while taking care of his or her children), or when substance use is physically hazardous (e.g., drives when intoxicated).

         (5) Important social, occupational, or recreational activities given up or reduced because of substance use.

(6) Continued substance use despite knowledge of having a persistent or recurrent social, psychological, or physical problem that is caused or exacerbated by the use of the substance (e.g., keeps using heroin despite family arguments about it, cocaine-induced depression, or having an ulcer made worse by drinking).

(7) Marked tolerance: need for markedly increased amounts of the substance (i.e., at least a 50% increase) in order to achieve intoxication or desired effect, or markedly diminished effect with continued use of the same amount. Note: The following items may not apply to cannabis, hallucinogens, or phencyclidine (PCP).

(8) Characteristic withdrawal symptoms.

(9) Substance often taken to relieve or avoid withdrawal symptoms.

b) Some symptoms of the disturbance have persisted for at least one month or have occurred repeatedly over a longer period of time.

2. Psychoactive substance abuse
   a) A maladaptive pattern of psychoactive substance use is indicated by at least one of the following:
      (1) Continued use despite knowledge of having a persistent or recurrent social, occupational, psychological, or physical problem that is caused or exacerbated by use of the psychoactive substance.
      (2) Recurrent use in situations in which use is physically hazardous (e.g., driving while intoxicated).
   b) Some symptoms of the disturbance have persisted for at least one month or have occurred repeatedly over a longer period of time.
   c) Never met the criteria for psychoactive substance dependence for this substance.

D. Although abuse of alcohol and nicotine technically belong in this category, they are being discussed in a separate chapter because both of these are legal drugs. The Surgeon General's Report (1984) reveals that about 30 percent of all deaths in the United States are premature because of the use of just these two dependence-producing drugs.

II. Prevalence

A. Prior to the 1960s the nonmedical use of drugs other than alcohol and tobacco was relatively low. (For example, only 1% of Americans aged 12 to 17 ever used marijuana and only 4% of those aged 18 to 25 had ever used this drug.)

B. In the late 1960s and early 1970s nonmedical drug use reached epidemic proportions (e.g., marijuana use in the 12- to 17-year-old population rose to 31% in 1979 and 68% of Americans aged 18 to 25 reported that they had used marijuana at least once. In 1978, nearly 11% of American high school seniors reported using marijuana every day of their senior year). In the years since, the rates of illicit drug use have leveled off, and in some cases, declined but none have fallen to the levels characteristic of the years before 1962.

C. Epidemiologic studies have shown that the onset of the nonmedical drug use is all but limited to the teenage years. The progression is as follows: drug use begins with alcohol (the gateway into recreational, nonmedical use of intoxicants for adolescence). This is followed by the use of marijuana (the gateway into the use of illicit drugs), and moves on to the nonmedical use of dependence-producing pharmaceuticals (many anxiety agents, analgesics, and hypnotics) and cocaine. The final step is to the most stigmatized and least commonly used drugs, such as heroin and phencyclidine.

D. Youths who do not use cigarettes and alcohol during their teenage years are virtually immune to the nonmedical use of other dependence-producing drugs (DuPont, 1985).

E. Most drug-dependent people become so by their association with other people who are also drug dependent. Their lives prior to substance use have usually been ones of unsatisfactory or marginal adjustments.

F. Medications that reduce pain, diminish anxiety, or produce euphoria may be taken by those who seek relief from physical or psychological symptoms or feelings of inadequacy.

III. **Etiology**

A. Many of the etiological and psychopathological factors found in substance use disorders are also associated with alcoholism (see next chapter).

B. There are a number of theories as to the cause of drug abuse.
1. Availability
This is considered the "sine quo non" for drug dependence. In other words, the drug has to be available before one can become addicted. Example of this would be the availability of all kinds of drugs in the ghetto and the availability of sedatives, narcotics, and psychoactive drugs in the medical community. (Yet, the majority of both of these communities do not take drugs. Thus, availability by itself does not fully explain drug dependency.)
2. Psychological
There is no single personality type who becomes drug dependent. According to *DSM*-III-R, personality disturbance and disturbance of mood are often present, and may be intensified

by the psychoactive substance use disorder. For example, antisocial personality traits may be accentuated by the need to obtain money to purchase illegal substances. Anxiety or depression associated with borderline personality disorder may be intensified as the person uses a psychoactive substance in an unsuccessful attempt to treat his or her mood disturbance.

In chronic abuse or dependence, mood lability and suspiciousness, both of which can contribute to violent behavior, are common (*DSM*-III-R).

There are numerous psychological theories (e.g., oral dependence is considered to be etiological in psychoanalytic theory, and some say drugs are used to control anger).

3. Socioeconomic
The incidence is highest in the lowest socioeconomic group and highest socioeconomic group, and lowest in the middle class.
4. Social (e.g., in dictatorships, disapproved drugs are kept out). Russia does not have a drug problem but has a serious problem with alcohol. Sweden and Japan have major problems with amphetamines.
5. Biologic (e.g., opiate addiction is thought to result from an endorphin deficiency).

C. Some people take drugs to overcome feelings of inferiority or inadequacy.
1. The individual who has a reduced tolerance to tension, feelings of inadequacy, and who feels under personal or social stress may take drugs.
2. The availability of drugs and other cultural factors may play a role. Physicians are apt to abuse narcotics and antianxiety agents, housewives are most likely to abuse sedatives and antianxiety agents; adolescents are most apt to abuse marijuana or other street drugs. (As a matter of fact, availability of drugs is the most common predisposing factor in substance use.)

D. Some take drugs mostly for the euphoric effect (e.g., cocaine or marijuana).

IV. **Psychopathology**
A. Persons who develop drug dependency have subnormal tolerance of tension and above-normal feelings of dependency.
B. Features of various personality disorders are often present in substance abusers. For example, some show traits of antisocial personality, others may show evidences of borderline personality or dysthymic disorder (chronic depression).
C. Some authorities believe that there is absence of a strong father figure in the developmental histories of people who become addicts.

V. Classes of pyschoactive substances

The following are some of the drugs, other than alcohol and nicotine, on which people can become dependent or which they can abuse.

A. Amphetamine or similarly acting sympathomimetic compound

This group includes all of the substances of the substituted phenylethylamine structure, such as amphetamine, dextroamphetamine, and methamphetamine ("speed"), and those with structures different from the substituted phenylethylamine that have amphetaminelike action, such as methylphenidate and some substances used as appetite suppressants ("diet pills"). These substances are typically taken orally or intravenously, although methamphetamine is frequently taken by nasal inhalation (like cocaine) (*DSM*-III-R).

1. Medical use
   a) They were first used in otolaryngology as a nasal decongestant.
   b) They were also prescribed to relieve fatigue or depression, to control appetite, or to produce wakefulness in those who had to perform tasks of long duration.
   c) There are far fewer legitimate medical indications for their use now, and they have come under much closer government supervision because of their widespread abuse.
   d) They are used in the treatment of hyperactive syndrome in children and in attention-deficit disorders.

2. Prevalence and course
   a) These drugs are stimulants and produce euphoria.
   b) Sometimes those dependent on sedatives for sleep take them to stay awake during the daytime.
   c) Many people obtain them illicitly.
   d) Acute paranoid psychosis may develop in people who abuse this group of drugs. A urine test for amphetamines is necessary to make the diagnosis of amphetamine intoxication, which may be clinically indistinguishable from acute paranoid schizophrenia.
   e) Occurs in approximately 2 percent of the adult population (*DSM*-III-R).
   f) Many develop abuse or dependence after first using an appetite suppressant.
   g) The amphetamine user often abuses or is dependent on other drugs to counteract unpleasant aftereffects of amphetamine intoxication.
   h) Psychological and behavioral changes include depression, irritability, anhedonia, anergia, and social isolation.

3. Patterns of use

   Many people develop amphetamine abuse or dependence after first using amphetamines or amphetaminelike compounds as appetite suppressants.

4. Associated features

   Often the user of amphetamine also abuses or is dependent on other drugs, which are taken in an attempt to counteract the unpleasant aftereffects of intoxication.

   Psychological and behavioral changes associated with amphetamine abuse and dependence include depression, irritability, anhedonia, anergia, and social isolation.

B. Cannabis

   1. This group includes all substances with psychoactive properties derived from the cannabis plant plus chemically similar synthetic substances (marijuana, hashish, and occasionally purified THC; they are almost always smoked).

   2. Cannabis or marijuana is a leaf that grows wild in most parts of the United States and South America.

   3. Medical use

      a) Cannabis was previously used as a treatment for tension headache, dysmenorrhea, and glaucoma.

      b) It was removed from the U.S. Pharmacopoeia in 1935.

      c) Generally, it has been prescribed only experimentally (e.g., it has been released for the treatment of glaucoma, and nausea and other side effects of anticancer drugs and anorexia nervosa).

   4. Patterns of use

      Many people regard this as a substance of low abuse potential, not appreciating its capacity to induce dependence. Dependence is usually characterized by daily or almost daily use. It is used in combination with other substances, particularly alcohol and cocaine. Psychological symptoms associated with cannabis dependency include lethargy, anhedonia, and attentional and memory problems.

   5. Course

      Chronic use produces the amotivational syndrome.

   6. Prevalence

      It is the most widely used illicit psychoactive substance in the United States. Approximately 5 percent of the adult population have used it at some time in their lives.

C. Cocaine

   1. Cocaine has a limited use in medical practice (e.g., as an anesthetic in certain types of nasal surgery).

   2. It produces euphoria, loquaciousness, elation, and grandiosity.

3. Sometimes produces somatic hallucinations, including formication (this sometimes is referred to as the "cocaine bug"), a tactile hallucination or illusion that insects are crawling on the body or under the skin.
4. Types
Several different types of coca preparations are used for their psychoactive properties: coca leaves (chewed), coca paste (smoked), cocaine hydrochloride powder (inhaled or injected), and cocaine alkaloid—"freebase" or "crack" (smoked). The most commonly used form in the United States is cocaine hydrochloride powder, which is usually inhaled through the nostrils, and then absorbed into the bloodstream through the mucous membranes.
5. Status
   a) Prior to the mid-1960s, cocaine was used primarily by heroin addicts and members of the hard core drug culture, whom Americans regarded as criminals. Thus, cocaine had little appeal or status.
   b) During the late 1960s and the early 1970s it began to be used by a broad segment of American society, when cocaine became viewed as similar to marijuana use. (Possession was illegal, but use was not viewed as criminal behavior.)
   c) Some feel the mass media played an important role popularizing cocaine and it developed an elite status. Perhaps the reduced availability of amphetamines was another factor in popularizing cocaine. Further, cocaine was viewed as "not addicting" because it did not induce physical dependence. (Currently, few still believe this.)
   d) It is increasingly reported as the primary drug of abuse among those seeking treatment for addiction in both the private and public sectors. However, this is misleading because all the drug abusers will claim cocaine dependency because it is "fashionable."
   e) Bromptom's solution is an oral pain-relieving medication for terminal cancer patients that contains methadone (or morphine), alcohol, and cocaine.
6. Patterns of use
Cocaine abusers often use barbituates, methaqualone, benzodiazepines, or alcohol to self-medicate for insomnia, agitation and irritability, which result from the cocaine use.

Cocaine abuse and dependence are associated with two different patterns of use: episodic, and chronic daily, or almost daily, use.

"Bingeing" is a common form of episodic use consisting of compressed time periods of continuous high dose use.

7. Psychological features

Cocaine can produce a broad range of psychological effects, ranging from acute anxiety to full-blown cocaine psychosis with paranoia and auditory or visual hallucinations.

Psychological and behavioral changes include depression, irritability, anhedonia, anergia, and social isolation. Sexual dysfunction, paranoid ideation, attentional disturbances, and memory problems may also occur.

8. Course
   a) Cocaine smoking and intravenous administration of cocaine tend to engender rapid progression from infrequent cocaine use to cocaine abuse or dependence, often within only a few weeks or months.
   b) Progressive tolerance of the desirable effects of the substance leads to use of increasing doses.
   c) With continued use there is a progressive diminution in pleasurable effects and a corresponding increase in dysphoric effects.

9. Prevalence

Cocaine abuse has reached epidemic proportions in this country. Current estimates suggest that 20 to 24 million Americans have experimented with cocaine. Four to five million people are considered to be regular users, and the amount of cocaine used in this country increases by 10 to 20 percent each year (Spitz and Rosecan 1987).

D. Hallucinogens
   1. Definition

   This group includes two types of substances, both of which have hallucinogenic properties:
      a) Substances structurally related to 5-hydroxytryptamine, for example, lysergic acid diethylamine (LSD) and dimethyltryptamine (DMT)
      b) Substances related to catecholamine (e.g., mescaline).
   2. Effect
      a) Most produce a reaction similar to hypomania and schizophrenic withdrawal (preoccupation with own thoughts and perceptions).
      b) Among the perceptual changes are subjective intensification of perceptions, depersonalization, derealization, illusions, hallucinations, or synesthesias (e.g., seeing colors when a loud sound occurs). These occur in a state of full wakefulness and alertness.
      c) These drugs can lead to serious psychological damage.

    d) Some of the adverse effects that have been reported from LSD use are

      (1) Long-term psychotic disorders

      (2) Panic from a reaction to the hallucinatory experiences ("bad trip")

      (3) Serious injury and even death from the delusional experiences (e.g., feelings of omnipotence or the feeling that one can fly)

      (4) Long-term intellectual and emotional disorientation

      (5) Flashback phenomenon, a reexperiencing of a trip without further use of the drug

3. Patterns of use

Most people are introduced to a hallucinogen by "experimenting" with the substance. Some find the hallucinosis extremely dysphoric and stop using the substance, whereas others enjoy the experience and continue its use.

4. Associated features

Hallucinogens are frequently contaminated with other drugs, such as PCP and amphetamine. In addition, users frequently smoke cannabis and abuse alcohol.

5. Course

The course is unpredictable and probably related to the nature of the underlying pathology that played a role in onset of its use. Most people rapidly resume their former life-style after only a brief period of abuse or dependence.

6. Prevalence

The use of hallucinogens as the predominant substance is extremely rare (*DSM*-III-R).

E. Inhalants

1. Included in this classification are disorders induced by inhaling, through the mouth or nose, the aliphatic and aromatic hydrocarbons found in substances such as gasoline, glue, paint, paint thinners, and spray paints. Less commonly used are the halogenated hydrocarbons found in cleaners, typewriter correction fluid, and spray-can propellants and other volatile compounds containing esters, ketones, and glycols.

2. Most compounds that are inhaled are a mixture of several substances that can produce psychoactive effects. Therefore, under most circumstances, it is difficult to ascertain the exact substance responsible for the disorder.

3. Several methods are used to inhale intoxicating vapors. Most commonly, a rag soaked with the substance is applied to the mouth and nose and the vapors are breathed in.

    The background of inhalant users is generally marked by considerable family dysfunction (as in school or work adjustment problems).

Generally, inhalants are used by quite young children, nine to thirteen years of age, generally with a group of peers who are likely to use alcohol and cannabis as well.

4. Users of inhalants nearly always use other psychoactive substances as well.
5. Younger children may use inhalants several times a week, often on weekends and after school. Severe dependence in young adults may involve varying periods of intoxication throughout each day.
6. Prevalance not known.

F. Opioid substances
   1. Abuse of or dependence upon opioids generally follows a period of "polydrug use."
   2. Course
      a) Once the pattern is established, substance procurement and the use generally dominate the individual's life.
      b) The course is a function of the context of the addiction; that is, the vast majority of persons who became dependent on heroin in Vietnam did not return to their addiction when back in the United States. In contrast, it is believed that most individuals who become dependent on opioids in the United States become involved in a chronic behavioral disorder, marked by remissions while in treatment or prison or when the substance is scarce, but relapses on returning to a familiar environment where these substances are available and friends or colleagues use these substances (*DSM-III*).
      c) In the United States, persons with opioid dependence have a high annual death rate (approximately 10 per 1,000).
   3. Case examples
      a) Thomas De Quincey (1785–1859), essayist and critic, reported his experiences in *Confessions of an English Opium Eater*. While still in college, he took his first opium to relieve the pain of facial neuralgia and several years later became a "regular and confirmed opium eater." Though he wrote "these troubles are passed," he actually remained an opium user for the rest of his life.
      b) Samuel Taylor Coleridge (1772–1834), who was the author of *The Rhyme of the Ancient Mariner, Kubla Kahn,* and *Christabel,* in his later years was dejected and became addicted to opium.

G. Phencyclidine or similarly acting arylcyclohexylamine compounds
   1. Phencyclidine is a white powder, commonly called PCP ("peace pill").
   2. Although available as a veterinary anesthetic, most of the illicit supply comes from home laboratories.

3. On the "street" it is called "angel dust."
4. It is sold in powder and tablet form, both in many colors.
5. It is often sprinkled on marijuana or parsley leaves and smoked in a "joint."
6. It may well be that the use of PCP is quite common among abusers of other drugs.
7. PCP is stronger than marijuana, perhaps more comparable to LSD.
8. The diagnosis of overdosage is frequently missed because the presenting symptoms often closely resemble those of an acute schizophrenic episode.
9. Some authorities feel that phenothiazines should not be used to manage a patient during the acute stage of overdose because of the anticholinergic potentiation.

H. Sedative, hypnotic, or anxiolytic substances
  1. Types

Hypnotics or "sleeping pills," include benzodiazepines such as flurazepam, triazolam, and temazepam, and other substances unrelated to benzodiazepines, such as ethchlorvynol, glutethimide, chloral hydrate, methaqualone, and the barbiturates. Benzodiazepines are also used for the treatment of anxiety and are the most commonly prescribed psychoactive medications (*DSM*-III-R).

  2. Although these psychoactive substances differ widely in their mechanisms of action, rates of absorption, metabolism, and distribution in the body, at some dose and at some duration of use, they are all capable of producing similar syndromes of intoxication and withdrawal. Substances in this category are usually taken orally (*DSM*-III-R).

  3. Patterns of use

There are two patterns.

    a) The person originally obtained the psychoactive substance by prescription from a physician for treatment of anxiety or insomnia, but gradually increases the dose in frequency of use on his or her own.

    b) A second pattern more frequent than the first that leads to the dependence involves young people in their teens and early twenties who, with a group of peers, use substances obtained from illegal sources. The initial objective is to obtain a "high" or euphoria on the substances used alone.

  4. Course

The most common course is heavy daily use that results in dependence. A significant number of people with dependence eventually stop using the substance and recover completely, even from the physical complications of the disorder (*DSM*-III-R).

5. Prevalence

Approximately 1.1 percent of the adult population have had sedative, hypnotic, or anxiolytic abuse or dependence at some time in their lives.

Epidemiologic data gathered over the last fifteen years show that the U.S. benzodiazepine use is not higher than that of other developed nations and that most patients who use these drugs do so with symptomatic relief and restraint in terms of amount, dose, and duration of treatment. On the other hand, the same data show that almost 2 percent of the adult population use these agents more or less chronically.

For many patients suffering from anxiety disorders, continued use of a benzodiazepine is preferable to enduring the underlying anxiety symptoms (DuPont, 1986).

VI. Treatment

A. Treatment of the underlying personality disorder
   1. This is often extremely difficult, because the substance abuser and the substance-dependent person, like the alcoholic, has reduced tolerance for tension.
   2. Psychotherapy
      a) Psychotherapy is of help in many cases.
      b) Support and reassurance are important.
      c) Group psychotherapy has been helpful in some cases.
B. Treatment of the drug dependence
   1. Self-help groups
   Groups such as AA or other groups composed of drug-dependent people are often the most helpful.
   2. Withdrawal
      a) At present, most withdrawal treatment is fairly abrupt and uses the principles of supportive treatment. Sometimes people who are intoxicated or stuporous are taken to detoxification centers or to hospitals.
      b) Supportive treatment involves
         (1) A detoxification period during which certain drugs are judiciously prescribed. The drugs include methadone (see below), chlordiazepoxide (Librium), diazepam (Valium), or phenobarbitol. They are continued for several days after the patient has discontinued using the abused drug.
         (2) Adequate diet and fluid intake.
         (3) Often, placement in "chemical dependency units" where patients are treated much like alcoholics. Such persons often need more "attention" than other patients.
         (4) A therapeutic, supportive, and reassuring attitude. The therapist avoids being judgmental or moralistic.

c) Methadone

Methadone (Dolophine) is the drug used to treat addicts of opiate and opiatelike agents. It is administered in two ways.

   (1) Methadone substitution

In this approach, the addict takes a regular dose of methadone, given orally, after which the methadone is progressively withdrawn over a period of a few days.

   (2) Methadone maintenance

In this method, the methadone is prescribed indefinitely.

   (3) Methadone withdrawal

Clonidine (Catapres) has been used with reported success in withdrawing people from methadone.

3. Therapeutic communities demanding total commitment from the patient are residential treatment programs that attempt to deal with the psychological causes of addiction by changing the addict's personality and character (not suitable for very many).

4. Rehabilitation of the drug-dependent person must be regarded as a long-term management problem. Refer to the next chapter, "Alcoholism," for information about follow-up treatment and rehabilitation after the patient leaves the hospital.

VII. Prognosis

A. The prognosis is often poor.

B. Relapses are common.

C. However, given someone who is well motivated and willing to regard his or her problem as a long-term one that must be dealt with consistently over a protracted period of time, the frequency of relapses can be reduced and the periods of abstinence can be lengthened.

D. Follow-up programs such as AA, halfway houses, and other various group settings have improved the remission rate.

VIII. Case examples

A. Medical addiction

Mrs. J., a forty-year-old housewife, had suffered from migraine headaches since puberty. They had gradually increased in frequency and severity. At thirty, she began taking codeine. For a few years, this gave some relief but for five years she had been taking demerol (a synthetic narcotic drug) in increasingly larger doses. At the time of admission to the hospital, she was using 500–600 mg of demerol per day (the usual dose is 50 mg). She was always very dependent on her mother. Even after her marriage, she never lived farther away from her mother than one block. She had always had a reduced tolerance for any kind of discomfort; for example, she required medication for painful menses, sinusitis, and other pain.

Although demerol was successfully withdrawn rapidly during her hospitalization, she was never fully able to face her underlying problems of dependency and unexpressed hostility. One month after discharge, she was again beginning to take demerol for her headaches.

In the foregoing case, note that the patient began taking drugs for a psychosomatic illness (migraine), that she had a reduced tolerance of discomfort, was very dependent, and was unable to express hostile feelings.

B. Self-administration

Mr. D. S., a twenty-three-year-old single male, was referred to the court's psychiatric consultant for evaluation after he had been placed in the county correctional facility for driving after suspension of his license and driving under the influence of drugs. These offenses occurred while he was awaiting trial on a charge of aggravated robbery.

He had received an undesirable discharge from the Marine Corps centering around his possession and use of marijuana, "at my own request." In addition, he reported, he had been court-martialed for disrespect to a noncommissioned officer and had received minor discipline for two other offenses. Concerning his use of drugs, he said that he was first "turned on" by marijuana about three years earlier, while serving with the Marines. From then until the time of the arrest that brought him to the attention of the court's consultant, he had used drugs extensively. He had used LSD and other hallucinogenic drugs, but gave these up after he began to have bad trips and flashbacks. He said that he had been hospitalized in Okinawa for four days for withdrawal of hallucinogenic drugs. He suffered minor withdrawal symptoms when he was jailed for the current offenses. Chiefly, he had been "mainlining" heroin, although he also used cocaine. Throughout this whole period, he had never tried to stop smoking marijuana, although he said that for periods of up to one or two months during the preceding four years he had been able to remain off other drugs. He also admitted that he had used "speed" intravenously. He said that his "habit" was costing him $100 to $120 a day.

Mental-status examination revealed him to be somewhat anxious and superficial, and he seemed to be trying to impress the examiner by his need to be released. He admitted feeling depressed in the past when his freedom was restricted, and also sometimes from the bad effects of drugs. Although he was lucid, appropriate, and free of psychotic mentation, he said that he was aware of paranoid ideation at times in the past when he was on drugs. He also admitted having hallucinatory experiences from LSD, mescaline and, on one occasion, from "Panama marijuana." In all of these instances, he had pleasant and vivid visual and auditory sensations. His later trips had a paranoid content and would last up to five hours. Needle scars were evident over the antecubital areas of both arms. Treatment in a hospital was recommended.

References

American Psychiatric Association. *Diagnostic and Statistical Manual of Mental Disorders*. 3d ed., rev. Washington, D.C., 1987.

DuPont, R. L. "Substance Abuse." *Journal of the American Medical Association* 256 (1986): 2114–2116.

———. "Substance Abuse." *Journal of the American Medical Association* 254 (1985): 2335–2337.

Eaton, M. T., Jr., M. H. Peterson, and J. A. Davis. *Psychiatry*. 4th ed. Garden City, N.Y.: Medical Examination Publishing Co., 1981.

Farnsworth, D. L., and F. J. Braceland, eds. *Psychiatry, the Clergy and Pastoral Counseling*. Collegeville, Minn.: Saint John's University Press, 1969.

Goodwin, D. W., and S. B. Guze. *Psychiatric Diagnosis*. 2d ed. New York: Oxford University Press, 1979.

Kaplan, H. I. and B. J. Sadock. *Comprehensive Textbook of Psychiatry/IV*. 4th ed. Baltimore: Williams & Wilkins, 1985.

Kolb, L. C., and H. K. H. Brodie. *Modern Clinical Psychiatry*. 10th ed. Philadelphia: W. B. Saunders Co., 1982.

Spitz, H. I., and J. S. Rosecan, eds. *Cocaine Abuse*. New York: Brunnel/Mazel, 1987.

There is no doubt that not to drink wine is a great deduction from life; but it may be necessary.

Samuel Johnson

A custom loathsome to the eye, harmful to thee brain, dangerous to the lungs, and in the black stinking fume thereof, nearest resembling the horrible Stygian smoke of the pit that is bottomless.

James I of England:
Counterblaste to tobacco, 1604

ALCOHOLISM AND NICOTINE DEPENDENCE

I. Introduction

Alcoholism and nicotine dependence are being discussed separately because both of these substances are legal and yet a recent report showed that about 30 percent of all deaths in the United States are premature because of the use of these two dependence-producing drugs. Additionally, "youths who do not use cigarettes and alcohol during their teenage years are virtually immune to the nonmedical use of other dependence-producing drugs." (Dupont, 1985)

II. Alcohol

A. Very likely, alcoholic beverages were discovered accidently in preliterate societies.

B. Although water was probably the original liquid used as an offering in religious worship, alcoholic beverages early replaced it. Red wine became the symbol of the blood of life and remains so in modern Christianity.

C. Subsequently, drinking—and drunkenness—passed from a state of religious rites to common practice.

D. The widespread use of alcohol seems to have commenced with the beginnings of Western industrial societies, but the consequences of its continued abuse were known much earlier. In the United States, in the eighteenth century, Benjamin Rush, one of the founders of American psychiatry, thought there should be a chain of asylums for inebriates around the country. In the late nineteenth century, a medical organization known as the American Association for the Study and Care of Inebriety was formed.

E. Of all the drugs people have used over the centuries to relieve pain and tension, facilitate socialization, or produce pleasure, it is apparent that alcoholic beverages are the most commonly used. Alcoholism remains one of the four major public health problems, along with mental illness, cancer, and cardiovascular disease.

III. Tobacco

According to the Encyclopaedia Britannica: "Tobacco was first cultivated by North and South American Indians and introduced into Europe by Christopher Columbus and other early explorers. The Indians used tobacco in ceremonies (for example, smoking a peace pipe) and believed it possessed medicinal properties.

Nicotine and related alkaloids furnished the narcotic effect of the substance.

Studies suggest that smoking begins from curiosity, desire to conform and need to achieve status and self-assurance as well as advertising that encourages smoking and, the example of parents. The habit seems to persist because it reduces tension and because it is thought to be pleasurable."

IV. Each of these substances will be discussed separately in the two following chapters.

ALCOHOLISM

I. Definition

A. Alcoholism is a disorder characterized by excessive use of alcohol to the point of habituation, overdependence, or addiction.

B. Many definitions of alcoholism have been formulated by various authorities, partly because of the complexity of the disorder and partly because of the divergent orientations of the investigators. Some have stressed operational aspects, whereas others have attempted to describe causal factors.

1. The World Health Organization regards excessive drinking to be any form of drinking that goes beyond traditional and customary use or ordinary compliance with the customs of the community. By the definition, alcoholics are those excessive drinkers whose dependence upon alcohol has attained such a degree that it causes a noticeable mental disturbance or interferes with their bodily and mental health, their interpersonal relationships, or their smooth and economic functioning.

2. *The Manual of Alcoholism* of the American Medical Association defines alcoholism as "an illness characterized by a significant impairment that is directly associated with persistent and excessive use of alcohol. Impairment may involve physiological, psychological, or social dysfunction."

3. E. N. Jellinek (1960) defines alcoholism as any use of alcoholic beverage that causes damage to the individual or society or both. He delineates five subgroups.

   a) *Alpha alcoholism*—a purely psychological, continual dependence upon the effects of alcohol, which is used to relieve bodily or emotional pain (sometimes called *problem drinking* or *thymogenic drinking*).

   b) *Beta alcoholism*—similar to Alpha with the added complication of physiological derangements, such as gastritis, neuritis, liver and vascular disease (sometimes called *somatopathic*).

   c) *Gamma alcoholism*—characterized by the traditional pharmacological criterion of addiction, including both tolerance (a diminished effect with repeated use) and dependency. This is the usual type of alcoholism seen in the United States, Canada, and other Anglo-Saxon and hard-liquor-drinking countries. It is the form most commonly seen in courts, large municipal hospitals, and correctional institutions (also known as *essential alcoholism*).

   d) *Delta alcoholism*—characterized by the inability to abstain from drinking for even short periods of time; continuous speed drinking. This is the usual type of alcoholism seen in wine drinking countries such as France (Also known as *inveterate drinking*).

   e) *Epsilon alcoholism*—characterized by paroxysmal drinking bouts, during which the alcoholic drinks for varying periods of time, ranging from days to weeks (also known as *periodic drinking* and formerly called *dipsomania*).

4. In *DSM*-III-R, three main patterns of chronic alcohol abuse or dependence are listed: regular daily intake of large amounts; regular heavy drinking limited to weekends; and long periods of sobriety interspersed with binges of daily heavy drinking lasting for weeks or months.

C. Alcoholics have lost the power of choice in the matter of their drinking, and their drinking interferes with their health, work, or personal relationships. Generally, one can say that persons are alcoholics if their drinking interferes in any way with their lives.

D. Earlier, technically, abuse of and dependence on alcohol belong in the chapter, "Psychoactive Substance Use Disorder," but for previously stated reasons is treated separately here.

II. Social drinking

A. Alcohol is widely used socially. Field surveys reveal that about 71 percent of Americans drink alcohol. The rates are generally higher in urban and industrial regions. Geographically, drinking is most prevalent in the Middle Atlantic states (88 percent) and least in the East South Central Region (33 percent).

B. Today, most drinking occurs in the home, whereas, in the past, three-quarters of all drinking occurred in bars, taverns, pubs, and restaurants.

III. Prevalence of alcoholism

A. It is difficult to accurately estimate the prevalence of alcoholism. Not everyone who occasionally becomes drunk (or even fairly often) can be considered an alcoholic. Drinking is considered pathological only when it is prolonged and excessive.

B. No adequate prevalence rates of alcoholism are available, partly because of the lack of agreement about the definition of the disorder.

C. One basis of current estimates uses the Jellinek definition and relates the prevalence to death from cirrhosis of the liver. Of the estimated 120 million people in the United States who drink alcohol, perhaps as many as 9 or 10 million of these could be considered alcohol dependent.

D. Other estimates are that one of every thirteen alcohol users becomes a problem drinker.

E. There are about five to six times as many male alcoholics as female alcoholics (probably because of the different role expectations of the two sexes). This ratio has remained fairly constant in the United States for many years, even though recent estimates suggest that the proportion of female alcoholics is increasing.

F. Much of the absenteeism in industry is related to alcoholism.

G. Alcoholism is an important factor in traffic accidents, and studies have indicated that about 50 percent of fatal accidents involve alcohol abuse. In general, courts are becoming much firmer in dealing with the driver who is under the influence of alcohol.

    H. Many alcoholics are unrecognized because their drinking is done secretly and their problem does not become manifest for a long time.

    I. Many very responsible people are alcoholics. This is often one of the reasons why spouses are reluctant to identify them as such.

    J. People with other kinds of emotional disorders are more predisposed to alcoholism; for example, some persons with bipolar disorder may use alcohol excessively.

IV. Sociocultural factors

    A. Functions of alcohol

    The many purposes for which various groups employ alcohol can be divided into four general categories. These purposes influence drinking patterns greatly.

        1. Religious (e.g., wine in Roman Catholic and Jewish services).

        2. Ceremonial (e.g., toasting the bride with champagne, drinking wine at the Bar Mitzvah ceremony).

        3. Utilitarian (e.g., in cooking, in medicines, as a psychic balm, and at business and social functions).

        4. Hedonistic (e.g., as a social lubricant and especially for the euphoria produced).

    B. Sociocultural studies reveal some interesting findings. Orthodox Jews who routinely use wine in association with religious rituals have a high incidence of drinking but a low rate of alcoholism. Asians, such as the Chinese, have a low rate of alcoholism. As ethnic groups become more acculturated in their behavior patterns in drinking, they are much more like their larger peer groups (an exception to this seems to be the Chinese, who apparently get a "flush" with the ingestion of small amounts of alcohol).

    C. Conversely, there are other nationality groups of high rates of alcoholism (and its complications). Among these are the Irish-Americans. Immigrating to this country created adjustment problems for the Irish who suffered economically, socially, and religiously. Also, this group tends to use alcohol for personal goals (the promotion of fun and pleasure, physical states of well-being, and the release of inner tension) rather than for social functions, and they have few, if any, strong sanctions against heavy drinking.

    D. Other studies have shown low incidence of alcoholism among first generation Italians, but this is not true of those in the third generation.

    E. Studies have indicated that if persons come from a Protestant background of strict abstinence drink, there is a relatively high likelihood that they will become problem drinkers.

    F. More men than women drink, and men drink larger amounts and more frequently. This sex difference in the rate of alcoholism is sometimes explained in terms of the different role expectations of the two sexes. There is less social pressure on women to drink, and they are expected to drink in fewer kinds of situations. Women do not have to prove their femininity by drinking. In addition, the negative social sanctions against female drunkenness are much greater than for male drunkenness.

G. Studies of industrial populations reveal that American industry numbers about 2 million alcoholics on its collective payroll, of whom 90 percent are in the 35 to 45 age group. The alcoholic's accident rate is twice that of others, and he or she loses 25 to 30 working days each year because of drinking. The direct costs of alcoholism include high rates of absenteeism and accidents, higher medical expenses, higher disability payments, and pension payments to alcoholics who retire prematurely. The indirect costs include low efficiency of employees with hangovers, slow-down in production, and adverse effects on safety standards and the morale of other workers. Some have referred to the alcoholic in the industrial setting as the "hidden half-man."

V. Etiology

A. Many theories about the etiology and psychopathology of alcoholism have been offered but the causes are not really known.

B. Generally, alcoholics show more depression, paranoid thinking, and aggressivity; they also have lowered self-esteem, lowered sense of responsibility, and self-control when compared to nonalcoholic populations. In the not-so-distant past, the public—including many physicians and other professionals—thought that an alcoholic was simply a weak person who lacked willpower and could really control his drinking if he wished to. Some naively assumed that alcohol itself was responsible and that if no alcoholic beverages were available, there would be no alcohol problem. (The eighteenth amendment to the U.S. Constitution was an attempt to solve the drinking problem on this basis.)

C. Most adults in the Western world drink alcohol but only one in twelve or less develop serious problems from drinking. There is no good explanation for this.

D. Although the cause of alcoholism is unknown, a number of risk factors have been identified. Included are:

1. Family history
There is little dispute that there is a strong family aspect to alcoholism. There is six times the incidence of alcoholism in children of families of which one parent is an alcoholic—but this may be an environmental factor rather than a genetic factor. However, children of alcoholics become alcoholic about four times more often than children of nonalcoholics and there is some evidence that this is true even if they are not raised by the alcoholic parents.

2. Genetics

The importance of genetics in vulnerability to alcoholism is supported by evidence from family, twin, and adoption studies in humans. Studies suggest that genetic influences are important in alcoholism and reflect multiple genes interacting with environment to produce a final level of risk. In this theory, no one is predestined to become an alcoholic but genetic factors increase or decrease this level of vulnerability toward this disorder (Schuckit 1985).

3. Sex.

Men are more frequently alcoholic than women in a ratio 3:1. Age.

Alcoholism develops later in women than in men.

4. Developmental factors

Childhood history of conduct disorder, attention deficit disorder, or both, apparently increases a child's risk of becoming an alcoholic, especially if there is alcoholism in the family.

5. Orientals develop a "flush," the basis for which is undoubtedly genetic. There is a lower alcoholism rate in the Orient than in the Western world.

6. In summary, alcoholism should probably be regarded as resulting from a complex interaction of psychological, sociocultural, biological, and possibly genetic factors. An eclectic and empirical approach to this problem is indicated.

VI. Symptoms

A. Efforts to establish diagnostic criteria for alcoholism have included definitions based on (1) the quantity imbibed, (2) the degree of loss of control, (3) social consequences, (4) psychophysiological and biochemical criteria, and (5) psychological factors.

B. There is a high incidence of various types of psychopathology among alcoholics. Included in these are depression, impulsivity, poor reality testing, struggle with dominance-submission issues, and activity-passivity conflict. None of these factors is specific for alcoholics.

C. There is no constellation of psychological factors that is uniquely specific for alcoholism per se. One can only say that a well-adjusted person is unlikely to drink regularly to excess and is even less likely to become an alcoholic.

D. Some alcoholics have symptoms of other emotional disorders (e.g., anxiety or depression).

E. Some alcoholics have symptoms of character defects (e.g., borderline antisocial or passive-aggressive personality).

F. Others seem to have no obvious symptoms apart from the excessive drinking.

G. Toxic effects may accompany alcoholism (see XIII this chapter).

H. Generally, alcoholics, in attempting to cope with their environment and their drinking, overuse the defenses of
1. Rationalization (that is, they give "reasons" to explain their drinking).
2. Denial (an inability or unwillingness to be able to admit to themselves that they have a drinking problem).
3. Projection (blaming factors outside of themselves for their drinking).
4. Dissociation.
I. Patterns
1. The patterns of drinking are usually of two types:
   a) Spree or periodic drinkers drink excessively for a period of time, alternating with periods of sobriety. Included in this group are those who plan drinking episodes carefully.
   b) Others are continual drinkers. Such alcoholics sip every day and although never obviously intoxicated, are nearly always under the influence of alcohol. Some alcoholics restrict their drinking to weekends (these are considered as a subtype of continual drinkers).
J. Some authorities divide alcoholism into three types:
1. Essential alcoholism
   Included here are those people who have drifted across the line from social drinking without any other obvious emotional problems. Also known as addictive drinking, compulsive drinking, and alcoholism simplex.
2. Symptomatic alcoholism
   The drinking is a symptom of a serious emotional disorder, such as anxiety disorder, affective disorder, or schizophrenic disorder.
3. Reactive drinking
   The drinking is in response to some particular emotional stress such as the death of a loved one; the alcohol helps the individual "work through" his or her feelings of grief.
K. Sheldon Bacon has given three criteria for determining the presence of alcoholism in individuals.
1. They not only ingest more alcohol, but in different ways from their appropriate associates.
2. So-called problems, especially of an intrapersonal and emotional nature, that are clearly related to the deviant use of alcohol emerge chronically.
3. There is a growing loss of rational, socially mature self-control over the ingestion of alcohol.

VII. Course

The progression into alcoholism often proceeds as follows:

A. The drinking is at first social and masquerades as a companionable or relaxing activity.

B. Then the drinkers turn to alcohol for escape from stress and anxiety and feelings of inadequacy.

C. Later, their self-control diminishes and their need for alcohol increases.

D. As control lessens, their work begins to suffer, and so also does their health, family and social relationships, and all other aspects of their lives.

E. Detection of alcoholism

Four clinical questions, CAGE, have proved useful in diagnosing alcoholism. These are:

1. Have you ever felt you ought to *Cut* down on your drinking?
2. Have people ever *A*nnoyed you by criticizing your drinking?
3. Have you ever felt bad or *G*uilty about your drinking?
4. Have you ever had a drink first thing in the morning to steady your nerves or get rid of a hangover (*E*yeopener)?

VIII. Alcohol-induced organic mental disorders (*DSM*-III-R).

A. Alcohol intoxication

The essential feature of this disorder is maladaptive behavioral changes due to recent ingestion of alcohol. These changes may include aggressiveness, impaired judgment, impaired attention, irritability, euphoria, depression, emotional lability, and other manifestations of impaired social or occupational functioning. Characteristic physiologic signs include slurred speech, incoordination, unsteady gait, nystagmus, and flushed face (*DSM*-III-R).

B. Alcohol idiosyncratic intoxication

This has also been called pathological intoxication. The essential feature of this disorder is a marked behavioral change—usually to aggressiveness—that is due to the recent ingestion of an amount of alcohol insufficient to induce intoxication in most people. There is usually subsequent amnesia for the period of intoxication. The behavior is atypical of the person when not drinking; for example, a shy, retiring, mild-mannered person, after one weak alcoholic drink, may become belligerent and assaultive.

C. Uncomplicated alcohol withdrawal

The essential features of this disorder are certain characteristic symptoms such as a coarse tremor of hands, tongue, or eyelids; nausea or vomiting; malaise or weakness; autonomic hyperactivity (such as tachycardia, sweating, and elevated blood pressure); anxiety, depressed mood, or irritability; transient hallucinations (generally poorly formed) or illusions; headache; and insomnia. These symptoms follow within several hours after cessation of or reduction in alcohol ingestion by a person who has been drinking alcohol for several days or longer.

D. Alcohol withdrawal delirium

The essential feature of this disorder is a delirium—reduced ability to maintain attention to external stimuli, disorganized thinking, as indicated by rambling, irrelevant, or incoherent speech, and at least two of the following: reduced level of consciousness; perceptual disturbances; misinterpretations, illusions, or hallucinations; disturbance of sleep-wake cycles with insomnia or daytime sleepiness; increased or decreased psychomotor activity; disorientation to time, place, or person; memory impairment. It usually develops within one week after a recent cessation of a reduction in alcohol consumption.

E. Alcohol hallucinosis

The essential feature of this disorder is an organic hallucinosis in which vivid and persistent hallucinations develop shortly (usually within 48 hours) after cessation of or reduction in alcohol ingestion by a person who apparently has alcohol dependence. The hallucinations may be auditory or visual. The auditory hallucinations are usually voices and, less commonly, unformed sounds such as hissing or buzzing.

In the majority of cases, the content of the hallucinations is unpleasant or disturbing. However, the hallucinatory content may be benign and leave the person undisturbed. The voices may address the person directly, but more often they discuss him or her in the third person.

F. Alcohol amnestic syndrome

The essential feature of this disorder is an amnestic syndrome (demonstrable evidence of impairment in both short- and long-term memory) apparently due to the vitamin deficiency associated with prolonged, heavy ingestion of alcohol. Alcohol amnestic disorder due to thiamine deficiency is also known as Korsakoff's syndrome.

1. Course

Alcohol amnestic disorder often follows an acute episode of Wernicke's encephalopathy, a neurologic disease manifested by confusion, ataxia, eye-movement abnormalities (gaze palsies, nystagmus), and other neurologic signs.

2. Wernicke's disease

Wernicke's syndrome is a rare disorder of central nervous system metabolism, associated with a thiamine deficiency and seen chiefly in chronic alcoholics. It is characterized by irregular eye movements, incoordination, impaired thinking and, often, sensory-motor deficit. Korsakoff's psychosis, with accompanying confabulation, commonly accompanies Wernicke's syndrome.

G. Dementia associated with alcoholism

The essential feature of this disorder is the development of a dementia, following prolonged and heavy ingestion of alcohol, for which all other causes of dementia have been excluded. In order to exclude transient effects of intoxication and withdrawal, this diagnosis should not be made until at least three weeks have elapsed since cessation of alcohol ingestion.

Features

1. Demonstrable evidence of impairment in short- and long-term memory.
2. At least one of the following:
   a) Impairment in abstract thinking.
   b) Impaired judgment.
   c) Other disturbances of higher cortical function, such as aphasia (disorder of language), apraxia (inability to carry out motor activities despite intact comprehension and motor function), agnosia (failure to recognize or identify objects despite intact sensory function), and "constructional difficulty" (e.g., inability to copy three-dimensional figures, assemble blocks, or arrange sticks in specific designs)
   d) Personality change.
3. The disturbance in 1 and 2 significantly interferes with work or usual social activities or relationships with others.

IX. **Treatment**
A. Treatment of the alcoholic can be considered under two headings:
   1. Treatment of withdrawal and the alcohol organic mental disorders.
   2. Treatment of the underlying personality disorder.
B. Treatment of underlying alcohol organic withdrawal and the organic mental disorder
   1. Treatment of acute alcohol organic mental disorder
      a) Those people who are unable to stop their drinking and have to be withdrawn from alcohol often have to spend time in the hospital or a detoxification center.
      b) Attention must be directed to the alcoholic's nutrition and electrolyte intake, but the use of intravenous fluids is usually not indicated.
      c) Adequate vitamin intake, especially thiamine and niacin, must be provided. These can be administered parenterally or orally, as indicated.
      d) Psychotropic drugs
         Medications are often useful in the management of withdrawal. A number of medications have been used, but perhaps the most commonly employed at the present time is chlordiazepoxide (Librium) in fairly substantial doses for several days; diazepam (Valium) may also be used instead.

If a withdrawal seizure (convulsion) is anticipated, an anticonvulsant such as Dilantin may be added.

e) Corticotropin

Used intramuscularly or intravenously, this drug has been helpful in some cases of acute hallucinosis or delirium tremens.

2. Treatment of the chronic mental disorders secondary to alcoholism

a) Hospitalization is sometimes necessary.

b) Maintenance of intake of fluids, vitamins, and nutrition is important.

c) Various psychotropic drugs may help to relieve certain symptoms. Antidepressants are used to relieve depression; antipsychotic agents are used if there is psychotic behavior.

d) Since the brain damage is irreversible, treatment is only palliative.

C. Treatment of the underlying personality disorder

1. Treatment of the personality disorder underlying the compulsion to drink is usually much more difficult than is hospital management of the acute organic mental disorders, especially since many alcoholics deny that their drinking problem exists and tend to resist intervention. Many alcoholics can be treated as outpatients if they present themselves during a period of sobriety. The physician can use certain medications to assist the patient in coping without alcohol. Most commonly employed drugs used to help the patient through the withdrawal period are chlordiazepoxide (Librium) and diazepam (Valium). These must be used with caution and for only a short period of time because of the possibility of creating dependence on them. Various other psychotropic drugs might be indicated when the physician finds there is another underlying psychiatric disorder.

2. Chemical dependency treatment centers

a) Estimates are that almost 95 percent of the treatment centers in the United States are based, at least loosely, on the "Minnesota model approach": 30-day impatient stay, abstinence, Alcoholics Anonymous-based inpatient treatment.

b) Patients in this program are in an extremely structured environment. They attend lectures and groups and individual counseling sessions all day and in the evenings there is another lecture or AA meeting.

c) Generally, outpatient programs are similar except the patients go home at night.

d) The overall approach, techniques, and methods have remained essentially the same for many years. Patients are provided with information about the disease of alcoholism and are also provided personal and emotional counseling.

e) The harsh confrontational approach once part of the treatment in the early days is no longer popular. In addition, there is a trend toward outpatient care, apparently as a result of younger persons and persons with families and jobs who are seeking treatment.

3. Pharmacological treatment

a) Disulfiram therapy

This is the antabuse treatment. Following its introduction in 1948, this therapy gained wide acceptance, but it, too, seems to have had only limited use in the treatment of alcoholism. The drug, tetraethylthiuram disulfide, when combined with alcohol, produces distressing vasomotor symptoms. No conditioned response is established. This is not an aversion therapy; the unpleasant effects are produced by mixing antabuse and alcohol. Patients must take the antabuse each day; if they stop for several days, they can drink alcohol without the distressing symptoms. Patients who receive this treatment must be in good physical health.

b) Tranquilizing drugs

Various types of psychotropic drugs are sometimes helpful in the management of alcoholism, either for facilitating psychotherapy or for mitigating anxiety or the symptoms of overindulgence. Neuroleptics are also used in the management of acute psychotic conditions related to alcoholic excesses. Among the tranquilizing medications that have been used in alcoholism are chlordiazepoxide (Librium), diazepam (Valium), chlorpromazine (Thorazine), and promazine (Sparine).

c) Aversive therapy

This was once widely used. The aim of treatment is to produce a conditioned response such that the odor or taste of alcohol will immediately lead to nausea and vomiting. The drugs used to set up such a response are emitine and apomorphine, both of which are emetics (agents that induce vomiting). This form of treatment is seldom used now.

4. Dual focus (or dual treatment) programs

In some communities there are special programs for the treatment of people with alcoholism or other substance use disorders, in association with another psychiatric disorder (i.e., schizophrenia, bipolar disorder, or other affective disorders, including depression). Many times these are not AA oriented but more likely to be based on the behavior modification model.

5. Psychotherapy
   a) Any psychotherapeutic approach must operate from the premise that alcoholism is a personality problem and not a moral one.
   b) The ideal treatment goal should be the elimination of the desire to drink, rather than restraint.
   c) It is also important to keep in mind that the alcoholic is usually a dependent person who often has hostile, anxious, and guilty feelings.
   d) Psychotherapy has had only limited success, one reason being that the uncovering of conflicts produces anxiety, whereas the alcoholic has a reduced tolerance for tension.
   e) Certain authorities emphasize the importance of "surrender" versus "submission" in any psychotherapeutic approach; that is, the alcoholics must *accept* the fact that they are alcoholics, and not just admit it.

6. Group therapy
   Group therapy is often useful in the treatment of alcoholics. Sometimes, but not always, such therapy is moderated by a professional person, such as a psychiatrist, clinical psychologist, or social worker.

7. Community resources
   a) Continued care following discharge from the hospital or a chemical dependency unit is crucial. It is true that a "supportive network" is needed by all alcoholics, but it is especially necessary for those who lack close personal relationships. It is also important to keep in mind that the family, or other people affected by the alcoholic's disorder, may also need assistance.
   b) There are many agencies and organizations concerned with this problem.
      (1) The National Institute on Alcohol Abuse and Alcoholism, P.O. Box 2345, Rockville, Maryland (part of the Alcohol, Drug Abuse and Mental Health Administration of the U.S. Department of Health and Human Services). This organization provides funds to encourage the development of programs and makes research grants to investigators and institutions studying the disorder. It also conducts educational programs at the national level and is a source of valuable information for those working in the field.

(2) Most states have a department for alcoholism or substance use disorder.

(3) In many communities there is an alcoholism information center that acts as the coordinator of available resources for the understanding and treatment of alcohol problems.

c) Alcoholics Anonymous (AA) is an informal worldwide fellowship of groups of alcoholics who help each other to stay sober and to remain abstinent. The basic philosophy is based on twelve steps and twelve traditions. The basic source of AA's strength is the relationship with God as the individual understands him. For those who fit well into formal group activity, this approach has proven effective in maintaining sobriety. Of all the available resources, it has easily been the most helpful. However, there are some who cannot accept this approach, particularly those who have difficulty accepting a personal God.

Various attempts have been made to explain why the program has been so useful. Some think the evangelistic theme and religious overtones are important; others view the program as a resocialization process. Most local AA groups have telephone listings and place referral information in the personal columns in the newspapers.

d) Alanon and Alateen are groups that help the "significant others" in the alcoholic's life. They often need help to understand the problem and also to help the recovering alcoholic to maintain his or her health and sobriety. These people are sometimes referred to as "near" or "coalcoholics."

e) Since the decriminalization of drunkenness and the enactment of the Uniform Alcoholism and Intoxication and Treatment Act of 1970, detoxification centers for the treatment of alcoholics have been established in many communities. One significant advantage of such a place is that it is usually tied into the therapeutic network for alcoholics.

f) Many communities have established various types of halfway houses where alcoholics who have no place to live may go to avoid a life-style that is conducive to drinking. Such halfway houses usually have various support groups, including local AA groups.

g) Many churches and religious groups sponsor other active programs. Among them are Calix, a group for Catholic alcoholics, and social agencies such as the Salvation Army. The local mental health association is also a possible source of information.

X. Prevention

A. Very little is known about the prevention of alcoholism, mainly because we know very little of its natural history or distribution of its psychosocial determinants.

B. Alcoholism, like mental illness, has been negatively viewed by the general public. However, in recent years there has been a greater acceptance of alcoholism as a disorder.

C. Alcoholism is one of the four major public health concerns in the United States (the others are mental disorders, cardiovascular disease, and cancer).

D. There is a need to identify and discover cases of alcoholism *early* if we are to make any progress in controlling this disorder. Case findings should be active rather than passive. Many of the community programs, including those in industry, have this orientation.

E. Research in social, psychological, and biological areas is a continuing need.

XI. Case examples

A. Alcoholism with hallucinations

J. P. C., a thirty-eight-year-old single man, was referred to the court's psychiatric consultant for evaluation after he had pleaded guilty to a charge of drunkenness, growing out of an incident in which he was arrested for behaving in a strange manner near a neighbor's apartment building. When questioned by the police who were called, he said he was looking for his sister who was in a tree. He said that he had dropped her child in a culvert and that he had retrieved the baby. He explained that his sister, while changing the baby's diaper, was snatched up into the tree. The man appeared to be intoxicated and admitted to the officers that he had been drinking.

When interviewed by the psychiatric consultant, he admitted that he had been drinking excessively for years. For about a week before his arrest, he was aware that he was "acting screwy," that is, imagining things, but whenever he ceased drinking temporarily, he hallucinated. For example, he recalled that he believed that two men had crawled through the transom of his room at a cheap downtown hotel. This was so real that he phoned the police to complain.

Following his arrest, he experienced other vivid hallucinations. For example, he thought there were cockroaches in his cell and that the jailer was throwing ants into his cell to eat the cockroaches. In addition, he was certain that he had seen his drinking companion in jail with him and he insisted, when he was bailed out by his brother, that the companion was still there (which was not true).

His background history revealed that he had been arrested about twenty times, mostly for drinking, including one arrest for drunken driving and another for petty theft committed while he was drinking. He had been hospitalized on three occasions for his drinking problem. He believed that his drinking had been a serious problem for a least thirteen or fourteen years and said, "It continually gets worse." He had been in Alcoholics Anonymous programs at various times but regarded it as a married man's organization and considered it populated by many people who were not really alcoholics.

In addition, he complained of nervousness, uneasiness, and anxiety, which he said antedated his first drinking. His Minnesota Multiphasic Personality Inventory profile revealed a high level of anxiety and indicated that he was worried, apprehensive, and tense.

He admitted to a very poor employment record over the years because of his drinking problem and had been unemployed for six months prior to his arrest. For approximately a year before that, he had worked as an unskilled laborer.

This case is one of severe, chronic alcoholism in which the person also has symptoms of an anxiety disorder. In addition, he experienced a bout of acute alcoholic hallucinosis, which brought him to the attention of the police. The prognosis is poor.

B. Alcoholism with depression

C. T., a fifty-two-year-old woman, was admitted to the hospital, at the request of her personal physician, for depression and a drinking problem. Her husband, who brought her to the hospital, reported that when he returned home from a business trip, he found his wife drunk and she said she was unable to control her compulsive drinking. Her physician was summoned and arrangements were made for her admission to the hospital.

Her background history revealed that she had always been a passive person and had difficulty with recurrent depressive feelings. She had made two suicide attempts, once with barbiturates, and, on another occasion, with carbon monoxide in her automobile. She had been hospitalized for psychiatric treatment on at least four other occasions.

Prominent among her symptoms while she was in the hospital were social uneasiness and the ease with which she could feel rejected. Feelings of dependency, inferiority, and inadequacy were also evident. She said that for a number of years while she was struggling with her depressed feelings and her compulsion to drink, she blamed her difficulty on her husband. About three or four years earlier, she had finally come to realize that the problem was within her and not the fault of her husband. She had gone to AA meetings a number of times but, because of her passivity, she did not follow through very faithfully.

In this case, alcoholism complicates a recurrent depressive reaction. She was placed on antidepressants and psychotherapy and was referred to a local AA group for supportive help. A follow-up evaluation, six months following her discharge from the hospital, revealed that she had done reasonably well and had had only three minor slips, when she drank a few beers over a one- or two-day period.

References

American Medical Association. *Manual on Alcoholism*. 3d ed. Chicago, 1977.

American Psychiatric Association. *Diagnostic and Statistical Manual of Mental Disorders*. 3d ed, rev. Washington, D.C., 1987.

Bacon, S. D. "The Interrelatedness of Alcoholism and Marital Conflicts." *American Journal of Psychiatry* 24 (1959): 153.

Campbell, R. J. *Psychiatric Dictionary*. 5th ed. New York: Oxford University Press, 1981.

Dupont, R. L. "Substance Abuse." *Journal of the American Medical Association* (1985): 2335–2337.

———. "Substance Abuse." *Journal of the American Medical Association* (1986): 2114–2116.

Goodwin, D. W., and S. B. Guze. *Psychiatric Diagnosis*. 2d ed. New York: Oxford University Press, 1979.

Jellinek, E. M. *The Disease Concept of Alcoholism*. Highland Park, N.J.: Hillhouse Press, 1960.

Keller, M. "The Definition of Alcoholism and the Estimation of Its Prevalence." In *Society, Culture and Drinking Patterns*, edited by D. D. J. Pittman and C. R. Snyder. New York: John Wiley & Sons, 1962.

Kirn, T. F. "Advances in Understanding of Alcoholism Initiate Evolution and Treatment Programs." *Journal of the American Medical Association* (1985): 1405–1412.

World Health Organization, Expert Committee on Alcohol, *First Report*. W. H. O. Technical Report Series, no. 84, Geneva, 1955.

Schuckit, M. A. "Genetics and the Risk for Alcoholism." *Journal of the American Medical Association* (1985): 2614–2617.

Nicotine
Dependence

I. Definition

A. Nicotine withdrawal

The essential feature of this disorder is a characteristic withdrawal syndrome due to the abrupt cessation of or reduction in the use of nicotine-containing substances (e.g., cigarettes, cigars, and pipes, chewing tobacco, or nicotine gum) that has been at least moderate in duration and amount. The syndrome includes craving for nicotine; irritability, frustration, or anger; anxiety; difficulty concentrating; restlessness; decreased heart rate; and increased appetite or weight gain (*DSM*-III-R).

B. Nicotine dependence

The most common form of nicotine dependence is associated with the inhalation of cigarette smoke. Pipe- and cigar-smoking, the use of snuff, and the chewing of tobacco are less likely to lead to nicotine dependence. People with this disorder are often distressed because of their inability to stop nicotine use (*DSM*-III-R).

1. Course

The course of nicotine dependence is variable. Most people repeatedly attempt to give up nicotine use without success.

2. Complications

The most common complications are bronchitis, emphysema, coronary artery disease, peripheral vascular disease, and a variety of cancers.

II. Treatment

A. The most effective treatment programs are those that combine the use of nicotine chewing gum in conjunction with a behavioral program.

B. Nicotine blockade therapy (Mecamylamine): attenuates the effect of nicotine and is safe at doses that affect cigarette smoking. This blockade strategy may prove helpful in a subpopulation of cigarette smokers.

References

American Psychiatric Association. *Diagnostic and Statistical Manual of Mental Disorders*. 3d ed., rev. Washington, D.C., 1987.

Henningfield, J.E. "Pharmacologic Basis and Treatment of Cigarette Smoking." *Journal of Clinical Psychiatry* 45 Golden 12 (December 1984): 24–33.

Hughs, J. R. and D. Hatsukami. "Signs and Symptoms of Tobacco Withdrawal." *ARCH Gen. Psychiatry* 63 (March 1986): 289–94.

Mankind is made up of inconsistencies, and no man acts invariably up to his predominant character.
The wisest man sometimes acts weakly and the weakest sometimes wisely.

Philip Dormer Stanhope, 4th Earl of Chesterfield: *Letters to his Son* **(1748)**

Adjustment Disorders

I. Definition

The essential feature of this disorder is a maladaptive reaction to an identifiable psychosocial stressor, or stressors, that occurs within three months after onset of the stressor, and has persisted for no longer than six months. The maladaptive nature of the reaction is indicated either by impairment in occupational (including school) functionng or in usual social activities or relationships with others or by symptoms that are in excess of a normal and expectable reaction to the stressor. The disturbance is not merely one instance of a pattern of overreaction to stress or an exacerbation of one of the mental disorders. It is assumed that the disturbance will remit soon after the stressor ceases or, if the stressor persists, when a new level of adaptation is achieved. This category should not be used if the disturbance meets the criteria for a specific mental disorder, such as a specific anxiety or mood disorder, or represents uncomplicated bereavement (*DSM*-III-R).

II. Stressors

A. The stressors may be single (e.g., an uncomplicated divorce) or multiple (e.g., marked business difficulties or marital problems). They may be recurrent, as with seasonal business crises, or continuous, as with chronic illness or residence in a deteriorating neighborhood.

B. The severity of the reaction is not completely predictable from the severity of the stressor. People who are particularly vulnerable may have a more severe form of the disorder following only a mild or moderate stressor, whereas others may have only a mild form of the disorder in response to a marked and continuing stressor.

III. Prevalence

A. This disorder is apparently common.

B. It may occur at any age.

IV. Course

By definition, this disorder begins within three months of onset of a stressor and lasts no longer than six months.

V. Types

This disorder may manifest itself in a number of ways; hence there are several different types, according to the predominant symptoms, and include:

A. Adjustment disorder with anxious mood
   This is manifested as symptoms of anxiousness, such as nervousness, worry, and jitteriness.

B. Adjustment disorder with depressed mood
   Predominant manifestation involves depressive symptoms such as depressed mood, tearfulness, and feelings of hopelessness.

C. Adjustment disorder with disturbance of conduct
   This is manifested chiefly in violation of the rights of others or of major age-appropriate societal norms and rules, (e.g., truancy, vandalism, reckless driving, fighting, defaulting on legal responsibilities).

D. Adjustment disorder with mixed disturbances of emotions and conduct
   The predominant manifestations of both emotional symptoms, such as depression or anxiety and a disturbance of conduct, such as those listed under C. above.
E. Adjustment disorder with mixed emotional features
   This disorder shows various combinations of depression and anxiety or other emotions.
F. Adjustment disorder with physical complaints
   The predominant manifestation is physical symptoms for example, fatigue, headache, backache or other aches and pains that are not diagnosable as specific Axis III physical disorder or condition.
G. Adjustment disorder with withdrawal
   The predominant manifestation is social withdrawal without significant depressed or anxious mood.
H. Adjustment disorder with work (or academic) inhibition
   Predominant manifestation here is an inhibition in work or academic functioning, occurring in a person whose previous work or academic performance has been adequate.
I. Adjustment disorder not otherwise specified
   This category is for disorders involving maladaptive reaction to psychosocial stressors that are not classifiable as specific types of adjustment disorder.

VI. Treatment
A. Some believe that because the stressor is clearly identifiable and the condition will have a spontaneous remission that psychotherapy or other kinds of treatment are not indicated.
B. Generally, treatment for disorders in this group is time limited. The goals are to remove the stressor if possible, to relieve symptoms and assist the person in achieving a level of adaptation that existed prior to the stressful event.
C. Psychosocial treatment methods most commonly recommended are:
   1. Individual psychotherapy, specifically, brief psychodynamic therapy focusing on the meaning of the stressful event to the individuals and its possible activation of underlying conflict. Supportive and or expressive psychotherapy may both be appropriate.
   2. Behavior therapy may be helpful.
   3. Group therapy, including self-help groups with others who have undergone similar stresses may be useful.
D. Psychopharmacological treatment
   Generally, psychotropic medications are not used in adjustment disorders because the condition is often self-limited and there is always the possible risk that the person may develop psychological or physical dependency on the agents.

However, in some cases antianxiety agents or perhaps antidepressant agents may be useful for short periods of time to help bring the stress under control, permitting the person to reerect his defenses or develop other means of coping.

VII. Case examples

A. A forty-four-year-old, single, female bank clerk was referred for psychiatric evaluation by her gynecologist because she complained of "depression alternating with nervousness." She described the depression as "heavy feelings associated with sadness" and described the nervousness as "tenseness in her arms, legs, and shoulders." She related that these symptoms had been present for about three months and were related to (1) a stressful work environment, and (2) a stressful living situation. Concerning her job, she reported that she was the oldest of twelve women in a "dead-end job," in an office where she felt "snubbed and ignored" by the younger women. In addition, she felt she had a moody supervisor.

When describing her living situation, she reported that she resided in one-half of a double house, where the family in the adjoining portion of the house had noisy children who disturbed her in the evening when she went home. Thus, she felt under stress both in her workplace and in her home.

She described herself as being shy and extremely sensitive and admitted it was difficult for her to forget hurts.

She always enjoyed good health, although about six months before the onset of her symptoms, she had undergone a hysterectomy for uterine fibroids and endometriosis. She had never experienced any nervous symptoms in the past.

This seemed to be an adjustment disorder with mixed emotional features (with depressed and anxious mood). She elected to explore feelings and the issues in a few psychotherapeutic sessions.

B. A thirty-eight-year-old male management engineer sought evaluation with a psychiatrist because of anxiety and dissatisfaction, which were secondary to divorce proceedings in progress at the time of his initial consultation.

He reported that he had been married fourteen years to a woman of the same age. He described her as a loving, unselfish person, but one who wanted to control. He said, "We were in competition, and without communication and without intimacy." He had decided on the divorce when his wife refused to join him in seeking counseling in an effort to work out their marital relationship.

There was no history of previous mental illness or emotional disturbance of any kind.

This seems to be an example of adjustment disorder with mixed emotional features (with anxious and depressed mood).

He was seeking counseling to aid him in adjusting to his divorce and to assist him in working out a continuing relationship with his two children.

References

American Psychiatric Association. *Diagnostic and Statistical Manual of Mental Disorders.* 3d ed., rev. Washington, D.C., 1987.

Goldman, H. H. *Review of General Psychiatry.* Los Altos, Calif.: Lange Medical Publications, 1984.

Kaplan, H. I., and B. J. Sadock. *Comprehensive Textbook of Psychiatry/ IV.* 4th ed. Baltimore: Williams & Wilkins, 1985.

Hence, loathed melancholy,
Of Cerberus and blackist midnight born,
In Stygian cave forelorn,
'Mongst horrid shapes, and shrieks and sights unholy!

John Milton: *L'Allegro* **(1632)**

Mood Disorders (Affective Disorders)

I. Introduction

   A. The main characteristic is a primary pervasive disturbance in mood.

   B. The affective disorders are characterized by pathologically elevated or depressed mood and should be regarded as existing on a continuum with normal mood. The mood changes, to depression or elation, differ from other mood swings chiefly in degree and duration. The change may occur without apparent cause, seem disproportionate, or persist too long.

   C. Many times the abnormality of activity, affect, and thought appear to have a plausible relationship to the immediate social environment. Any concomitant disturbances in thought or behavior are appropriate to the mood.

   D. Mood disorders, chiefly depression, are the most common disorders seen in outpatient practice. They are the principal disorders associated with suicide.

   E. Generally, when people speak of depression, they are referring to the *emotion* of feeling sad, blue, or unhappy (i.e., dysthymia). When clinicians speak of depression they are usually referring to a *syndrome* or mental disorder of depression consisting of many symptoms and signs, including anorexia, anhedonia, hopelessness, insomnia, and dysthymia.

   F. Much recent research has been concerned with these disorders. Many improvements have been developed in various drug treatments, including the tricyclic antidepressants, monoamine oxidase inhibitors, lithium, and some of the newer classes of antidepressant medication (for details, see the chapter, "Treatment in Psychiatry: Pharmacological and Somatic Treatment").

II. Terms (or, terminology)

   IN *DSM*-III-R, the following terms are used in the classification of mood disorders.

   A. *Mood syndrome* (depressive or manic) is a group of mood and associated symptoms that occur together for a minimal period of time. (For example, major depressive syndrome is defined as a depressed mood or loss of interest of at least two weeks' duration accompanied by several associated symptoms, such as weight loss and difficulty concentrating.) Mood syndromes can occur as part of a mood disorder, as part of a nonmood psychotic disorder (for example, schizoaffective disorder, or as part of an organic mental disorder, for example, organic mood disorder).

   B. *Mood episode* (Major depressive, manic, or hypomanic) is a mood syndrome that is not due to a known organic factor and is not part of a nonmood psychotic disorder (e.g., schizophrenia, schizoaffective disorder, or delusional disorder). For example, a major depressive episode is a major depressive syndrome (as defined above) in which it cannot be established that an organic factor initiated and maintained the disturbance, and the presence of a nonmood psychotic disorder has been ruled out.

C. *Mood disorder* is determined by the pattern of mood episodes. For example, the diagnosis of major depression is made when there have been one or more major depressive episodes without a history of a manic or unequivocal hypomanic episode.

III. Classification of mood disorder

A. Cases of mood disorder really fall along a continuum varying from mild, short-lived, subclinical depressions and elations on one end, to severe delusional depressions and delirious manias on the other.

B. In *DSM*-III-R the mood disorders are classified as follows:

1. Bipolar disorders

   The essential feature is the presence of one or more manic or hypomanic episodes (usually with a history of major depressive episodes). There are two bipolar disorders.

   a) Bipolar disorder, in which there is one or more manic episodes (usually with one or more major depressive episodes).

   b) Cyclothymia, in which there are numerous hypomanic episodes and numerous periods with depressive symptoms.

   c) "Bipolar II" disorders with hypomanic and full major depressive episodes are included in the residual category of bipolar disorder NOS.

2. Depressive disorders

   a) Major depression, in which there is one or more major depressive episodes.

   b) Dysthymia, in which there is a history of a depressive mood more days than not for at least two years and in which during the first two years of the disturbance the condition did not meet the criteria for a major depressive episode. In many cases of dysthymia, there are superimposed major depressions (*DSM*-III-R).

IV. Degrees of depression

A. A depression is a normal human emotion. Such "normal" depression is characterized by feelings of sadness, disappointment, despair, frustration, or unhappiness. It is a universally experienced emotion and is not considered abnormal.

B. Grief (uncomplicated bereavement)

   Bereavement is a normal, appropriate, affective sadness in response to a recognizable external loss. It is realistic and appropriate to what has been lost; it is self-limiting and gradually subsides. It seldom leads to serious disorder in one's personal life.

The reaction to the loss may not be immediate, but rarely occurs after the first two or three months. The duration of "normal" bereavement varies considerably among different cultural groups (*DSM*-III-R).

C. Major depressive disorder

The etiological factor is less obvious than normal grief or the depression is more severe or persists unduly long. The situation that occasions the reaction is often more of a precipitating event than a causal factor. The individual usually realizes that the response is excessive but does not recognize the underlying cause.

Depression can range from mild to profound in which the patient may lose contact with reality, develop delusions, and may be of serious suicidal risk. Such a person is often said to be psychotic.

V. **Descriptive types of depression**

A. Aside from the official diagnostic classification of the various depressive disorders, certain clinical types of depression are often described.

B. It should be kept in mind that depression is really a syndrome and that modern researchers suggest multiple etiologies (a spectrum disorder).

C. Symptom complex (subtypes)

Among the descriptive subtypes that have been described are the following:

1. Primary-secondary affective disorders
   a) *Primary affective disorders* are those that occur in persons who have never had an episode before or whose only previous psychiatric illnesses were episodes of depression or mania.
   b) *Secondary affective disorders* occur in persons who have had other psychiatric illnesses (e.g., schizophrenia or alcoholism) or who have suffered an affective disorder related to a medical condition.

2. Bipolar-unipolar dichotomy
   a) The *bipolar* group consists of patients who have had both depressive and manic episodes.
   b) The *unipolar* group consists of those who have only had depressive episodes.
   c) Genetic studies indicate that persons with a bipolar affective disorder have families with a greater frequency of a similar illness and are more likely to develop hypomanic responses to administration of the tricyclic antidepressants.

3. The psychotic-neurotic dichotomy
   a) This distinction has lost its importance in recent years.
   b) The frequency of depressions of psychotic proportions has greatly decreased in recent years. Perhaps this is in part accounted for by the fact that people with signs of depression receive early treatment; hence, the fully developed psychotic syndromes described in the past do not occur. More recent use of the term psychotic has become synonymous with severe impairment of social and personal functioning. But even using this criteria, psychotic depressions are relatively infrequent in current clinical practice.
4. Endogenous-reactive dichotomy
   a) This subdivision of depression is based on whether or not the depression seemed to develop "from within" (endogenous) or was related to life events (reactive).
   b) Those who have endogenous depressions usually show a central group of symptoms including psychomotor retardation, early morning awakening (terminal insomnia), weight loss, guilt, and unreactivity. It is more likely to occur in older patients, and people with endogenous depressions show more stable nonneurotic premorbid personality.
   c) Those with reactive depression show a correlation with light stress.
   d) Recent studies suggest that a valid definition of endogenous depression is one in which the endogenous group is characterized by the following:
      (1) A greater family history of depression
      (2) A lower family history of alcoholism
      (3) A lower family history of antisocial personality
      (4) Older age
      (5) Higher scores on symptom severity indexes
      (6) Less frequent, nonserious suicide attempts
      (7) A lower prevalence of divorce or marital separations
      (8) Fewer life events
      (9) Less premorbid personality disorders
      (10) Better social support
      (11) Less cognitive distortion
      (12) A higher frequency of neuroendocrine or other biologic abnormalities
      (13) A better response to somatic therapy
      (14) A poorer response to psychotherapy

5. Agitated-retarded dichotomy

This subdivision is based on whether or not the symptoms include

a) Uneasiness, mental perturbation, and motor restlessness (agitation).

b) Slowing down of mental and physical activity (retardation).

6. Early versus late onset

This includes, "pure" versus "spectrum" depression, involutional depression, chronic characterological depression, and hysteroid dysphoria.

D. Life events and stress as precipitating factors

1. Not all persons who experience loss and separation subsequently develop depression.

2. Loss and separation are demonstrable in only about a quarter of people with depressions.

3. Loss and separation may precipitate a wide variety of psychiatric conditions.

4. Predisposing factors, as well as precipitating factors, must be taken into account. Genetic factors (e.g., in the bipolar affective disorder) or early life experiences may render the individual sensitive to losses or separations.

E. Melancholia

1. This is a term used since ancient times to refer to a severe form of depression.

2. In *DSM*-III-R, the term major depressive episode, melancholic type, refers to a severe depression that includes anhedonia (loss of pleasure), lack of reactivity to usually pleasurable stimuli, depression regularly worse in the morning, early morning awakening (terminal insomnia), psychomotor retardation or agitation, significant anorexia, weight loss, no significant personality disturbance before the first major depressive episode, one or more previous major depression episodes followed by complete or nearly complete recovery and previous good response to specific and adequate somatic antidepressive therapy.

3. Involutional melancholia

a) The term *involutional melancholia* was used to describe a depression of initial onset occuring during the involutional years (40–55 in women and 50–65 in men), with symptoms of marked anxiety, agitation, restlessness, somatic concerns, hypochondriasis, occasional somatic or nihilistic delusions, insomnia, anorexia and weight loss (Brown et al. 1984).

b) This disorder characteristically occurred in an obsessive-compulsive personality (narrow range of interests, difficulty adjusting to change, limited capacity for sociability and friendship, rigid adherence to a strict ethical code, etc.).

c) Such patients who experience the first depressive episode in the involutional period have more somatic symptoms and hypochondriasis.

d) This diagnosis was excluded in *DSM*-III and *DSM*-III-R and a recent study (Brown et al. 1984) does not support the clinical picture of the previous outlined involutional melancholia. However, even if involutional melancholia does not stand as a separate entity, it may be useful to recognize that elderly patients may present a somewhat different clinical picture from that of their younger counterparts (Brown et al. 1984).

F. Seasonal affective disorder (SAD)

This term is new in *DSM*-III-R. Diagnostic criteria for seasonal pattern are: a regular temporal relationship between the onset of an episode of bipolar disorder or recurrent major depression and a particular sixty-day period of the year; full remission or change from depression to mania or hypomania also occurred within a particular sixty-day period of the year; there have been at least three episodes of mood disturbance three separate years that demonstrated the temporal seasonal relationship; seasonal episodes of mood disturbance outnumbered any nonseasonal episodes of such disturbance that may have occurred by more than three to one (*DSM*-III-R).

G. Atypical depression

This term originally referred to a depressive syndrome responsive to a monoamine oxidase inhibitor (MAOI). It does not really describe a discrete or homogeneous group of patients. Rather, it describes a variety of nonendogenously depressed patients. Some reports have emphasized the importance of atypical neurovegetative signs (e.g., increased sleep and increased appetite); however, others have stressed the coexistence of anxiety symptoms, generalized or phobic anxiety or panic disorder; and others described atypical depression as being nonendogenous or neurotic depression. Atypical depression has a chronic course if there's no treatment intervention. Although MAOI antidepressants are considered to be specific for this condition, tricyclic antidepressants are now considered useful. (The MAOIs seem to have a special efficacy for atypical depression with prominent anxiety or panic attacks.) Atypical depression is not an official *DSM*-III-R diagnosis.

VI. Suicide

A. Introduction
1. Since the possibility of suicide is frequently raised by depressive disorders of all types, it is considered here.
2. However, it should be kept in mind that suicide is not exclusively limited to people with such diagnoses. Nearly everyone has had death wishes and suicidal thoughts but only the suicidal ruminate about them.
3. The number of suicidal attempts is much smaller than the number of people who have contemplated suicide, and the percentage of successful suicides is even smaller. It is variously estimated that attempts are five to fifty times more common than successes (the most common estimate seems to be ten attempts for every successful suicide).

B. Prevalence
1. Suicide is the tenth major cause of death in the United States (officially 50,000 people kill themselves each year; however, an estimate of 100,000 would probably be a more realistic figure). These figures do not include unconsciously motivated "fatal accidents" or numerous other self-destructive behaviors, such as alcoholism. Among white males, aged fifteen to nineteen, it is the second major cause of death.
2. Throughout the world, the annual number of suicides is equivalent to the population of Edinburgh, Scotland, and the number of people who try to kill themselves each year is equal to the population of London or Los Angeles.
3. There is an increase in the suicide rate for succeeding generations; the later the generation one is in, the more likely he or she will die from suicide.
4. Some studies indicate that it is rare for people to make more than one suicide attempt.
5. Although more attempts are made by women in the United States, more men are successful. (Completed suicides are twice as high for men, although attempted suicides are twice as high for women.)
6. Sociocultural influences
   a) Suicide is less common in Catholic countries, such as Ireland, and more common in Japan, Germany, Denmark, and Switzerland.
   b) Cultural attitudes toward suicide, death, and afterlife seem to play a role.
7. Suicide prevention centers have apparently not affected the suicide rate.

C. Psychodynamic factors
   1. Most authorities believe that suicide rarely results from a single cause. Several factors may be operant in a cumulative way.
   2. Any serious loss may be a possible etiological factor (e.g., loss of a loved one, a job, money, health, beauty, independence).
   3. The anniversary of an important event (e.g., the death of a loved one) may initiate a suicide attempt.
   4. Karl Menninger regarded suicide as self-murder. In *Man against Himself,* he also described other self-destructive behavior that stops short of suicide (invalidism, alcoholism, self-mutilation, and accident proneness).
   5. Beck was not able to substantiate the earlier dynamic formulation of internalized aggression.
   6. Schneidman and Faberow (1961) have classified people who commit suicide into four general groups:
      a) Those who view suicide as a means to a better life or as a means of saving reputation
      b) Those who are psychotic and commit suicide in response to delusions or hallucinations
      c) Those who commit suicide as revenge against a loved person
      d) Elderly and infirm people who use suicide as a release from pain
   7. What prods a person from contemplation to action is not really known.
   8. Some authorities feel that suicide attempts are motivated by
      a) A wish for revenge
      b) Feelings of hopelessness
      c) Fantasies of reunion (anniversary suicide)
      d) Thus, suicide contains a wish to kill as well as a wish to die. Hostility toward rejecting persons, presumed or actual, may motivate individuals to attempt to kill themselves and thus make the rejecting person feel guilty.
D. Danger signs
   1. History of previous suicide attempts or threats
   2. Suicide note
   3. Psychotic reactions with suspiciousnes, paranoid delusions, or panic
   4. Chronic illness (especially the attitude toward the illness)
   5. Alcoholism or drug dependency
   6. Advancing age, especially in men
   7. Recent surgery or childbirth
   8. Hypochondriasis
   9. Unaccepted homosexuality

E. Evaluation of suicidal risks

Most suicidal patients will admit their intentions to a physician. When estimating the possibility that a person will attempt suicide, the following questions are helpful.

1. Have you thought of suicide?
2. Have you thought of what way you would take your life?
3. Have you already made preparations?
4. Do you trust yourself?

VII. **Symptoms of affective disorders**

A. Depression

1. The chief clinical complaints of patients with depression are psychological.

a) The mood is either depressed or possibly, in children or adolescence, irritable; or loss of interest or pleasure in almost all activities. The person will usually describe feeling sad, hopeless, discouraged, "down in the dumps," or some other colloquial equivalent.

(1) The vast majority of depressed patients complain of this.

(2) Behavior is consistent with the verbally expressed depression. But sometimes the presence of the depressed mood can be inferred from the person's sad or depressed appearance.

(3) A small number of patients do not spontaneously complain of depression, but the disorder is manifested as two other symptom complexes. Such covert depression may appear as

(a) Chiefly hypochondriacal symptoms

(b) Neurasthenic symptoms of exhaustion, fatigue, or weakness

(4) A few cases are "smiling depression."

(5) Pleasurelessness (anhedonia) or loss of interest is often present. Previous interests no longer gratify the patient. A depressed person may not complain of this but it will be manifested to family members and friends as his withdrawal from socializations and neglect of avocations.

(6) Adolescents often show negativistic or "acting-out" behavior. These are sometimes referred to as "behavioral correlates" and include running away from home, school problems, vandalism, verbal assaultiveness, physical assaultiveness, petty theft, major theft, forgery, dealing in illicit drugs, property break-ins, sexual promiscuity, extortion, lying, gambling, court

involvement, teasing, taunting or abusing domestic animals, sadistic actions, masochistic actions, fire setting, assault with weapon, substance abuse, and so forth.

(7) Elderly patients often show symptoms of impaired memory and disorientation (not due to organic factors and termed "pseudodementia"); an exaggerated indifference to one's surroundings without actual mental impairment.

b) Anorexia

Most depressed patients suffer loss of appetite and often lose weight. A small number, usually adolescents, have increased appetite (bulimia).

"Atypical" depressed patients exhibit hyperphagia.

c) Insomnia

Most patients experience some type of sleep disturbance. This may involve difficulty falling asleep (initial insomnia), difficulty remaining asleep (middle insomnia), or early morning awakening (terminal insomnia). A few, usually adolescents, sleep excessively (hypersomnia). It may be manifest as sleeping for longer periods of time than usual, daytime sleepiness, or taking excessive naps. Patients with "atypical" depression also have hypersomnia. Sometimes a sleep disturbance, rather than a depressed mood or anhedonia, is the main symptom.

d) Psychomotor retardation or psychomotor agitation

Depressive patients may appear retarded or agitated.

(1) Retarded depressions are manifested by decreased activity.

(a) Slowed speech, increased pauses before answering, soft or monotonous speech, and verbal frugality

(b) Inactivity: slowed body movements. In stuporous depression, the patient may be mute, immobile, and severely regressed.

(2) Agitated depressions are manifested by increased psychomotor activity.

(a) Restlessness, inability to sit still, jitteriness, pacing, handwringing, pulling or rubbing hair, skin or clothing

(b) Difficulty in concentration—the patients report that thinking is slowed down or that their minds are blank, and they often complain of loss of memory.

e) Sense of worthlessness

This may vary from lowered self-esteem with accompanying feelings of inadequacy and incompetence and poor self-concept, or the patient may reproach himself/herself for underlying feelings that are exaggerated, or this guilt may be expressed as an excessive reaction to either current or past feelings, or, a sense of worthlessness or guilt may be of delusional proportions (*DSM*-III-R).

f) Difficulty in concentrating, slowed thinking, and indecisiveness are frequent. The patient may complain of memory difficulties; this is more a function of inability to concentrate because of the depressed affect.

g) Thoughts of death (not just the fear of dying) are common. Many times the person feels that he or she may be better off dead. There may be suicidal thoughts with or without a specific plan or suicidal attempts.

2. Associated features

a) Anxiety, irritability, or obsessive rumination may occur.

b) When hallucinations are present their content is usually consistent with a predominant mood (mood congruent). Less commonly the hallucinations or delusions are unrelated to the mood disturbance (mood incongruent).

3. Somatic symptoms

a) These may be manifested as a mild physiological response of any body system, hypochondriacal preoccupation, definite physical symptoms, or somatic delusions.

b) Often it is the somatic symptom that first concerns the patients and leads them to seek medical examination. This is especially true of elderly depressed patients.

c) Thus, depressed persons may complain of any one of a variety of physical complaints, such as headache, cramps, nausea, constipation, or indigestion.

4. Depression as a syndrome

a) A depressed patient usually has a constellation of the above-mentioned symptoms, but does not manifest all of them.

b) Thus, we may speak of three depressive syndromes:

(1) Ideational depressions (depressed mental content and few if any physical or motor symptoms)

(2) Retarded depressions

(3) Agitated depressions

B. Mania

1. Generally, the essential feature of a manic episode is an elevated euphoric, expansive, or irritable mood. Associated symptoms include inflated self-esteem or grandiosity (which may be delusional), decreased need for sleep, pressure of speech, flight of ideas, distractibility, increased involvement in goal-directed

activity, psychomotor agitation and excessive involvement in pleasurable activities that have a high potential for painful consequences that the person often does not recognize (*DSM*-III-R). This diagnosis is made only if it cannot be established that an organic factor initiated and maintained the disturbance (*DSM*-III-R).

2. In addition, other symptoms may be prominent.
   a) Inflated self-esteem or grandiosity
   b) Decreased need for sleep
   c) Loquaciousness or pressure of speech
   d) Flight of ideas or racing thoughts
   e) Distractibility
   f) Increase in goal-directed activity (in one of several areas, socially, work or school, or sexually) or psychomotor agitation
   g) Excessive involvement in pleasurable activities that have a high potential for painful consequences (e.g., unrestrained buying sprees, foolish business investments, or sexual indiscretions).

3. Absence of organic factor that might initiate a manic episode (toxic or metabolic factors).

VIII. Course
A. Depression
   1. Depressive episodes
      a) The onset is variable, with symptoms developing over a period of a few days to weeks.
      b) Many depressive episodes are self-limiting and remit without specific treatment.
      c) With treatment, the duration of episodes has been reduced from several months to a few weeks.
      d) It is estimated that at least half of the individuals with a major depressive episode will eventually have another one.
      e) It should be kept in mind in dealing with depressive people that one can usually be optimistic that the depression will remit.
   2. Chronic depression
      a) About 15 percent of depressive disorders run a chronic course.
      b) The patients continue to experience depressed mood, sleep disturbances, and various bodily symptoms.
B. Manic episodes (or elations)
   1. Most patients with manic episodes also have depressions.
   2. Before the advent of the psychotropic drugs (neuroleptic agents, antianxiety agents, lithium) and electroconvulsive therapy, the episodes were usually longer.
   3. Manic episodes are frequently recurrent.

4. Before the introduction of lithium, only about 25 percent of manic patients had a single episode.
5. The prophylactic administration of lithium therapy often prevents further attacks.

C. Diagnostic categories
   1. Depressive disorders
      a) Major depression, recurrent or major depression, single episode. The essential feature is one or more major depressive episodes without a history of either a manic episode or unequivocal hypomanic episode (unipolar depression).
         (1) Although some people have a single episode, estimates are that over 50 percent will eventually have another major depressive episode (major depression, recurrent).
         (2) People with the recurrent type of the illness are more likely to develop bipolar disorder (see later).
         (3) The course of recurrent depression varies from episodes separated by many years of normal functioning, or those having "clusters of episodes," and others who have increasingly frequent episodes as they grow older.
      b) Dysthymia (or depressive neurosis)
         (1) Central feature is the chronic disturbance of mood involving depressed mood (or possibly an irritable mood in children or adolescents), for most of the day more days than not, for at least two years (one year for children and adolescents).
         (2) The following associated symptoms may be present (*DSM*-III-R):
            (a) Poor appetite or overeating
            (b) Insomnia or hypersomnia
            (c) Low energy or fatigue
            (d) Low self-esteem
            (e) Poor concentration or difficulty making decisions
            (f) Feelings of hopelessness
         (3) Other predisposing factors
             Chronic, nonmood Axis I or Axis III disorder (e.g., anorexia nervosa, somatization disorder, psychoactive substance dependence, rheumatoid arthritis). Such cases are referred to as secondary types. Cases unrelated to any preexisting condition are called primary types.
         (4) There are no clear boundaries between dysthymia and major depression.
         (5) This disorder often begins in early life and hence is referred to as a depressive personality.

2. Bipolar disorder (mixed; manic; depressed)
The essential feature is one or more manic episodes usually accompanied by one or more major depressive episodes.
    a) Course
        (1) Manic episode is usually the initial episode that leads to hospitalization.
        (2) Often a manic or depressive episode is followed immediately by a short episode of the opposite kind ("rapid cycling").
        (3) Cases of bipolar with mixed or rapid-cycling episodes are much more often chronic.
        (4) Familial pattern: occurs at a much higher rate in first-degree biological relatives of people with bipolar than in the general population.
    b) Prevalence
    0.4 percent to 1.2 percent of the adult population.
    c) Sex ratio
    Equally common in males and females (unlike major depression, which is more common in females).
    d) Both manic and depressive episodes may be intermixed or rapidly alternate every few days (mixed bipolar disorder).
3. Cyclothymia
This is a chronic mood disturbance of at least two years' duration (one year for children and adolescents), involving hypomanic episodes and numerous periods of depressed mood or loss of interest or pleasure of insufficient severity or duration to meet the criteria for major depressive or a manic episode. The boundaries between this disorder and bipolar are not well defined. Some consider cyclothymia a mild form of bipolar disorder.
    a) Course
    Usually a chronic course without clear onset. Oftentimes the person develops bipolar disorder.
    b) Prevalence
    0.4 percent to 3.5 percent.
    c) Sex ratio
    Equally common in males and females.
    d) Onset
    Usually begins in adolescence or early adult life.

IX. **Prevalence**
    A. Depression is a very common symptom. It is at least ten times as prevalent as schizophrenia. Severe depression affects fully 2 percent to 3 percent of the world's population—some 100 million individuals—and recent figures indicate that this figure is probably an understatement.

B. In the United States alone, some 10 to 14 million people are estimated to be afflicted by moderate or severe depression. Other estimates are that 15 percent of Americans experience depressive episodes.

C. Its "ripple effect" extends in varying degress to family members, friends, and work associates.

D. For every severely or moderately depressed person who has been diagnosed as such, there are many more ill who have not been diagnosed or treated.

E. Depression occurs two to four times more frequently in women than in men. As noted earlier, bipolar disorder afflicts both sexes equally.

F. In the past, it was thought that manic-depressive disease was a disorder of the upper-middle and the upper classes, but subsequent investigators have found no relationship between social class and bipolar affective disorders.

X. Etiology

Any consideration of the etiology of affective disorders must take into account genetic and biological factors, environmental stress and life events, psychodynamic factors, and social factors.

A. Genetic factors

1. There is an increased frequency of affective illness, particularly bipolar affective illness or disorder, in the relatives of affectively disordered patients. Generally, these studies indicate that families with histories of unipolar illness are at risk for unipolar disease, and families with histories of bipolar disorder are more at risk for bipolar disorders.

2. Studies show a concordance of 72 percent for monozygotic (identical) twins and 14 percent for dizygotic twins in the incidence of manic-depressive disorder.

3. Depression also occurs in families and studies indicate that relatives are also at greater risk for other types of disorders: alcoholism, panic disorders, and phobias (suggesting that these disorders belong to the same "genetic cluster" or "depressive spectrum").

4. Studies also support the use of a bipolar-unipolar classification.

B. Biological factors

Certain biological factors, other than genetic, seem to be important.

1. Catecholamine hypothesis

According to this theory, a deficiency of norepinephrine leads to depression, and overactivity of norepinephrine leads to mania (this theory is incomplete for mania).

2. The biogenic amine permissive hypothesis holds that a functional underactivity of serotonin is necessary for every affective disorder. But the level of norepinephrine determines whether elation or depression exists.

3. The adrenergic-cholinergic imbalance hypothesis maintains that the ratio of acetylcholine to catecholamines in the brain is low in mania and high in depression.
4. The electrolyte-membrane potential disturbance theory asserts that depression is accounted for in part by an accumulation of intracellular sodium.

C. Environmental stress and life events
1. Most clinical psychiatrists believe there is a relationship between the onset of depression and environmental stress. Some believe that such events play the major role.
2. Some recent research confirms a relationship between stressful environmental factors (e.g., death or losses) and the onset of depression.

D. Psychodynamic factors
1. In the past, it was believed that the dependent person with a low self-esteem and a strong superego was more prone to depression. Subsequent clinical findings have not supported the existence of a single personality type or constellation of personality traits.
2. In the past, it was assumed that hostility turned inward was important in the development of the depression. Although this dynamic formulation enjoys wide clinical acceptance, research does not support it.
3. Some regard mania as a "running away from" depression.
4. At present, the psychodynamic hypotheses are chiefly of empirical value, assisting the therapist to formulate a therapeutic program.
5. From a pragmatic viewpoint, it is perhaps useful to regard the major affective disorders as genetically determined ones, but that specific psychodynamic factors interpreted as "loss" can act as precipitants of episodes of mania or depression. However, once started, the episode does not respond to interpretation and thus the person usually requires treatment with medication or electroconvulsive therapy. However, once the episode is controlled with appropriate medication or ECT, psychotherapy may be helpful in dealing with the secondary consequences of the illness and will foster avoidance of precipitants or help the individual cope with contributing underlying psychological problems.
6. Most psychosocial theories of depression involve loss of self-esteem. This loss can also trigger mania. It should be remembered that successful events may also trigger depression (e.g., "promotion depression").

XI. Treatment

A. Depression

There are many effective treatments for the depressive disorders, including drugs, various psychotherapy modalities, and electroconvulsive therapy. A pluralistic approach seems indicated.

1. Pharmacological therapy

   a) Although direct stimulants, primarily the amphetamines, were used by physicians for the treatment of depression for many years, the modern pharmacological treatment of depression dates back to the early 1950s, when the tricyclic antidepressants and the monamine oxidase inhibitors were introduced.

   b) Of the three types of antidepressant agents available—direct stimulants, the monoamine oxidase inhibitors (MAOI), and the tricyclic antidepressants—the last are by far the most commonly employed. Generally, they are effective and act by blocking the neuronal uptake of amines into the presynaptic nerve endings. MAOI antidepressants are drugs of choice for treating atypical depression (especially with panic attacks).

   c) Recently, some different classes of antidepressants have been introduced and are gaining popularity. Among these are amoxapine (Asendin), maprotiline HCL (Ludiomil), trimipramine maleate (Surmontil), trazodone HCI (Desyrel) and most recently, fluoxetine hydrochloride (Prozac)—a blocker of serotonin uptake. Generally, the effectiveness of these is similar to the effectiveness of tricyclics and it is the side effect profiles that often determine which drug is prescribed.

   d) Sedatives and antianxiety agents (generally, benzodiazepines) are prescribed for coexisting symptoms of anxiety and tension.

   e) Neuroleptics (e.g., the phenothiazines, thioxanthenes, butyrophenones) are also used if psychotic symptoms are present. They are sometimes helpful in treating depressed people with agitation.

2. Electroconvulsive therapy

   Remission rates with this treatment are 85 percent plus (in contrast to 70 percent plus with tricyclic antidepressants), although it is much less frequently prescribed since the advent of the antidepressant medications.

3. Psychotherapy

   a) A number of treatment modalities may be used with acutely depressed patients. Most respond to some type of supportive treatment (for details, see the chapter, "Treatment in Psychiatry: Psychotherapy").

b) Most important in the psychotherapeutic management of the acute depressive episode is that the therapist be available and active.

c) A word of caution: advice should be used very sparingly. One usually does not know all the nuances of the situation under consideration, and further, the depressed individual does not want advice, but rather someone to listen with respect, understanding, and without criticism.

d) Frequently depressed patients present themselves as markedly dependent. This is a feeling that must be handled delicately because they frequently are ambivalent about such strivings. (As one author has said: "Dispense hope, not saccharin.")[1] Also, it should be remembered that most depressions remit (the advantage of treatment is that it shortens the periods of depression).

e) Appropriate and prompt attention should be paid to suicidal issues. Sometimes hospitalization may be necessary not so much because of the actual suicidal potential but more because the depressed person has no networks of supportiveness.

4. Hospitalization
   a) Most depressed patients can be treated outside of the hospital.
   b) Patients with severe depressions, suicidal urges, or medical conditions that require extensive evaluations should probably be hospitalized.
   c) With modern treatment approaches, the average stay is less than a month.

5. Clinical treatment
   In clinical practice, most patients are treated with a combination of psychotherapy and medication.

6. Maintenance therapy
   For those with recurrent episodes or chronic symptoms, maintenance therapy consisting of antidepressants or other neuroleptics, as appropriate, plus supportive psychotherapy seems to be effective. Lithium is often used (see treatment of mania, below).

7. Dexamethasone Suppresion Test (DST)
   Recent studies have suggested some clinical value to the use of this test. It is theorized that in normal individuals the administration of dexamethasone suppresses cortisol secretion (from the hypothalamus). In some depressed patients, dexamethasone often does not suppress cortisol secretion. It is usually considered that patients with *endogenous* types of depression fail

1. J. S. Maxmen, *Essential Psychopathology* (New York: W. W. Norton and Co., 1986).

to suppress their cortisol after their DST. A positive DST is also found in nondepressed patients and a negative DST in depressed ones. Generally this test lacks sufficient sensitivity and specificity for a place in the *routine* assessment of depression.

B. Mania

    1. Persons with hypomania, or mild elations, can often be treated as outpatients.

    2. Hospitalization is indicated for patients who are acutely manic. Aside from specific treatment for the episodes, patients need to be protected from the social consequences of their expansive behavior and poor judgment.

    3. Pharmacological therapy

        a) Lithium carbonate shortens periods of elation and helps prevent attacks of either depression or elation when administered as part of a maintenance program. (Lithium citrate as a liquid may be prescribed for people who have difficulty swallowing tablets or for whom there is some suspicion they may be "cheeking" their lithium.)

        b) Neuroleptics, especially the phenothiazines, thioxanthenes and the butyrophenones are effective in controlling the maniacal symptoms. In clinical practice, since it usually takes several days for lithium to become effective, lithium and phenothiazines, (e.g., Thorazine or Mellaril) or a butyrophenone (e.g., Haldol) or, Thiothixine (e.g., Navane) are prescribed simultaneously. When the elation comes under control, the phenothiazine or butyrophenone is gradually withdrawn.

    4. Occasionally, when the episode does not respond to drugs, electroconvulsive therapy is prescribed.

C. Bipolar disorders

    1. The goal is to prevent recurrences of acute episodes, relieve chronic low-grade disturbing symptoms, and improve the patient's adjustment.

    2. The most effective clinical approach seems to be combined drug therapy and psychotherapy.

    3. Pharmacological therapy

        a) Lithium carbonate, other neuroleptic drugs, and supportive psychodynamic psychotherapy are often combined.

        b) Antidepressants must be administered judiciously to people who have manic episodes, since it is possible to precipitate an elation in the course of long-term maintenance therapy.

        c) Some recent studies indicate that the combining of lithium with either Tegretol or Verapamil is useful in the management of "rapid-cycling" bipolar disorder.

4. Occasionally, electroconvulsive therapy is used on a maintenance basis to prevent relapses. Such treatment is given at intervals of four, six, or eight weeks for several months or years. It has proved effective in some cases that have not responded to direct maintenance alone.

XII. Organic mood syndrome

A. In *DSM*-III-R, a separate category is listed for mood disturbances due to specific organic factors.
B. The essential feature is a prominent and persistent depressed, elevated, or expansive mood, resembling either a manic episode or a major depressive episode, which is due to a specific organic factor.
C. The clinical phenomenology of this syndrome is similar to that of manic or major depressive episode described earlier in this chapter.
D. Etiology

This is usually caused by toxic or metabolic factors (e.g., reserpine, methyldopa, and some of the hallucinogens are apt to cause a depressive syndrome). Certain endocrine disorders, such as hyper- and hypothyroidism and hyper- and hypoadrenocorticalism, may produce either depressive or manic episodes. Carcinoma of the pancreas is sometimes associated with depression (possibly due to neuro peptides in the gastrointestinal tract that are identical to those found in the brain). Viral illness may also cause a depressive illness. Structural disease of the brain, such as may result from hemispheric strokes, is a common cause of organic mood syndrome.

XIII. Case examples

A. Major depressive disorder, single episode

Mrs. S., a thirty-five-year-old housewife, was admitted to the hospital complaining of nausea, vomiting, crying, and depression. Her symptoms had begun four months earlier, following an incident that should have made her feel hostile toward her husband. However, because of guilt related to an extramarital affair a few years earlier, she was unable to express her hostile feelings and these became redirected against herself and produced the depressive symptoms.

On admission, she appeared depressed and cried rather easily when discussng her illness and her husband. There was no obvious psychomotor retardation, but she did complain of some difficulty in concentration. In the hospital, she ate poorly and had difficulty sleeping. She responded promptly to treatment and has remained free of symptoms for several years.

This patient had a single depressive episode, with symptoms common to most depression, namely, depressed mood, difficulty in concentration, disturbance of appetite and sleep, and somatic symptoms.

B. Major depressive disorder, recurrent

Mr. N., a fifty-five-year-old accountant, was admitted to the hospital with a severe depression, which had begun following the accidental injury of his son nine months earlier. He showed marked psychomotor retardation, refused to eat, and was mute most of the time. When he did speak, he expressed delusions of worthlessness, hopelessness, and nihilism. His history revealed three previous episodes of depression, beginning at age twenty. Only the first attack had been severe enough to require hospital treatment. During the other episodes, he was able to work, but with reduced efficiency. He was described as a quiet, shy, conscientious, sensitive person who worried unduly about his work and family.

This is a case of major depressive disorder characterized by several episodes of depression and an absence of personality deterioration between attacks. The marked psychomotor retardation, the muteness, the refusal to eat, and the delusions characterize the last attack as a stuporous depression.

C. Manic disorder, single episode

A forty-three-year-old married man was admitted to a closed psychiatric unit at the request of his family, after "uncontrolled" behavior. On admission, he was agitated, hyperactive, uncooperative, out of touch with reality, and had flight of ideas and rambling incoherent speech. He angrily ordered the nurses around. These symptoms had developed over a period of a few weeks, during which he was on strike. He first became insomniac and drank excessively.

Physical and laboratory examinations were normal. A brain scan was reported as within normal limits. He responded to treatment, including lithium and Haldol.

He had never had any previous affective symptoms. His family history revealed one sister who had schizophrenic disorder.

It was not clear whether his excessive alcoholic intake was causal or symptomatic of the manic episode. At any rate, this seems to be an example of a single manic episode.

D. Bipolar disorder

Mr. S., a forty-one-year-old attorney, was admitted to the hospital in an acute manic episode. He was extremely hyperactive, distractible, irritable, and demanding. He had a marked flight of ideas and expressed hostility toward his wife for what he described as infidelity. Eight years earlier, he had developed a depressive episode following his wife's severe infectious disease, and since that time he had developed manic symptoms every spring and depressive symptoms every fall. Prior to the onset of his illness, he was described as perfectionistic, egotistical, and outgoing. Between episodes, he practiced law with above-average skill and showed no evidence of personality deterioration.

This is a classical case of manic-depressive illness. The patient's behavior on admission—elated mood, flight of ideas, and increased activity—was typical of acute mania. Note, also, the absence of personality deterioration between attacks.

E. Other examples of bipolar disorder
　　1. John Ruskin (1819–1900), writer, critic, artist, and author of *Modern Painters,* was an example of a bipolar disorder, swinging from elation to misery, always sensitive and always expressive.

2. Vincent W. Van Gogh (1853–1890), Dutch painter, suffered from mood swings, alternating between profound depression and extreme exuberance. On Christmas Eve, 1888, he cut off part of his left ear and in July 1890, he committed suicide.

References

Aarons, S. F. et al. "Atypical Depression: A review of Diagnosis and Treatment. *Hospital and Community Psychiatry* 36 (March 1985): 275–82.

American Psychiatric Association. *Diagnostic and Statistical Manual.* 3d ed., rev. Washington, D.C., 1987.

Brown, R. P. et al. "Involutional Melancholia Revisited." *American Journal of Psychiatry* 141(January 1984): 24–28.

Kaplan, H. I., and B. J. Sadock. *Comprehensive Textbook of Psychiatry.* 4th ed. Baltimore: Williams & Wilkins, 1985.

Kolb, L. C., and H. K. H. Brodie. *Modern Clinical Psychiatry.* 10th ed. Philadelphia: W. B. Saunders Co., 1982.

Maxmen, J. S. *Essential Psychopathology.* New York: W. W. Norton and Company, 1986.

Nicholi, A. M., Jr., ed. *The Harvard Guide to Modern Psychiatry.* Cambridge: Belknap Press of Harvard University, 1978.

Schneidman, E. S. "Suicide." In *Comprehensive Textbook of Psychiatry,* edited by A. M. Freedman, N. I. Kaplan, and B. J. Sadock, vol. 2, 2d ed.Baltimore: Williams & Wilkins, 1976.

Schneidman, E. S., and N. L. Faberow. *A Cry for Help.* New York: McGraw-Hill, 1961.

Zimmerman, M., W. Coryell, B. Pfohl, D. Stangl. "The Validity of Four Definitions of Endogenous Depression." *Archives of General Psychiatry* (March 1986): 234.

We are prone to the malady of the introvert, who, with the manifold spectacle of the world spread out before him, turns away and gazes only upon the emptiness within. But, let us not imagine that there is anything grand about the introvert's unhappiness.

Bertrand Russell: *The Conquest of Happiness* (1930)

Schizophrenic Disorders

I. Historical notes

A. The syndromes that are now classified as schizophrenia have been recognized for at least 3,400 years, although in the past they have carried varying labels.

B. Greek physicians in the fifth century B.C. termed it *dementia* and distinguished it from mania and melancholia.

C. In 1683, Thomas Willis reported a patient whose personality had changed in early life.

D. Benedict Augustin Morel (1860) introduced the term *demence precoce* to describe psychosis in a fourteen-year-old boy.

E. E. Hecker (1871) described *hebephrenia* as a progressive psychotic illness of rapid onset in adolescence.

F. K. Kahlbaum (1874) described *catatonia,* or *tension insanity,* and assumed it to be a symptom of some organic brain disease. His description was of a condition characterized by muteness, immobility, waxy flexibility, and so forth.

G. Emil Kraepelin (1896), believing that all of the above syndromes were related, classified them into one group called *dementia praecox.* He reserved the diagnosis for a relatively small group of psychotic patients whose prognosis was poor.

H. Adolph Meyer (1906) theorized that dementia praecox was a type of reaction to environmental experiences (*parergastic reaction*).

I. Eugen Bleuler (1911) coined the term *schizophrenia* to emphasize the "splitting" of the personality (from the Greek *schizo,* "to split"; and *phren,* "mind"). He recognized that dementia praecox does not always lead to deterioration but he regarded it as a syndrome, a group of disorders.

J. Jacob Kasan (1933) described *schizoaffective psychosis.*

K. G. Langfeldt (1949) described *reactive schizophrenia,* or *schizophreniform psychosis* and emphasized a relatively good prognosis and good response to treatment.

L. Paul Hoch and P. Polatin (1949) described *pseudoneurotic schizophrenia* to apply to those patients whose defense mechanisms seemed neurotic but on close investigation showed basic schizophrenic mechanisms. Symptomatically they showed pan anxiety and pan neurosis.

II. Definition

A. The APA glossary defines schizophrenia as a large group of disorders, usually of psychotic proportion, manifested by characteristic disturbances of language and communication, thought, perception, affect, and behavior, which last longer than six months. Thought disturbances are marked by alterations of concept formation that may lead to misinterpretation of reality, misperceptions, and sometimes to delusions and hallucinations. Mood changes include ambivalence, blunting, inappropriateness, and loss of empathy with others. Behavior may be withdrawn, regressive, and bizarre. The clinical picture is not explainable by any of the organic mental disorders.[1]

B. *DSM*-III-R describes the essential features as "the presence of characteristic psychotic symptoms during the active phase of the illness and functioning below the highest level previously achieved (in children or adolescents, failure to achieve the expected level of social development), and a duration of at least six months that may include characteristic prodromal or residual symptoms. At some phase of the illness schizophrenia always involves delusions, hallucinations, or certain characteristic disturbances in affect and the form of thought. The diagnosis is made only when it cannot be established that an organic factor initiated and maintained the disturbance. The diagnosis is not made if the symptoms are due to a mood disorder or schizoaffective disorder" (*DSM*-III-R).

    1. Clinical criteria include:

        a) Functioning below a highest level previously achieved in such areas as work, social relations, and self-care.

        b) Characteristic symptoms involving multiple psychological processes including: content and form of thought, perception, affect, sense of self, volition, impaired interpersonal functioning and relationship to the external world and psychomotor behavior.

        c) For elaboration on these descriptions, see VII. Symptoms.

III. Prevalence

A. It is estimated that the prevalence rate of schizophrenia in the United States is between 0.6 percent and 3.0 percent of the population.

B. Thus, approximately 1.2 to 6 million Americans are presently schizophrenic.

C. Although schizophrenic disorders affect a small percentage of the population, patients with these disorders occupy a significant proportion of mental hospital beds.

D. According to Freedman et al., somewhere between 460,000 to 940,000 people will need treatment annually for this disorder.

E. It is most prevalent between the ages of fifteen and fifty-four.

IV. Conceptions of schizophrenia

A. Emil Kraepelin believed that dementia praecox resulted from injury to the germ plasm or from some metabolic disorder, which caused autointoxication. Thus, he thought of it as an organically caused disease. He was the first to include hebephrenic, catatonic, and paranoid reactions under one category.

---

1. American Psychiatric Association, *A Psychiatric Glossary*, 6th ed. (Washington, D. C., 1988).

B. Eugen Bleuler's concept was broader than Kraepelin's. Although he believed this illness to be primarily of physical origin, he did consider certain secondary symptoms (such as delusions, hallucinations, and mannerisms) to be psychogenic (an indicative attempt at adaptation to the primary disturbance). He emphasized the "splitting of the various mental functions" (i.e., the coexistence of disharmonious complexes). He regarded the formal mechanism underlying schizophrenic symptoms as the loosening of association.

C. Adolph Meyer regarded this as a maladaptive reaction ("the accumulation of lifelong faulty habits of adaptation in the setting of an inferior psychobiological endowment"). That is, he saw it as a habit disorganization. He emphasized longitudinal (versus cross-sectional) psychological factors.

D. Sigmund Freud regarded schizophrenia as withdrawal and regression associated with a weak ego, a return to early narcissism (e.g., the libido is withdrawn from external objects and directed toward the ego).

E. Carl Jung believed that schizophrenia arises when the psyche is unable to rid itself of a complex and can no longer adapt to the surroundings. Thus, separation from reality results. He thought that delusions, hallucinations, and other schizophrenic symptoms were due to an autochthonous complex (i.e., a group of ideas that, because they were disturbing, were removed from consciousness and maintained in an independent existence).

F. Harry Stack Sullivan regarded schizophrenia as the indirect outcome of unhealthy interpersonal relationships between the child (who later becomes schizophrenic) and the parents.

G. Emil Kraepelin and Eugen Bleuler are the two progenitors of the modern concept of schizophrenia.

V. Etiology

A. The etiology of schizophrenia is not clearly understood.
  1. Conflicting findings by different investigators lead to the belief that schizophrenia is really several different disorders.
  2. Others describe two major types: (1) "process," which does not respond to treatment, has a poor prognosis, and is probably biologically determined, and (2) "reactive," a remitting type that has a more favorable prognosis and is probably related to experiential factors.

B. Theories of etiology can be divided into
  1. Biological
  2. Sociocultural
  3. Experiential, or psychological

C. Biological theories

There seems little doubt that biological factors play a role in the cause of schizophrenia. What factors are significant and the importance of the role remain controversial.

1. Genetic predisposition

a) Some studies suggest a genetic factor in schizophrenic disorders. However, many authorities who believe that there is some genetic predisposition also believe that subsequent factors (biological, psychological, social, or experiential), are necessary for the production of a schizophrenic disorder.

b) Studies indicate that children of schizophrenic parents are much more likely to develop the disorder than the general population. The expectancy of schizophrenia in children of one schizophrenic parent is 16 percent versus 0.85 percent for the general population. In families where both parents are schizophrenic, the expectancy in the children is 40 percent.

c) Kalmann's (1953) studies of twins also suggest a genetic factor.

(1) Among monozygotic (identical) twins, if one is schizophrenic, 85 percent of the other twins will also be.

(2) Among dizygotic (fraternal) twins, the correlation is 14 percent, about the same as among other siblings.

d) On the basis of presently available information, we cannot label schizophrenia a hereditary disease, but it does seem that a hereditary predisposition is present in many, if not all cass.

2. Biochemical predisposition

a) There has been a remarkable increase in our knowledge of brain biochemistry and psychopharmacology in recent years.

b) Biochemical abnormalities are present in many if not all the cases.

c) There are two main groups of theories about the basic biochemical factors in schizophrenia. These are

(1) Transmethylation hypothesis

Harley-Mason theorized that, since many hallucinogens are methylated substances, an accumulation of methylated substances might occur in schizophrenia. Methylated indoleamine has been found in the blood and urine of schizophrenics.

(2) Dopamine hypothesis
    (a) Schizophrenia is assumed to reflect a defect in dopamine-mediated brain systems.
    (b) Amphetamines, which stimulate release of catecholamines, can also produce psychotic symptoms that resemble schizophrenia and exacerbate psychotic symptoms of acute schizophrenia.
    (c) The class of antipsychotics (phenothiazines) most effective in treating schizophrenic symptoms acts to inhibit or block dopamine-mediated transmissions. (Although altered levels of dopamine are not considered a "cause" of schizophrenia, they do seem to be implicated in the manifestation of symptoms. Also, such drugs are equally effective in reducing psychotic symptoms and other types of psychosis.)

D. Sociocultural theories
1. There is a high density of schizophrenics in urban ghettos and other underprivileged areas of the city. This finding has led to two contradictory theories.
    a) The "downward-drift" theory states that schizophrenics drift to such areas because they are socially and economically incompetent.
    b) These areas "breed" schizophrenics because they are populated by people laden with severe socioeconomic problems. In other words, the schizophrenic has never experienced achievement.
2. Many studies confirm the association of schizophrenia and lower socioeconomic class. Social and economic limitations prevent the achievement of fundamental gratification, thus poverty and crowding may be factors that produce greater stress and reduce flexibility in the choice of personal response to stress.
3. There is a higher incidence of broken homes in the lower socioeconomic areas.

E. Experiential, or psychological, theory
1. Psychoanalytic theories
    a) Freud emphasized the role of sexual regression in the development of the illness.
    b) Melanie Klein emphasized the importance of early mother-child relationships.
    c) Harry Stack Sullivan emphasized the patient's deeply disturbed interpersonal relationships, rather than the intrapsychic mechanisms emphasized by Freud and Klein.

d) Gregory Bateson suggested that repeated exposure to double-bind experiences makes the potential schizophrenic perceive the entire environment as a double bind.

VI. Psychopathology

A. Most psychiatrists regard schizophrenic disorder as regression (see the Freudian concept, above, and the section on regression in the chapter, "Adaptations to Anxiety").

   1. There is withdrawal of interest from the environment and loss of interest in objects and other persons.

   2. According to psychoanalytic theory, this is regression to a level at which schizophrenics, like infants, are incapable of distinguishing themselves from the environment (i.e., regression to primary narcissism).

B. Those having paranoid delusions are also overusing the mechanism of projection (see "Adaptations to Anxiety").

C. The prepsychotic personality is often schizoid (introverted), schizotypal, or borderline.

D. Precipitating factors may or may not be evident, and their effect varies with the individual's vulnerability. They are evident in the so-called reactive types of schizophrenia.

E. The onset may be gradual, occurring in the absence of obvious precipitating factors, as in so-called process schizophrenia.

VII. Symptoms

A. Since our present-day concept of this disorder includes varying clinical types, it is difficult to present a "typical" cluster of symptoms.

B. Bleuler

   1. Bleuler (1950) described four main symptoms: disturbance of association; disturbance of affect; autism; and heightened ambivalence. These are often called the "four A's."

     a) Disturbance of association is looseness of association (cognitive slippage or derailment). In schizophrenic speech, successive ideas appear to be unrelated or only slightly related to each other.

     b) Disturbances of affect usually take the form of flatness, bluntness, or inappropriateness.

     c) Autism is fantasy and daydreaming that substitutes for reality.

     d) Heightened ambivalence is exaggeration of coexisting opposite feelings or emotions for the same person, thing, situation, or goal.

   2. In addition, Bleuler believed that the main accessory or secondary symptoms need to be present. In severe or advanced cases they are usually found. They are delusions, hallucinations, and ideas of reference. Ideas of reference include feelings of thought control and feelings of influence.

C. According to *DSM*-III-R, the essential features of this group of disorders are
  1. Presence of characteristic psychotic symptoms during the active phase of the illness.
  2. Functioning below the highest level previously achieved in such areas as work, social relationships, and self-care and a duration of at least six months.
  3. Characteristic symptoms involving multiple psychological processes.
     a) Content of thought
        The major disturbance involves delusions that are multiple, fragmented, or bizarre.
        (1) Persecutory and referential delusions.
        (2) Delusions of thought broadcasting (belief that one's thoughts are broadcast to the external world).
        (3) Thought insertion (belief that one's thoughts are not one's own but inserted into the mind).
        (4) Thought withdrawal (belief that thoughts have been removed from one's head).
        (5) Delusions of being controlled (belief that one's feelings, impulses, thoughts, or actions are imposed by external force).
        (6) Somatic, grandiose, religious, and nihilistic delusions—less common.
     b) Form of thought
        A disturbance in the form of thought is frequently present ("formal thought disorder").
        (1) Most commonly this is manifest as loosening of associations (cognitive slippage), in which ideas shift from one subject to another completely unrelated or only obliquely related subject.
        (2) When loosening of association is severe, speech may become incoherent and incomprehensible.
        (3) There also may be poverty of content of speech (that is, conveys little information because it is vague, overly abstract, or stereotyped).
        (4) Less common disturbances include neologisms, perseveration, clanging, and blocking.
     c) Perception
        The major perceptual disturbances are varieties of hallucinations.
        (1) Although these occur in all modalities, the most common are auditory hallucinations, frequently involving voices the individual perceives as coming from outside the head.

        (2) Tactile and somatic hallucinations are much less common.

        (3) Visual, gustatory, and olfactory hallucinations may occur (but always raise the possibility of the presence of an organic mental disorder).

d) Affect

        (1) Blunting, flattening, or inappropriateness are common.

        (2) Antipsychotic drugs have effects that may appear similar to affective blunting and affective flattening.

e) Sense of self

        (1) The sense of self that gives the normal person a feeling of individuality, uniqueness, and self-direction is frequently disturbed.

        (2) This is sometimes referred to as a loss of ego boundaries and is frequently manifested by extreme perplexity.

f) Volition

        (1) Disturbance in self-initiated, goal-directed activity, which may grossly impair work or other role functioning.

        (2) This may take the form of inadequate interest or drive or inability to follow a course of action to its logical conclusions.

        (3) Ambivalence regarding alternative courses of action can lead to near cessation of goal-directed activity.

g) Relationship to the external world

        (1) Frequently there is a tendency to withdraw from involvement with the external world and become preoccupied with egocentric illogical ideas and fantasies in which objective facts are obscured, distorted, or excluded.

        (2) Severe forms of this condition are referred to as "autism."

h) Psychomotor behavior

Various disturbances in psychomotor behavior are observed.

        (1) A marked decrease in reactivity to the environment.

        (2) The individual may appear unaware of the nature of his or her environment (as in catatonic stupor).

        (3) The individual may maintain a rigid posture, resisting efforts to be moved (as in catatonic rigidity).

        (4) The individual may make apparently purposeless and stereotyped, excited motor movements (as in catatonic excitement).

(5) The individual may voluntarily assume inappropriate or bizarre postures (as in catatonic posturing).

(6) The individual may resist and actively counteract instructions or attempts to be moved (as in catatonic negativism).

(7) In addition, there may be mannerisms, grimacing, or waxy flexibility.

i) Associated features

Almost any symptom can occur as an associated feature.

(1) Perplexed, disheveled, or eccentric grooming and appearance may occur.

(2) Symptoms can include abnormalities of psychomotor activity, for example, pacing, rocking, or apathetic immobility.

(3) Frequently, there is poverty of speech.

(4) Ritualistic or stereotyped behavior associated with magical thinking may occur.

(5) Dysphoric mood is common and may take the form of depression, anxiety, anger, or a mixture of these.

(6) Depersonalization, derealization, ideas of reference, and illusions are often present, as are hypochondriacal concerns.

(7) Usually there is no disturbance in sensorium.

VIII. Types

Because of the varied clinical picture, cases are classified into different clinical types depending upon the predominant symptomatology. In *DSM*-III-R, the following phenomenological subtypes are described:

A. Catatonic type

The essential feature is marked psychomotor disturbance, which may involve stupor, negativism, rigidity, excitement, or posturing. Sometimes there is rapid alternation between the extremes of excitement and stupor (*DSM*-III-R).

1. The five different types of catatonic symptomatology described in *DSM*-III-R are

a) Catatonic stupor or mutism

Characterized by marked decrease in reactivity to environment, reduction of spontaneous movements and activity, or mutism.

b) Catatonic negativism

Characterized by an apparently motiveless resistance to all instructions or attempts to be moved.

c) Catatonic rigidity

Characterized by maintenance of a rigid posture against efforts to be moved.

d) Catatonic excitement

Characterized by excited motor activity, apparently purposeless and not influenced by external stimuli.

e) Catatonic posturing

Characterized by voluntary assumptions of inappropriate or bizarre posture.

2. Onset and course

The onset of catatonic schizophrenia is usually sudden, and the course is usually short.

3. Prognosis

Good for recovery from the episode, but guarded about future recurrences.

4. Case example, catatonic stupor

Miss J., a thirty-nine-year-old secretary, was brought to the hospital by her two sisters because her behavior had been bizarre for a week. She was described as a quiet, reserved person who had few friends and preferred to remain by herself. Although she danced occasionally, she was generally shy in the company of men. She had no symptoms of emotional illness until seven days earlier, when she suddenly began to abstain from food. Five days later she expressed religious delusions, became self-condemnatory, refused to go to bed at night, and demanded to see a priest at 3:00 A.M. A few hours later, she was admitted to a general hospital and given intravenous feedings because of her refusal to eat. She would not remain in bed and left the hospital against advice. At home she continued to refuse food. Finally, her sisters sought her admission to the hospital.

On admission she was negativistic, refusing food, medication, and nursing care. She was mute most of the time, and when she did speak she expressed religious delusions and hallucinations. She postured, that is, assumed uncomfortable postures for long periods, and exhibited waxy flexibility, that is, her extremities would remain in positions in which they were placed.

She recovered from this episode after a course of electroconvulsive therapy and was discharged to her home at the end of one month. A few weeks later, the symptoms recurred. This second episode also responded rather promptly to treatment, and she was discharged after six weeks. She has remained well for several years.

The characteristic features in the foregoing case of catatonic stupor are the sudden onset of negativism, mutism, posturizing, and waxy flexibility; the good response to treatment in both instances; and the prepsychotic schizoid personality.

5. Case example, catatonic excitement

P. H., a twenty-year-old college student, was brought to the hospital in restraints by the police. His illness had become manifest the previous day, when he began expressing delusions of grandeur and persecution. He left his fraternity house without telling anyone where he was going and remained away all night. About two hours before admission, the police were summoned to pick him up in a nearby suburb because of bizarre behavior characterized by agitation, assaultiveness, and disrobing. Before the onset of his illness he was described as conscientious, compulsive, and meek. He resisted accepting responsibility and had an "inferiority complex."

On admission he was uncooperative, mute, belligerent, agitated, and assaultive. He refused food, medications, and nursing care, and was careless of his excreta. After a series of electroconvulsive treatment, he became cooperative and calm. Treatment was continued in another hospital to which he was transferred in order to be nearer his parents.

Mutism, negativism, agitation, assaultiveness, and violent behavior characterized this case as catatonic excitement.

    6. Periodic catatonic type

    This is a rare form of episodic catatonia that is related to shifts in the individual's metabolic nitrogen balance. Maintenance on neuroleptic drugs prevents recurrence.

B. Disorganized type

Also called *hebephrenic,* after Hebe, the Greek goddess of youth.

    1. The essential features are marked incoherence, marked loosening of associations, or grossly disorganized behavior, flat or grossly inappropriate affect, fragmentary, unsystematized delusions or hallucinations with an incoherent theme.

    2. Associated features include grimacing, mannerisms, hypochondriacal complaints, extreme social withdrawal, and other oddities of behavior.

    3. It is usually associated with extreme social impairment and poor premorbid personality, insidious onset, and chronic course without significant remissions.

    4. Case example

Mary, a twenty-one-year-old stenographer, was brought to the hospital by the police, who had been called after she had entered a strange residence at 1:00 A.M. in response to an uncontrollable urge to urinate. She had always been a shy, introverted, and intensely religious girl. Three years earlier, after high school graduation, she had had a "nervous breakdown" that required six months' hospitalization. She showed improvement following that treatment, but still seemed shy and self-contained, and behaved inappropriately at times.

Three days before her second admission to the hospital she became restless, sleepless, and spent the night on her knees in continuous prayer. The following morning she seemed elated and became upset by several commonplace incidents. She started out for work, but in response to a "voice" went instead to religious services at a nearby church. The second night was likewise spent in continuous prayer. The following morning, she again started out for work but became confused and returned home. The evening preceding admission, she boarded a bus to attend church but became confused "because my friend Anne prayed that I would get mixed up" and she left the bus far from church. She wandered about aimlessly, finally entering the strange residence at 1:00 A.M.

On admission she was obviously disturbed. She was preoccupied with religious and moral ideas and said that God was talking to her through the newspapers, radio, and television. She repeatedly misidentified the ward personnel as apostles, disciples, and other biblical characters. Her affect was euphoric and inappropriate. She was physically active, making frequent changes in posture and moving about the room aimlessly. She was unkempt and continously disrobed.

Despite a three-month stay in the hospital, during which time she received thirty electroconvulsive treatments, there was no sustained improvement in her behavior and she was committed to a state hospital for prolonged care.

In this case, note the schizoid premorbid personality, the rather definite onset of psychotic symptoms in adolescence, the obvious emotional disturbance at the time of admission, the bizarre nature of her symptoms, and her bizarre delusions and hallucinations.

C. Paranoid type
   1. The essential feature is preoccupation with one or more systematized delusions or with frequent auditory hallucinations related to a single theme.
   2. Symptoms characteristic of catatonic and disorganized types are absent.
   3. Associated features include unfocused anxiety, anger, argumentativeness, and violence.
   4. The onset is abrupt and usually occurs in adult life, later than the other subtypes.
   5. Case example

   Mrs. L., a thirty-year-old housewife, was brought to the hospital by her family because she had behaved strangely for the preceding seven months. The behavior was characterized by withdrawal, inappropriate mood, preoccupation with religious ideas, and delusions that her husband and the family physician were "trying to poison the food." In preschool years she had been overly attached to her mother, but she subsequently became so interested in outdoor activities that she was considered a tomboy.

   In the hospital, she was markedly suspicious of the entire staff, accusing them of poisoning her food, talking about her, gambling, and so forth. She said she received messages from Christ, whose voice came to her over the radio. Much of the time she was withdrawn, but at times she talked readily though inappropriately. Her affect was flattened.

   Following a course of electroconvulsive therapy, she improved, and returned home. Eighteen months later, the same symptoms recurred and she was readmitted to the hospital. Though the second episode was more refractory to treatment, she did improve sufficiently to return home after eight months.

D. Undifferentiated type

The essential features are

1. Permanent psychotic symptoms (delusions, hallucinations, incoherence or grossly disorganized behavior) that cannot be classified as catatonic, disorganized or paranoid, or

2. Meets the criteria for more than one category

E. Residual type

1. This category is for those who have at least one episode of schizophrenia. The clinical picture that occasioned the evaluation or admission to clinical care is without permanent psychotic symptoms, though signs of the illness persist.

2. This is equivalent of the category, *in partial remission.*

3. Examples of persistent symptoms are emotional blunting, social withdrawal, eccentric behavior, and persistent but inconspicuous delusions or hallucinations—but not accompanied by strong affect.

4. The course is either chronic or subchronic.

IX. **Cultural influences**

A. Records suggest that the incidence of schizophrenia in this country has probably remained essentially unchanged during the past century, perhaps even longer.

B. Cultural factors, however, have had an influence on the relative frequency and character of schizophrenic symptoms.

C. Prior to the publication of *DSM*-III-R, there had been a classification of simple schizophrenia. Such cases are probably now classified as schizoid personality or schizotypal personality.

D. Catatonic forms of schizophrenia seem less frequent.

E. Schizophrenics are less aggressive than they were a quarter of a century ago, perhaps in part because of the early prescription of antipsychotic medications that reduce assaultive and antisocial behavior.

F. Although paranoid reactions have increased, delusions of grandeur, witchcraft, and other magic have become less frequent, whereas ideas of being hypnotized or influenced by electronics or radiation have increased.

G. The content of delusions has become more realistic and plausible.

X. **Course and prognosis**

A. Schizophrenia was once regarded as a progressive disorder with a poor or hopeless prognosis.

B. As can be noted from the *DSM*-III-R classification, episodic types of the disorder are now recognized. These are many times followed by symptom-free periods, long periods of remission. Occasionally, individuals have been observed to have a single mild schizophrenic or (schizophrenic like) attack, without any recurrence.

C. As noted earlier, schizophrenic disorders can occur either in attacks or as a progressive disease; thus, we speak of "reactive" and "process" schizophrenic disorder.

D. However, it still must be regarded as a tenacious disorder.

E. Currently, there is more optimism about arrest and recovery in this illness, chiefly because of the favorable effect of psychotropic drugs.

F. In general, however, the prognosis is guarded.

G. Certain criteria have become more or less accepted for prognosticating the outcome of any case of schizophrenic disorder.

  1. The following are considered favorable prognostic signs:
- a) Sudden or acute onset
- b) Conspicuous precipitating factors
- c) Catatonic symptoms
- d) The presence of affective symptoms, that is, depression or elation; perhaps these cases are more properly classified as schizoaffective disorders in the present nomenclature
- e) The presence of confusion
- f) The history of a good previous social adjustment
- g) Married schizophrenics have a better outlook than single, divorced, or widowed ones
- h) Stable employment (the schizophrenic has a job to which to return)
- i) Cooperativeness (the patient cooperates with the treatment regime)
- j) An empathic therapist

  2. The following are considered unfavorable signs:
- a) History of previous episodes
- b) Schizoid or schizotypal premorbid personality
- c) Absence of conspicuous precipitating factors
- d) Family history of mental illness
- e) Persistence of the symptoms for more than one year
- f) The presence of sustained emotional withdrawal, aloofness, and shallow or inappropriate affect, which makes the patient less cooperative about taking maintenance medication
- g) Onset in childhood or early puberty (recovery is unlikely)

XI. Treatment of schizophrenia

A. Since schizophrenia is probably a heterogenous group of disorders and etiology is incompletely understood, the treatment has been largely empirical.

B. The type of treatment depends upon the type and severity of the disorder. It can be divided into
  1. Milieu therapy
  2. Various psychotherapies (psychoanalytic, supportive, and behavior)

3. Somatic (electroconvulsive therapy)
4. Chemotherapy (antipsychotic drugs)

C. Milieu therapy

The exact plan varies according to the individual needs of the patient. Included are:

1. Various inpatient hospital programs

   Although some schizophrenics can make a marginal adjustment extramurally, hospitalization is frequently indicated, at least for a period of time. Partial hospitalization has been found useful in recent years.

2. Various outpatient arrangements, individually arranged. These include:

   a) Various living arrangements, such as halfway houses, apartments, board-and-care facilities, foster homes, and family care.

   b) Vocational arrangements, such as sheltered workshops, day activity centers, and vocational rehabilitation placements.

D. Psychotherapeutic treatment

1. Psychoanalytic psychotherapy (see the chapter "Treatment in Psychiatry: Psychotherapy").

2. In general, therapists should be active and positive in their approach.

3. Establishing a relationship may be difficult because of the schizophrenics's distrust and inability to become close.

4. The patient's ability and willingness to collaborate in treatment often is largely determined by the bond that forms in the doctor-patient relationship.

5. Behavioral therapy is mostly based on the operant conditioning of B. F. Skinner. The value of this kind of treatment has yet to be determined and should be regarded as in the experimental stage.

6. Supportive therapy

E. Somatic therapy (electroconvulsive therapy)

Its status is uncertain, although it has been successfully used in two types of cases, those that have not responded to drugs and acute attacks.

F. Psychosurgery is a rare form of treatment (see the chapter, "Treatment in Psychiatry").

G. Megavitamin therapy

This treatment involves the administration of large doses of niacin. Major controlled studies indicate that niacin is no better than a placebo.

H. Chemotherapy (antipsychotic agents)
   1. Antipsychotic agents—there are a large number of these, including the phenothiazines, the thioxanthenes, the dibenzoxaze-pines, (eg. Loxapine), the butyrophenones, and the indolones (see appropriate section in the chapter "Treatment in Psychiatry").
   2. Intramuscular injections of long-acting phenothiazines (such as Prolixin Decanoate) or butyrophenones (Haldol Decanoate) may be necessary until the patient becomes cooperative. Or, it may be necessary, in those patients who find it easier, to receive an injection once every two to four weeks, rather than to take oral or injected medications daily.
   3. It should be kept in mind, however, that a large percentage (two-thirds or more) of schizophrenics do not comply with the drug regime after discharge.
   4. Maintenance therapy may be necessary.
      a) In many cases, drugs can eventually be discontinued.
      b) However, a significant number of patients relapse when antipsychotic agents are withdrawn.
I. Combined psychotherapy and drug therapy
   Antipsychotic drugs plus "the therapeutic alliance" seem helpful to most schizophrenics.
J. The most effective treatment program is usually one combining psychotropic, psychotherapeutic, and milieu therapy.
K. Results of treatment
   1. About one-third of the patients will do relatively well.
   2. One-third will become hard-core failures.
   3. The remainder will occupy an intermediate status.

References

American Psychiatric Association. *Diagnostic and Statistical Manual of Mental Disorders*. 3d ed., rev. Washington, D.C., 1987.

Arieti, S. *Interpretation of Schizophrenia*. New York: Basic Books, Inc., Publishers, 1975.

Bleuler, E. *Dementia Praecox or the Group of Schizophrenias*. New York: International Universities Press, 1950.

Eaton, M. T., Jr., M. H. Peterson, and J. A. Davis. *Psychiatry*. 4th ed. Garden City, N.Y.: Medical Examination Publishing Company, 1981.

Freedman, A. M., H. I. Kaplan, and B. J. Sadack. *Modern Synopsis of Comprehensive Textbook of Psychiatry*. Baltimore: Williams & Wilkins, 1976.

Goldman, H. H. *Review of General Psychiatry*. Los Altos, Calif.: Lange Medical Publications, 1984.

Goodwin, D. W., and S. V. Guze. *Psychiatric Diagnosis*. 2d ed. New York: Oxford University Press, 1979.

Kalman, F. J. *Heredity and Health and Mental Disorder*. New York: W. W. Norton & Co., 1953.

Kaplan, H. I., and B. J. Sadock. *Comprehensive Textbook of Psychiatry/IV*. 4th ed. Baltimore: Williams & Wilkins, 1985.

What is madness: To have
erroneous perceptions and to
reason correctly from them.

Voltaire: "Madness," in
Philosophical Dictionary (1764)

Delusional (Paranoid) Disorders

I. Introduction

A. This category was labeled paranoid disorder in *DSM*-III.

B. Since in this disorder delusions are the primary symptom and the term *paranoid* has multiple other meanings, the term *delusional disorder* is used.

II. Definition

A. The essential feature of this disorder is the presence of a persistent, nonbizarre delusion that is not due to any other mental disorder, such as schizophrenia, schizophreniform disorder, or a mood disorder.

B. Organic factor as an etiological determinant must also be excluded (*DSM*-III).

C. Apart from the delusion or its ramifications, there is no obvious or odd behavior.

III. Types

A. Common delusional themes are

1. Erotomanic

The central theme is an erotic delusion that one is loved by another, usually of a higher status, such as a famous person, or a superior at work. It usually concerns idealized romantic love and spiritual union rather than sexual attraction. Efforts to contact the object of the delusion, through telephone calls, letters, gifts, visits, and so forth, are common.

2. Grandiose

These delusions center around the person's conviction that he or she possesses great unrecognized talent or insight or has made some important discovery. They seem to represent a regression to an earlier phase of development in which children regard themselves as omnipotent. An example is Cervantes' *Don Quixote* who roamed the world righting wrongs and tilting windmills— his combat against the villainous foe. Grandiose delusions may have a religious content and sometimes people with this delusion can become leaders of religious cults.

3. Jealous

The jealousy is usually more persistent and profound than normal jealousy. There is usually some grain of truth in the pathological jealousy, but the constructs on which it rests are based on inadequate evidence. The delusionally jealous person may find bits of "evidence" to substantiate his delusion. Shakespeare's Othello becomes furiously jealous of his innocent wife, Desdemona, and his loyal lieutenant, Michael Cassio, and executes Desdemona with his own hands. When he learns of her innocence, he judges and executes himself.

4. Persecutory

This is the most common type. The paranoid person feels conspired against, cheated, spied upon, followed, poisoned or drugged, maliciously maligned, harassed, or obstructed in the pursuit of long-term goals (*DSM*-III-R). Sometimes the focus of the delusion is some injustice that must be corrected (querulous paranoia).

    5. Somatic

Such delusions can take one of several forms: most common ones involve beliefs that the person emits a foul odor from his or her skin, mouth, rectum, or vagina; there's an infestation of insects on his or her skin; he or she has an internal parasite; certain parts of the body are misshapen or ugly; or certain parts of the body are not functioning.

    6. Litigious

This is not listed in *DSM*-III-R as a type of delusional disorder. Such people's delusions produce disputatiousness, contentiousness, fondness for litigation, or proneness to engage in lawsuits.

B. Delusions in such disorders usually involve a single theme or a series of connected themes. Aside from the delusional system, there are no signs of mental disorder in the paranoid person. There is no withdrawal or regression (as in the schizophrenic disorders), or any affective changes (as in affective disorders or schizoaffective disorders).

IV. Prevalence

A. Delusional disorders are relatively uncommon (0.03% of the population).

B. Immigration, emigration, deafness, and other severe stresses may predispose to this disorder.

V. Psychopathological factors

A. The main causes are believed to be psychological (experiential).

B. There is overuse of denial and projection as defenses against underlying conflicts, feelings of insecurity, repudiated impulses, and other conflictual factors.

C. In the grandiose type, there is also overuse of rationalization. The behavior may be a response to a need to improve self-esteem or to enhance prestige.

D. Paranoid, schizoid, or avoidant personality may be more likely to develop this disorder.

E. The individual may form a projective defense structure (the paranoid system) in response to conscious and unconscious perceptions of himself or herself as weak and inadequate ("power anxiety," according to Ovesey and others).

F. In the shame-humiliation theory, the individual develops a series of defenses eschewing underlying shame and assigning blame to others for any underlying failure (Colby).

G. Sex ratio

Delusional disorders are apparently somewhat more common in females, with the exception that in forensic cases most are males.

VI. Treatment

A. Treatment of patients in this category would be similar to management of people with paranoid delusions in other diagnostic groups.

B. Most of these people make at least marginal adjustments outside of the hospital and, hence, treatment attempts would focus on treatment within the community.

C. The therapist who can accept the delusional person and at the same time, clearly indicate nonagreement with the delusional system may be of value in a supportive way to the patient. The therapist who is not skilled in dealing with such an individual may run the risk of becoming a part of the patient's delusional system.

D. Various neuroleptic drugs, especially the phenothiazines, butyrophenones, thioxanthenes, may be of some help in modifying the patients' delusional preoccupations or in assisting them to adapt more comfortably.

E. Sometimes management of such disorders is determined more by the needs of society than by the needs of individual patients.

F. Few patients eventually require institutionalization.

References

American Psychiatric Association. *Diagnostic and Statistical Manual of Mental Disorders.* 3d ed., rev. Washington, D.C., 1987.

Kaplan, H. I., and B. J. Sadock. *Comprehensive Textbook of Psychiatry.* 4th ed. Baltimore: Williams & Wilkins, 1985.

There is no great genius without some touch of madness.

Seneca: *Moral Essays*
(8 B.C.–A.D. 65)

Psychotic Disorders Not Elsewhere Classified

I. Introduction

This class is for disorders that cannot be classified as organic mental disorder, schizophrenia, delusional disorder or mood disorder with psychotic features.

II. Brief reactive psychosis (*DSM*-III-R)

A. The essential feature is sudden onset of psychotic symptoms of at least a few hours, but no more than one month's duration, with eventual return to premorbid level of functioning.

B. The psychotic symptoms appear shortly after one or more events that, singly or together, would be markedly stressful to almost anyone in similar circumstances. Precipitating event(s) may be any major stress, such as the loss of a loved one or the psychological trauma of combat.

C. Invariably there is emotional turmoil.

D. Behavior may be bizzare; there is often suicidal or aggressive behavior; affect is often inappropriate.

E. Age at onset
Usually begins in adolescence or early adulthood.

F. Predisposing factors
Preexisting psychopathology may predispose to the development of this disorder; individuals with paranoid, histrionic, narcissistic, schizotypal, or borderline personality disorder are thought to be vulnerable to the development of this disorder.

III. Schizophreniform disorder (*DSM*-III-R)

A. The essential features are identical with those of schizophrenia, with the exception that the duration, including prodromal, active, and residual phases, is less than six months.

B. It is classified outside the category of schizophrenia because the evidence linking schizophreniform disorder to typical schizophrenia remains unclear. There is consistent evidence that people with symptoms of less than six months' duration have a better outcome than those with a more prolonged disturbance.

C. The diagnosis is made under two conditions: (1) an episode of illness of less than six months' duration from which the person has already recovered; and (2) a person who is symptomatic but has been this way for less than six months (qualified as "provisional").

IV. Schizoaffective disorder (*DSM*-III-R)

A. This diagnosis has been used in many different ways since it was first introduced.

B. The approach taken in *DSM*-III-R emphasizes the temporal relationship of schizophrenic and mood symptoms.

C. The description of schizoaffective disorder appears to have tentative validity from prognostic treatment and family studies as delimiting an entity that appears to be distinct from mood disorder.

D. Course

Some suggestion that there is a tendency toward a chronic course but with a prognosis somewhat better than for schizophrenic disorder, but less good than mood disorder.

V. Induced psychotic disorder

A. Definition

The essential feature of this disorder is a delusional system that develops in a second person as a result of a close relationship with another person who already has a psychotic disorder with prominent delusions. The delusions are at least partly shared. Usually, if the relationship with the primary person is interrupted, the delusional beliefs in the second person diminish or disappear.

B. Previously known as shared paranoid disorder or foilie à deux, or communicated psychosis. It was also sometimes called double insanity or psychosis of association.

C. Gralnick, who reviewed the English literature and reported on one hundred and three cases in 1942, defined it as a "psychiatric entity characterized by the transference of delusional ideas or abnormal behavior from one person to one or more others who have been in close association with the primarily affected patient."

D. This is a rare condition, first described in 1877 by Laseque and Falret.

E. Psychopathology

1. A. A. Brill described the essential psychological process as unconscious identification.

   a) There is a communication of delusional ideas from one person to another (both of whom have been closely associated for a long period of time).

   b) It frequently involves a parent and child, husband and wife, or two sisters.

   c) The identification is a mutual phenomenon.

   d) Nothing is ever accepted by the secondary partner that is ego-alien. That is, the delusional material from the primary partner must resemble the unconscious fantasies and fit the defense mechanisms of the secondary partner.

   e) The identification in *foilie a deux* may be more akin to identification with the aggressor. As this was described by Anna Freud, identification with the aggressor is a defensive maneuver that protects the ego against real or feared aggression by allowing the individual to share in the power of the feared one.

2. The interdependence of the two partners is extreme; the identification is carried out in order to avoid a separation, which would be unendurable.

3. Heredity may be a predisposing factor.

4. Both persons usually have a long history of poor adjustment.
5. There is close physical association between the two, who have usually lived in relative isolation and often in poverty.
6. The dominant partner is usually brighter.
7. In the prepsychotic relationship, the dominant partner is strongly dependent on the secondary partner and has few outside sources of gratification.
8. The dominant (primary) partner in the relationship is usually the one who has the primary psychotic disorder. The recipient (the secondary partner) of the induced delusions is often submissive, seclusive, and suspicious (i.e., schizoid), but develops these symptoms secondarily.
9. Since the disorder is usually characterized by delusions, the mechanism of projection is also operating. Because the primary partner is afraid of giving up the relationship, emerging hostility toward the secondary partner cannot be expressed directly. The defense used is the projection of the hostility onto an outsider in the form of paranoid delusions. The result is a paranoid psychosis.

F. Treatment
1. Separation of the two involved individuals.
2. Psychiatric treatment directed at the dominant person (primary partner), who has the primary psychotic symptoms. Treatment modalities should be those recommended for the patient's particular paranoid condition, and may include psychotherapy, neuroleptics, hospitalization, and maybe even electroconvulsive therapy.
3. The disorder of the recipient (secondary partner) may clear up without formal treatment, following separation from the primary psychotic partner.

G. Case Example

A. T., a sixty-one-year-old single man, and V. T., his fifty-seven-year-old single sister with whom he had lived for many years, were referred to the court's psychiatric consultant for evaluation after they had both been found guilty of violation of the city fire ordinance on a number of occasions. Their offense consisted in hoarding a number of combustible items and trash in their home and on their premises. Neighbors complained, and the fire-prevention bureau, after repeatedly warning them about the combustible nature of the rubbish and other materials, filed a complaint.

The man, upon examination, showed flattened affect and was silly and inappropriate. He showed signs of schizoid behavior, including introversion, lack of verbal spontaneity and blocking, and was overly sensitive and suspicious. The schizoid and paranoid elements in his personality also became evident in the presentence study, where it was learned that he tended to place much of the blame for the collection of rubbish on his sister. His Minnesota Multiphasic Personality Inventory profile was clearly psychotic, showing elevations of the scales on the right-hand side.

The sister, at the time of the examination, seemed very frightened and kept asking if her brother could be present during the interview so he could "support me." She seemed preoccupied with her fantasy, but denied that she had hallucinations or delusions. She was evasive and defensive and had a number of "reasons" for hoarding trash in their home. From her description, she and her brother would collect a number of items and then spend much time going over them to try sorting out things that might have some value. Whenever she was questioned in detail about what valuable items might be in the trash or why the trash continued to accumulate, she would say, "You are trying to upset me."

Our conclusion was that the brother was the one primarily ill, that he had a paranoid, schizophrenic reaction, and that his sister had the same psychotic illness but, because she was the passive, submissive, suggestible one, she had developed it secondarily, through induction.

References

American Psychiatric Association. *Diagnostic and Statistical Manual of Mental Disorders*. 3d ed., rev. Washington, D.C. 1987.

Gralnick, A. "Foilie à Deux. The Psychosis of Association." *Psychiatric Quarterly* 16 (1942): 230.

Kaplan, H. I., and B. J. Sadock. *Comprehensive Textbook of Psychiatry/ IV.* 4th ed. Baltimore: Williams & Wilkins, 1985.

Nicholi, A. M. *The Harvard Medical Guide to Modern Psychiatry*. Cambridge: Harvard University Press, 1978.

Pulver, S. E. and M. Y. Brunt. "Deflection of Hostility and Foilie à Deux." *Archives of General Psychiatry* 5(1961): 257–65.

Now the time has fled—the world is strange,
something there is of pain and change;
My books lie closed upon the shelf;
I miss the old heart in myself.

**A student: Adelaide Proctor
(19th Century)**

ORGANIC MENTAL SYNDROMES AND DISORDERS

I. Definition

According to *DSM*-III-R, a distinction is made between organic mental syndromes and organic mental disorders.

A. *Organic mental syndrome* is used to refer to a constellation of psychological or behavioral signs and symptoms without reference to etiology (e.g., organic anxiety syndrome, dementia).

B. *Organic mental disorder* designates a particular organic mental syndrome in which the etiology is known or presumed (e.g., alcohol withdrawal delirium, multi-infarct dementia).

In the *DSM*-III-R classification the term *disorder* is used when an organic mental syndrome is associated with an Axis III physical disorder or condition, as in organic delusional disorder due to a brain tumor.

C. The essential feature of all these disorders is a psychological or behavioral abnormality associated with transient or permanent dysfunction of the brain.

II. Characteristics

A. Organic mental disorders are a heterogeneous group; therefore, no single description can characterize them all. The differences in clinical presentation reflect differences in the localization, mode of onset, progression, duration, and nature of the underlying pathophysiologic process.

B. The fundamental process is the (presumed) destruction or damage of neurons (nerve cells).

C. It is this damage, rather than the quality of the destructive process, that is responsible for the typical clinical picture.

D. Strictly speaking, damage to the brain does not fully account for the occurrence of the abnormal behavior. Psychological and sociocultural factors also play a role.

1. Psychological factors
These include: (a) previous personality; (b) the manner in which the person previously coped with environmental stresses and internal conflicts; and (c) the manner of dealing with the organic deficit, which is determined by the person's adjustive patterns and coping mechanisms.

2. Sociocultural factors
These include: (a) the demands of the environment; (b) the psychosocial setting in which the illness develops; (c) the person's cultural background; and (d) the presence or absence of support from family and others.

E. The reactions in organic mental disorders might be regarded as being released by the brain damage and superimposed upon it.

F. The most common organic mental syndromes are delirium, dementia, intoxicaton, and withdrawal.

III. Prevalence

A. Organic mental disorders are common and may occur at any age.

1. Some, such as primary degenerative dementia of the Alzheimer type are found in late life.

2. Others, such as Pick's disease (a presenile focal degenerative disease of the brain affecting the cerebral cortex, particularly the frontal lobes) are found in the late middle life.

3. Others, resulting from head injuries, are more commonly found in early life.

4. Organic brain syndromes associated with infectious diseases, psychoactive substance abuse, or alcohol abuse, may occur at almost any age.

B. Variable incidence

1. Some organic mental disorders seem to be increasing in frequency, as, for example, primary degenerative dementia of the Alzheimer's type; normotensive hydrocephalus (a nonabsorptive communicating type of hydrocephalus that develops in the absence of a demonstrable lesion). These are increasing because of the aging of the population.

2. Others are decreasing in frequency as, for example, the organic mental brain disorder associated with syphilis of the central nervous system (general paresis).

IV. Etiology

A. Any condition that causes cerebral tissue impairment may lead to organic mental disorder.

B. Among the potential causes of organic mental disorder are[1]

1. Endocrine dysfunction
   a) Thyroid disease
   b) Parathyroid disease
   c) Adrenal dysfunction
   d) Hypoglycemia

2. Metabolic and electrolytic abnormalities
   a) Liver disease
   b) Kidney disease
   c) Lung disease
   d) SIADA acidosis, alkalosis
   e) Wilson's disease
   f) Porphyria

3. Nutritional and deficiency states
   a) Vitamin deficiencies such as thiamin, niacin, and vitamin B-12
   b) Iron deficiency
   c) Pernicious anemia

1. G. C. Peterson, "Organic Brain Syndrome," *Psychiatric Clinics of North America* 1(1)(April 1978):21.

4. Drugs and medications
    a) Alcohol
    b) Various sedatives
    c) Anticholinergic drugs
    d) Steroids
    e) Amphetamines
    f) Antihypertensive drugs
5. Toxic conditions
    a) Heavy metal such as lead, mercury, arsenic, thalium
    b) Solvents
    c) Organophosphates
6. Infections
    a) Brain abscess
    b) CNS syphilis
    c) Meningoencephalitis
    d) Pneumonia
    e) Septicema
7. Post-traumatic reactions
    a) Subdural hematoma
    b) Normotensive hydrocephalus
    c) Contusion
8. Degenerative and "slow viral" diseases
    a) Alzheimer's disease
    b) Pick's disease
    c) Amyotropic lateral sclerosis
    d) Huntington's disease
9. Vascular disorders
    a) Hypertension
    b) Cerebral embolism and thrombosis
    c) Cerebral atherosclerosis
    d) Congestive heart failure
10. Neoplastic disorders
    a) Primary brain tumor
    b) Metastic cancer
11. Other causes
    a) Intractible seizures
    b) Status petit mal
    c) Remote effects of carcinoma
C. The most common organic brain disorders seen in clinical practice are the dementias, occurring in the geriatric population.

V. Symptomatology
A. There is usually some evidence of an organic factor from the history, physical, neurological, or laboratory examinations. For example, cerebral concussion or contusion in patients with skull fractures; paralysis, paresis, reflex or sensory changes in patients with brain tumors; urinary or blood chemistry changes in people who have had heavy

metal poisoning; spinal fluid changes in patients with deliria caused by infectious illnesses; evidence of cerebral atrophy on computerized cranial tomography (CT scan) in patients with degenerative diseases such as Alzheimer's, Pick's, or senile dementia; history of excessive alcoholic intake in persons with dementia associated with chronic alcoholism; history of exposure to some industrial toxin in a person with toxic delirium.

B. The symptomatology associated with the various organic brain syndromes (modified from *DSM*-III-R)

   1. Delirium (acute brain syndrome)

      All the symptoms listed below develop over a short period of time, fluctuate rapidly, and are evidenced by physical, neurological, or laboratory examinations, or by a history of specific organic factors.

      a) Reduced ability to maintain attention to external stimuli

      b) Disorganized thinking, as indicated by rambling, irrelevant, or incoherent speech

      c) At least two of the following:

         (1) Reduced level of consciousness (e.g., difficulty keeping awake during examination)

         (2) Perceptual disturbances: misinterpretations, illusions, or hallucinations

         (3) Disturbances of sleep-wake cycle with insomnia or daytime sleepiness

         (4) Increased or decreased psychomotor activity

         (5) Disorientation to time, place, or person

         (6) Memory impairment

   2. Dementia (may be reversible, e.g., normotensive hydrocephalus)

      a) Demonstrable evidence of impairment in short- and long-term memory

      b) At least one of the following:

         (1) Impairment in abstract thinking, as indicated by inability to find similarities and differences between related words and concepts, and other similar tasks

         (2) Impaired judgment, as indicated by inability to make reasonable plans to deal with interpersonal, family, and job-related problems and issues

         (3) Other disturbances of higher cortical function, such as aphasia (disorder of language), apraxia (inability to carry out motor activities despite intact comprehension and motor function), agnosia (failure to recognize or identify objects despite intact sensory function), and "constructional difficulty" (e.g., inability to copy three-dimensional figures, assemble blocks, or arrange sticks in specific designs)

(4) Personality change, that is, alteration or accentuation of premorbid traits
c) The disturbance in a and b above significantly interferes with work or usual social activities or relationships with others.
d) Not occurring exclusively during the course of delirium
e) Either (1) or (2):
(1) There is evidence from the history, physical examination, or laboratory tests of a specific organic factor (or factors) judged to be etiologically related to the disturbance.
(2) In the absence of such evidence, an etiologic organic factor can be presumed if the disturbance cannot be accounted for by any nonorganic mental disorder (e.g., major depression accounting for cognitive impairment).
3. Amnestic syndrome
a) Demonstrable evidence of impairment in both short- and long-term memory disturbance, in the absence of dementia or delirium
b) Not occurring exclusively during the course of delirium, and does not meet the criteria for dementia (i.e., no impairment in abstract thinking or judgment, no other disturbances of higher cortical function, and no personality change)
c) There is evidence from the history, physical examination, or laboratory tests of a specific organic factor (or factors) judged to be etiologically related to the disturbance
4. Organic delusional syndrome (delusions predominate)
a) Prominent delusions
b) Evidence from physical examination, laboratory tests, or a history of a specific organic factor
5. Organic hallucinosis (hallucinations predominate)
a) Persistent or recurrent hallucinations in a state of full wakefulness and alertness
b) There is evidence from the history, physical examination, or laboratory tests of a specific organic factor (or factors) judged to be etiologically related to the disturbance
6. Organic mood syndrome
a) Prominent and persistent depressed, elevated, or expansive mood
b) There is evidence from the history, physical examination, or laboratory tests of a specific organic factor (or factors)
7. Organic anxiety syndrome
a) Prominent, recurrent, panic attacks or generalized anxiety
b) There is evidence from the history, physical examination, or laboratory tests of a specific organic factor (or factors) judged to be etiologically related to the disturbance

8. Organic personality syndrome
    a) A persistent personality disturbance, either lifelong or representing a change or accentuation of a previously characteristic trait, involving at least one of the following:
        (1) Affective instability (e.g., marked shifts from normal mood to depression, irritability, or anxiety)
        (2) Recurrent outbursts of aggression or rage that are grossly out of proportion to any precipitating psychosocial stressors
        (3) Markedly impaired social judgment (e.g., sexual indiscretions)
        (4) Marked apathy and indifference
        (5) Suspiciousness or paranoid ideation
    b) There is evidence from the history, physical examination, or laboratory tests of a specific organic factor (or factors) judged to be etiologically related to the disturbance.
    c) This diagnosis is not given to a child or adolescent if the clinical picture is limited to the features that characterize attention-deficit hyperactivity disorder.
9. Intoxication
    a) Development of a substance-specific syndrome due to recent ingestion of a psychoactive substance. (*Note:* More than one substance may produce similar or identical syndromes.)
    b) Maladaptive behavior during the waking state due to the effect of the substance on the central nervous system (e.g., belligerence, impaired judgment, impaired social or occupational functioning).
    c) The clinical picture does not correspond to any of the other specific organic mental syndromes, such as delirium, organic delusional syndrome, organic hallucinosis, organic mood syndrome, or organic anxiety syndrome.
10. Withdrawal
    a) Development of a substance-specific syndrome that follows the cessation of, or reduction in, intake of a psychoactive substance that the person previously used regularly.
    b) The clinical picture does not correspond to any of the other specific organic mental syndromes, such as delirium, organic delusional syndrome, organic hallucinosis, organic mood syndrome, or organic anxiety syndrome.
11. Organic mental syndrome not otherwise specified are syndromes that do not meet the criteria for any of the other organic mental syndromes and in which there are maladaptive changes during the waking state, with evidence, from either physical examination, laboratory tests, or history, of a specific organic factor that is judged to be etiologically related to the disturbance, should be diagnosed organic mental syndrome NOS. Examples include the

"neurasthenic" picture associated with early Addison's disease and unusual disturbances of consciousness or behavior occurring during seizures.

C. Organic mental disorders
1. Organic mental disorders may be grouped into three categories:
    a) Disorders related to aging of the brain
    b) Disorders due to an ingestion of a substance
    c) Organic mental disorders whose etiology or pathophysiologic process is an Axis III physical disorder or condition, or is unknown.
2. Among the dementias arising in the senium and presenium is primary degenerative dementia of the Alzheimer type. (It should be remembered that the definitive diagnosis of this condition is dependent on histopathologic findings.) The second type of dementia due to aging is multi-infarct dementia.
    a) In Alzheimer disease the dementia is of insidious onset with a generally progressive deteriorating course, whereas with the multi-infarct dementia, the dementia has a course characterized by stepwise deterioration with "patchy" distribution of deficit.
    b) Evidence from history, physical examination, or laboratory tests of significant cerebrovascular disease (recorded on Axis III) and has focal neurologic signs and symptoms.
3. Psychoactive substance-induced organic mental disorder can be produced by any of the psychoactive substances listed in the chapter, "Psychoactive Substance Use Disorders," which include alcohol, amphetamines, caffeine, cannabis, cocaine, hallucinogens, inhalants, nicotine, opioids; phencyclidine (PCP) or similar acting arylcyclohexylamines; and various sedatives, hypnotics, or anxiolytics.

VI. Treatment
A. Treatment depends upon the underlying etiology. Treatment is directed at the underlying mental, medical, or neurological disorder.
B. Certain medications are prescribed. For example, phenothiazines are prescribed for agitation accompanying senile behavior; benzodiazepines, during the withdrawal period from various substance use disorders; and vasodilators, for patients who have vascular disorders of the brain. In many of these cases, only the smallest dose should be used, since patients with brain syndromes are frequently quite sensitive to these drugs.
C. Management of the patient's behavior frequently involves repeating simple explanations and giving help with orientation, as well as frequently adopting a reassuring attitude.
D. Patients who have deliria do better with constant light. Shadows and darkness increase their illusions and frighten them.
E. Some patients need protection from harming themselves or others.

VII. Case examples

A. Case examples, withdrawal

A thirty-five-year-old man was admitted to the hospital for a leg injury. He gave a history of alcoholism dating back to age eighteen and said that he had been drinking at least one pint of whiskey daily for several months prior to admission.

The morning following admission, the nurses noted that he seemed confused and could not give the correct date or the name of the hospital. By late afternoon he appeared anxious and swept his hand along his torso and extremities as if brushing something off. On inquiry, he admitted to "seeing" tiny green animals crawling over his body. By late evening he was very excited and fearful, especially if left by himself in the darkened room. He was transferred to the psychiatric ward, where he recovered from the acute psychotic episode after two days.

In this case, note the history of substance use disorder (chronic alcoholism), the sudden onset of disorientation, mood change, and the vivid, visual hallucinations. Note also the rapid recovery from the acute episode.

B. Case example, delirium

A seventy-four-year-old man developed symptoms of enlarged prostate, or benign prostatic hypertrophy (frequent urination, nocturia, dysuria, and urinary retention). The urinary retention became so severe that he had to be hospitalized.

Two days after admission, he became confused, disoriented, and unruly. He had visual hallucinations (e.g., he saw his son outside his hospital room) and was delusional (he was paranoid about some of the nurses and at times thought he was God). Examination revealed a markedly enlarged prostate gland and an elevated blood urea nitrogen (indicative of uremia). Following surgical resection of the enlarged prostate, his uremia cleared up and his mental symptoms disappeared.

Note that his symptoms were produced by uremia and disappeared when this was cleared up by treating the underlying cause of the uremia.

C. Case example, primary degenerative dementia, presenile onset

A forty-eight-year-old woman was brought to the hospital by her son, who said she was disoriented, showed poor judgment, was difficult to manage, and behaved in a childish manner. The onset of symptoms was noted two years earlier, when she first complained of impaired memory for recent events and forgot some of the routine tasks associated with her job as a receptionist. Very shortly after, she showed poor judgment in dealing with people and made obscene remarks to her colleagues. Because of this behavior, she was fired. At home, she progressively deteriorated: she became slovenly in dress, careless of excreta, and markedly disoriented. At the time of admission, she was incapable of carrying out even simple household tasks.

Examination revealed her to be completely disoriented about time and place. Recent and remote memory were totally defective. She was apathetic, disinterested, and passively cooperative. At times she seemed to be responding to auditory hallucinations. Physical and neurological examinations were essentially negative. A pneumoencephalogram (X-ray examination of the skull after replacing the cerebrospinal fluid with air) revealed findings compatible with generalized cerebral atrophy. She was transferred to a state hospital where her behavior progressively deteriorated.

Note the typical organic symptoms and their progressive nature, a result of the permanent and progressive cerebral atrophy. This generalized cerebral atrophy, occurring in middle life, is called Alzheimer's disease. The pathological changes in the brain are similar to those found in senile dementia.

D. Case example, primary degenerative dementia, senile onset

A seventy-six-year-old widow was admitted to the hospital complaining of memory loss and hallucinations. She had been well until about a year earlier, when her family first noticed that she was forgetful and had trouble remembering the date. Shortly, she began complaining about strange noises in her apartment. The family was not especially concerned by this complaint because they knew that one of her neighbors had frequent parties and that another kept a dog and other pets in his apartment. About four months before admission, the patient began complaining that her next-door neighbor was a gangster and accused him of shooting someone in the apartment. One week before admission, she went to the manager of the apartment building and complained about the people who were walking through her closed doors and windows. Her family was summoned and they brought her to the hospital.

Examination revealed her to be grossly disoriented about time and place. Both recent and remote memory were impaired. She had visual hallucinations (e.g., she saw dogs in her room) and was mildly suspicious of the staff. Physical and neurological studies were negative except for X-ray evidence of mild rheumatoid arthritis. After a few weeks, her hallucinations and delusions cleared up and she recognized that she had experienced a psychotic episode. At the time of her discharge two months later, she was still disoriented about time and had a fair amount of recent memory impairment. However, she was able to return to her apartment and adjust with only minimal supervision.

This is primary degenerative dementia, senile onset. Note the onset in late life of behavioral changes in the absence of any specific positive physical, neurological, or laboratory findings. The "improvement" following hospitalization is not unusual in this type of reaction although, as in this case, there is usually some residual permanent brain damage (disorientation and memory loss persisted after discharge).

References

American Psychiatric Association. *Diagnostic and Statistical Manual of Mental Disorders.* 3d ed., rev. Washington, D.C., 1987.

Goodwin, D. W., and S. B. Guze. *Psychiatric Diagnosis.* 2d ed. New York: Oxford University Press, 1979.

Kaplan, H. I., and B. J. Sadock. *Comprehensive Textbook of Psychiatry/* *IV.* 4th ed. Baltimore: Williams & Wilkins, 1985.

Kolb, L. C. *Modern Clinical Psychiatry.* 10th ed. Philadelphia: W. B. Saunders Co., 1982.

Peterson, G. C. "Organic Brain Syndrome in Symposium on Brain Disorders." *Psychiatric Clinics of North America* 1:21.

False facts are highly injurious to the progress of science, for they often endure long; but false views, if supported by some evidence, do little harm, for everyone takes salutory pleasure in proving their falseness.

Charles Robert Darwin: *Descent of Man* (1871)

Assessment of the Psychiatric Patient

I. Purposes of assessment

A. Assessment procedures play an important role in establishing a working diagnosis and planning a treatment program for a psychiatric patient.

B. Systematic assessment contributes to establishing the probable etiology and course of the patient's disorder, designing the form of intervention, predicting and monitoring response to treatment, evaluating results of treatment, and following up the patient when intervention is terminated.

II. Areas of investigation

Assessment procedures elicit information about the following areas of the patient's condition and experience.

A. Current psychological functioning and symptom formation

B. Current life situation and sources of stress

C. Personal history, including critical developmental incidents

D. Family history

E. Personality structure and defenses (psychodynamics)

F. Strengths, competencies, and abilities

G. Relationships and sources of support

III. Methods of assessment

A. The interview

1. The interview is the most widely used assessment technique in psychiatric practice.

2. The interview provides not only factual information about the patient, but also an opportunity to observe such personal characteristics as appearance, manner, speech, and mode of interpersonal response.

3. Interviews with informants other than the patient provide independent information that may corroborate the patient's report or indicate important omissions and inconsistencies. This source of information is particularly important when patients may be without insight, delusional, confused, or otherwise inaccessible or uncooperative.

4. In psychiatric interviewing, the following points of inquiry are usually included:

   a) The presenting complaint
   b) History of present illness
   c) Nature of previous adjustment
   d) Family and marital history
   e) Educational, social, and occupational history
   f) Past medical history

5. A number of general and specialized structured interview formats are available, including some specially designed to assess *DSM*-III-R Axis II, IV, and V dimensions.

B. Mental-status examination

The mental-status examination is a special form of assessment often conducted in conjunction with the history-taking interview. (Refer to section on symptom formation in mental disorders.) It provides the following kind of outline for recording the interviewer's descriptions of the patient's behavior.

1. Attitude, manner, and behavior
   a) Appearance, dress, facial expression, activity, posture, and demeanor are noted.
   b) Disturbances include deviations of degree of activity, mannerisms, distortions of motility, and uncooperativeness.

2. Mental content
   a) This consists of the thoughts, concerns, and trends that are uppermost in the patient's mind.
   b) Disturbances of content include delusions, hallucinations, obsessions, and phobias.

3. Sensorium and intellect
   a) The degree of the patient's awareness and the level of his or her functioning are assessed.
   b) Disturbances of orientation, memory, retention, attention, information, and judgment can be elicited with standardized questions and test materials.

4. Stream of thought (as manifest in stream of speech)
   a) This includes the quantitative and qualitative aspects of the patient's verbal communication.
   b) Disturbances include over- and underproductivity, disconnectedness, unintelligibility, and incoherence.

5. Emotional tone
   a) This includes the patient's report of subjective feelings (mood or affect) and the examiner's observations of facial expression, posture, and attitude.
   b) Disturbances include both quantitative deviations (elation, depression, apathy) and incongruence (disagreement among the patient's subject report, behavior, and mental content).

6. Insight

   This means the degree to which the patient can appreciate the nature of his or her condition and the need for treatment.

7. Instruments

   Instruments have been developed to standardize the mental-status examination.
   a) The Mental Status Schedule is an example of such an instrument. A trained interviewer, guided by a standard interview schedule, administers the tests and scores the responses at intervals during the session.

b) The Inpatient Multidimensional Psychiatric Scale provides a systematic way for rating the behavior of severely disturbed psychiatric patients.

C. Physical and neurological examination
A routine physical and neurological examination is an essential part of general psychiatric assessment. Special diagnostic and laboratory procedures are used when organic impairment is suspected.

IV. **Psychological testing**
The development of psychological measurements of human characteristics has provided many tools for psychiatric assessment.

A. Variability from person to person is a commonly acknowledged aspect of many characteristics of human behavior. Psychological testing is based on the assumption that this variability can be measured.

B. Technically, a test is a systematic way to compare the behavior of two or more persons.

C. The development, administration, and interpretation of the tests most widely used in psychiatric assessment require special skill and training. The American Psychological Association has established ethical standards for the distribution and use of psychological tests.

D. Criteria for evaluation of psychological tests. Although psychological tests vary in content, purpose, and range of application, they are generally evaluated by the following criteria:

1. *Reliability,* the consistency with which a test measures what it proposes to measure.

2. *Validity,* the accuracy with which a test fulfills its purpose of prediction, selection, or classification.

3. *Standardization,* the establishment of responses of reference groups so that individual performance may be compared with the performance of an appropriate group.

E. Other characteristics of tests

1. Individual versus group
Some tests can be administered to only one person at a time (individual tests); others are administered to a number of persons at one time (group tests).

2. Standardization of administration
Tests vary in the degree to which the tester must follow a prescribed procedure.

3. Objectivity
Tests vary in the degree to which interpretation is required in the scoring of responses. An objective test is one whose scoring minimizes differences among different scorers.

4. Form of response
Some tests require a specific form of response (e.g., true–false); others permit open-end responses (e.g., sentence completion).

F. There are various kinds of psychological tests. In the ensuing sections, we shall describe the most important of the following types:
   1. Intelligence tests
   2. Personality tests
      a) Objective personality tests
      b) Projective techniques of measuring personality
   3. Vocational and educational tests
   4. Neuropsychological tests
   5. Behavioral assessment

V. Intelligence tests

A. The "intelligence" measured by intelligence tests is considered to be a general, relatively stable capacity to learn and deal effectively with one's environment.
B. Intelligence is assumed to be normally distributed in the population.
C. The results of intelligence tests are frequently reported in terms of an IQ (intelligence quotient) score.
   1. The IQ score indicates the position of a person's intelligence test performance relative to the average performance of his or her age group. The average IQ is 100.
   2. The commonly used classification of intelligence measures includes:
      a) Very superior, IQ 130 or more
      b) Superior, 120–129
      c) Bright-normal, 110–119
      d) Average, 90–109
      e) Dull-normal, 80–89
      f) Borderline, 70–79
      g) Mental defective, 69 or less.[1]
D. In psychiatric practice, the intelligence test is used to
   1. Aid in establishing the diagnosis of mental retardation.
   2. Assess the effects of brain damage.
   3. Assess effective intellectual performance in psychiatric disorders.
   4. Define a patient's intellectual resources for educational and vocational adjustment.
   5. Define efficiency of application of intellectual resources (e.g., when limited by anxiety, depression, etc.).
   6. Show patterns of performance, which are viewed as expressions of personality characteristics by some clinicians.

---

1. The American Association of Mental Deficiency and *DSM*-III-R list four categories of mental retardation: mild (IQ 50–69), moderate (IQ 35–50), severe (IQ 20–35), and profound (IQ 20 or below). The IQ limits are, of course, approximate.

E. Since intelligence is, to a substantial degree, defined culturally, tests of intelligence reflect competencies and achievements that are considered important for success in the culture. Interpretations of test results should be made with full consideration of the appropriateness of the test for the particular person who is tested.

F. Major intelligence tests in current usage
  1. The New Revised Stanford-Binet (1960)
     a) Widely used, individually administered intelligence test for children and for the assessment of mental retardation.
     b) Serves as the standard for comparison with other tests of intellectual ability.
     c) Composed of various tasks and problems organized by year levels arranged from two years to superior adult.
     d) The problems successfully solved at each year level are totaled and the sum is expressed as a Mental Age Score and has an IQ score equivalent.
     e) Test has proved useful in the prediction of school achievement.
     f) Examples of types of tasks include vocabulary, memory span for digits, words and sentences, reasoning, comprehension, copying geometric figures, and so forth. Verbal ability is strongly emphasized.
     g) Test is of limited usefulness with adults because it was standardized primarily with children and is composed of tasks that are more appropriate for children.
     h) The test of choice for reliable assessment of the extreme ranges of intelligence, both low and high.
  2. The Wechsler Adult Intelligence Scale (WAIS)
     a) The most widely used individually administered intelligence test for adults and the standard against which other adult intelligence tests are compared.
     b) Composed of a series of subtests organized into a verbal scale and a performance scale.
     c) Verbal subtests are information, comprehension similarities, arithmetic, digit span, vocabulary.
     d) Performance subtests are picture arrangements, picture completion, block design, object assembly, digit symbol.
     e) The test yields three IQ scores: Verbal Scale IQ, Performance Scale IQ, and Full Scale IQ.
     f) Differences between verbal and performance IQ scores may sometimes be of diagnostic value. Many hypotheses have been proposed about ways in which patterns of subtest scores might be related to specific diagnoses, but no widely accepted pattern analysis has been developed.

g) There are three other forms of the Wechsler Intelligence Scale:

    (1) Wechsler-Bellevue Form I, which is now rarely used.

    (2) Wechsler-Bellevue Form II, which is the retest instrument for the WAIS.

    (3) Wechsler Adult Intelligence Scale, Revised (WAIS-R). In the administration of this recently developed form, each Verbal subtest is alternated with a Performance subtest rather than administering the total Verbal Scale first and then the Performance Scale as was the procedure with the other forms.

h) Two forms of the test have also been developed for children.

    (1) The Wechsler Intelligence Scale for Children (WISC-R) is a 1974 revision of the original WISC. It is designed for children ages five to fifteen and is the most widely used intelligence test for children.

    (2) The Wechsler Preschool Primary Scale of Intelligence (WPPSI) has been developed for children ages four to six-and-one-half.

    (3) Special individually administered intelligence tests have been devised for use with illiterate, blind, deaf, and other handicapped persons who would not be accurately tested on the standard tests.

    (4) Group tests

        (a) Large numbers of paper-and-pencil group tests of intelligence are available and are used primarily in schools and personnel departments in business and industry.

        (b) Although these tests generally yield IQ scores, it may be more meaningful to reserve the use of the term IQ for the results of individually administered intelligence tests.

VI. Personality tests

A. There is a great variety of personality measures that differ in form, content, purpose, and interpretation.

B. Some personality measures are attempts to assess personality traits or characteristics, others are attempts to reveal a pattern of personality dynamics (e.g., motives, defenses, conflicts).

C. Personality measures can be divided roughly into objective tests and projective techniques.

VII. Objective personality tests

A. Objective tests usually take the form of questionnaires or rating scales; the subjects respond to the items according to how characteristic they are of their experience and behavior.

B. Tests are administered and scored in a standardized way; the results are expressed in numerical scores.
C. Since objective tests are a form of self-report, they are open to faking and dissimulation. However, their ease of administration permits the testing of large numbers of persons by staff other than special clinical personnel.
D. The Minnesota Multiphasic Personality Inventory (MMPI) is the most widely used objective personality test in psychiatric practice in the United States. It consists of 566 true–false items.
   1. Validity scales
      There are four special scales that are scored to indicate response tendencies and test-taking attitudes that might make interpretations of the test doubtful.
   2. Clinical scales
      a) Responses are scored in terms of correspondence to the responses of diagnosed psychiatric groups. The clinical scales can be scored for hypochondriasis, depression, hysteria, psychopathic deviate, paranoia, psychasthenia, schizophrenia, and mania.
      b) Two other scales, masculinity-femininity and social introversion, are typically used in connection with the clinical scales.
   3. Other scales
      In addition to the clinical scales, many research scales have been developed for special purposes or to measure other personality characteristics (e.g., dependency, ego-strength).
   4. Interpretation
      Interpretation of the test is based on the pattern of scores. In recent years, standardized interpretations have been developed for common patterns. Computer programs can now be used to score the test and produce analyses of the profiles of the scores.
   5. Evaluation
      A sizable literature (more than six thousand articles and books) has been developed around the MMPI. Reviews of this literature indicate that the test is sufficiently reliable and valid for many applications.
   6. The MMPI is currently undergoing its first revision and restandardization.
E. Other objective personality tests in clinical use
   1. Although hundreds of personality tests and scales have been developed to evaluate and extend particular theories of personality or for other research purposes, most of them are not directly useful as diagnostic or descriptive instruments in clinical practice.

2. Other multiple-scale objective tests that have been found useful in psychiatric practice include the following:
   a) Cattell's Sixteen Personality Factor Scale (16 PF)
   b) The Differential Personality Inventory (DPI) developed by Jackson and Messick
   c) The Millon Multiaxial Clinical Inventory (MMCI)
   d) Gough's California Psychological Inventory (CPI)
   e) The Myers-Briggs Type Indicator, which is based on Jung's theory of personality types
3. None of these tests has as yet rivaled the wide range of clinical application and research of the MMPI, but they may prove to be valuable additions to clinical assessment techniques.

VIII. Projective techniques of measuring personality

A. Characteristics of projective measures
   1. The term *projective* implies that the patients "project" their personalities into the responses they make.
   2. The materials of most projective methods are unstructured or ambiguous; thus, they require that the patient organize them in some imaginative way.
   3. The patients have considerable freedom in their responses.
   4. It is assumed that the way the patients respond reveals emotional and motivational factors that are characteristic of them, though perhaps unconsciously.
   5. The interpretation of the responses is subjective and is usually based on the theoretical assumptions of the interpreter. This leads to less consistent interpretation than is obtained with objective tests.
   6. Both the administration and interpretation of projective tests require special training and experience.

B. The Rorschach method
   The Rorschach is the best known and most widely used of the projective techniques.
   1. History
      a) Hermann Rorschach, a Swiss psychiatrist, initiated the use of inkblots for diagnostic and descriptive purposes. His students introduced the Rorschach test to the United States. Beginning in the 1930s, the United States became the major source of research on the Rorschach.
      b) Several systems, or approaches to the test, have been developed. Among the best known systems are those of Samuel Beck, Marguerite Hertz, Bruno Klopfer, Zygmut Piotrowski, and David Rapport, together with Roy Schafer.

    c) There have been many differences of opinion and controversies among these systematizers. Each system has its own position on administration, scoring (including scoring symbols), and interpretation, but there are some general similarities among them.

    d) J. E. Exner has integrated the various approaches into a comprehensive system of scoring and interpretation.

2. Administration

    a) The materials consist of ten "inkblots." Although there are differences in instructions from system to system, in general, patients are asked to describe what each one looks like. They may offer as many responses to each card as they wish.

    b) Following the administration of the test, the examiner questions the subject about the response made, asking him or her to indicate the location on the inkblot that prompted the response, and to say what about the blot (e.g., shape, color, texture) contributed to the response. Again, there are some differences among the five approaches as to how much detail and elaboration are elicited in this inquiry.

3. Scoring

Responses are scored according to

    a) Content (e.g., human, animal, object, X ray).

    b) The area of the blot included in the content (whole blot or a particular section of it).

    c) The characteristics of the blot (e.g., color, shading, and shape) that determined the content.

4. Interpretation

    a) Interpretation is based on the assumed personal significance of the responses, as well as on characteristic ways in which the patients organize their responses.

    b) Theories about Rorschach responses relate such factors as location, use of color, texture, and movement as well as content and sequence to personality characteristics, psychopathology, and special strengths.

    c) In all five systems, interpretation rests heavily on psychoanalytic theory. The Klopfer system is strongly Jungian in its interpretive emphasis.

5. Evaluation

A tremendous literature (more than six thousand articles and books) pertaining to the Rorschach has developed. The complexity of the technique (administration, scoring, and interpretation) and the existence of different systematic approaches to the test have made research difficult. Although some of the research has been rigorous, much of it has not met high standards

of research design. Reviews of the Rorschach literature over the years have consistently raised serious questions about the reliability and validity of this instrument.
C. Thematic Apperception Test (TAT)
　1. This test consists of twenty illustrations. The patient is asked to tell a story about the content of each picture.
　2. Stories are interpreted in terms of their themes, the handling of motivational states, the resolution of conflicts, the ways in which interpersonal relations are presented, and the extent to which patients identify themselves with the characters they describe.
　3. Several complete methods of scoring have been developed. They require special training.
D. Other projective techniques
　1. A large number of other techniques, involving word association, sentence completion, drawing, and storytelling have been devised.
　2. They have in common the assumption that imaginative productions and fantasy yield important clues to personality.

IX. **Vocational and educational tests**
A. Since the problems faced by some patients involve vocational maladjustment and dissatisfaction, vocational testing can contribute important information to a total treatment program. In general, vocational tests are of two types, measurements of aptitude and measures of interests.
B. Aptitude tests
　1. Available tests measure a variety of special aptitudes and abilities such as clerical ability, mechanical ability, spatial reasoning, hand-and-finger dexterity, and rate of manipulation.
　2. Norms permit comparison of individual scores with scores of representative occupational groups.
C. Achievement tests
　1. Achievement tests, which measure the outcome of learning experiences, can yield useful information on the level and extent of a person's attainment of educationally based skills.
　2. Achievement tests can be classified in three general categories:
　　a) Survey batteries that contain various individual subject matter or skill tests
　　b) Specific subject or area tests
　　c) Diagnostic tests that are designed to help determine someone's strengths and weaknesses in particular areas.
　3. There is an extremely large variety of achievement tests, most of which are designed for classroom use or that require the administrative and interpretive skills of an educational specialist.

4. Although achievement cannot usually be explored in detail in most psychiatric assessment, some appraisal of achievement is useful, since level of achievement is often involved in referral.
5. A useful achievement test for psychiatric assessment is the Wide Range Achievement Test (WRAT).
    a) WRAT scores indicate a person's current level in word recognition, spelling, and arithmetic computation.
    b) The WRAT helps determine weaknesses in areas that are essential as background for academic learning, and results can suggest the need for further evaluation and remediation.
D. Interest tests
    1. Interest tests permit the comparison of the individual's interests with the interests of persons representative of a number of professions and occupations.
    2. The most commonly used vocational interest test for adults is the Strong-Campbell Interest Inventory (SCII).
    3. The correlation of the individual's interests with those of representative members of particular occupations has been shown to be strongly related to job satisfaction.
E. Professional and managerial tests
    1. The assessment of aptitude for professional and managerial occupations is more complex.
    2. It involves the assessment of a variety of factors, including information, intellect, personality, attitudes, and interests.
    3. These tests are not considered as valid as the simpler tests of aptitudes and interests.

X. Neuropsychological tests
A. The assessment of intellectual deficit and the differentiation of organic brain conditions is often a problem in psychiatric diagnosis.
B. More accurate assessments of deficits due to brain damage can be made if earlier test scores, with which present performance can be compared, are available. This is seldom possible.
C. There are some tests that compare performance that is more sensitive to brain damage (e.g., abstract reasoning), with performance that is less affected (e.g., vocabulary).
D. Other tests have been designed to assess specific aspects of brain function such as memory, perception, language use, and motor coordination.
E. Neuroscientists and cognitive scientists have been making rapid advances in the localization of brain activity and the assessment of cognitive functioning. Techniques that have been developed for research purposes may also have great value in the clinical assessment of neurological deficits and potential for recovery.

XI. Behavioral assessment

A. The increase in the application of behavioral concepts and methodology to clinical practice has been accompanied by the elaboration of techniques of assessing behavior.

B. In behavioral assessment, emphasis is placed on the objective description of behavior and on the environmental events and contexts that were antecedent and consequent to the behavior being investigated.

C. Although some behavioral assessment is similar to traditional methods of investigation, the purpose is to elicit information about characteristic reactions to situations with a minimum of inference, rather than to elicit information about psychodynamic determinants.

D. The emphasis on objective-descriptions of current behavior makes behavioral assessment useful to the eclectic practitioner.

E. Techniques of behavioral assessment include:

1. Interviewing
   a) The interview is used to obtain self-reported information about problem behavior and the circumstances that influence it.
   b) The interview also provides an opportunity to raise and test hypotheses about the events that may interfere with or support attempts to modify the patient's behavior.

2. Inventories and scales
   a) Self-reported information can be obtained with questionnaires and "behavior-and-situation" checklists.
   b) A large and continually increasing number of special-purpose devices has been developed and information about reliability and applicability is accumulating.

3. Observation
   a) Both direct and indirect techniques have been used to obtain information about behavior.
   b) Although indirect methods are preferred because they do not, in themselves, influence behavior, they may not be feasible in most clinical situations.

4. Simulation
   a) This technique is also called role playing.
   b) "Real-life" situations are constructed, and patients are asked to assume a role.
   c) By observing how the role is played, the therapist is enabled to observe the patient's characteristic modes of response.
   d) Investigation of similarities in behavior in natural and simulated situations suggests that there is a fair degree of consistency.

5. Assessment of therapeutic change
    a) All the methods described in this section contribute to the modification of problem behavior by directing the patient's attention to the frequency with which it occurs and the contexts in which it is most likely to occur.
    b) Self-observation and simulation provide the patient as well as the therapist with opportunities to modify and monitor changes in behavior.
    c) In behavior therapy, the problems are formulated in terms of behavior that is to be altered. Thus, techniques of behavioral assessment can be used to determine the frequency and consistency of behavioral change and, thus, provide an index of success of treatment.
6. The integration of data from various assessment sources may yield a more comprehensive analysis of patient behavior, which emphasizes behavioral interrelationships rather than focusing on specific classes of behavior.

XII. Trends in psychiatric assessment

A. While emphasis in the use of assessment remains on establishing a diagnosis and providing a personality description of the patient, attention is now also given to defining problems and developing a program of intervention.
B. Emphasis is also shifting from the assessment of psychopathology or deficiencies to an inclusion of areas of competency.
C. Insofar as much behavior seems to be influenced by special characteristics of the environment, more attention is being paid to the assessment of situations and the way the person responds to and influences them.
D. As patients play a more active role in their own treatment and management, self-assessment procedures assume importance.
E. Assessment is becoming an essential component of therapeutic intervention, from its initial stages through follow-up.
F. In the multiaxial classification proposed in *DSM*-III-R, assessment is not only of symptoms (Axis I), personality (Axis II), and physical disorders (Axis III), but also of experiential and situational sources of stress (Axis IV) and competence or level of adaptive functioning (Axis V).
G. Assessment is conducted by each discipline of adjunctive therapies (e.g., occupational therapy, art therapy, etc.) and by nursing. The problems of each patient are identified, sometimes through structured tests and tasks (as in occupational therapy) and sometimes through observing the patient's characteristics, movements, and ways of relating to others (as in movement therapy and nursing). Interventions and possible rehabilitation and growth plans are then developed.

H. Programs and institutions are now assessed, so that the progress of the individual patient is viewed in relation to the effectiveness of programs in medical and social institutions.

References

American Psychiatric Association. *Diagnostic and Statistical Manual of Mental Disorders.* 3d. ed., rev. Washington, D.C., 1987.

American Psychological Association. *Standards for Educational and Psychological Tests and Manuals.* Washington, D.C., 1974.

Cronbach, L. *Essentials of Psychological Testing.* New York: Harper & Row, 1960.

Hersen, M., A. E. Kazdin, and A. S. Bellack, eds. *The Clinical Psychology Handbook.* New York: Pergamon Press, 1983.

Kaplan, H. I. and B. J. Sadock eds. *Comprehensive Textbook of Psychiatry/IV.* 4th ed. Baltimore: Williams & Wilkins, 1985.

Kendall, P. C., and J. D. Norton-Ford. *Clinical Psychology.* New York: John Wiley & Sons, 1982.

Kleinmuntz, B. *Personality and Psychological Assessment.* New York: St. Martin's Press, 1982.

The light that a man receiveth by counsel from another is drier and purer than that which cometh from his own understanding and judgement, which is ever infused and drenched in his affections and customs.

Francis Bacon, "Of Friendship," *Essays,* 1625

Treatment In Psychiatry: Psychotherapy

I. Introduction

A. Although reference has been made to types of treatment throughout the chapters on the various clinical syndromes, in this and the following two chapters the major modes of treatment available in psychiatry will be presented.

B. In the presentation on etiology in the first chapter of the outline, attention was given to possible causative factors. The possible sources were loosely classified as:
   1. Psychological and developmental
   2. Social and environmental
   3. Biological

C. Similarly, treatment can be classified according to the presumed causative factors that are being treated.
   1. Individual psychotherapy presumes the importance of factors in the personality dynamics and experiential history of the patient.
   2. Group, family, activity and expressive therapies presume the importance of factors in the social relationships and social communications of the patient.
   3. Pharmacological and somatic therapies presume the importance of genetic, physiological, and neural factors.

D. This chapter will be concerned with individual psychotherapy and the following two chapters will be concerned with group, family, and adjunctive therapies and pharmacological and somatic therapies, respectively.

II. Definition

A. In the broad sense, many things that are done to or for a patient may have a psychotherapeutic effect.

B. As defined in the more traditional sense in *A Psychiatric Glossary,* psychotherapy is "a process in which a person who wishes to relieve *symptoms* or resolve problems in living or is seeking personal growth enters into an implicit or explicit contract to interact in a prescribed way with the psychotherapist."[1]

C. Traditionally, distinctions have been drawn between the practice of psychotherapy and the practice of counseling in terms of differences in professional training of practitioners, type of patient or client treated, and setting in which treatment takes place. Currently, these distinctions are somewhat blurred or have been defined in terms of licensing and certification practices of individual states.

III. Types of psychotherapy

A. The types of therapy covered in this chapter are those that involve a one-to-one relationship between therapist and patient. Group and family therapies will be treated in the next chapter.

---

1. American Psychiatric Association, *A Psychiatric Glossary,* 6th ed. (Washington, D.C., 1988).

B. There are many variants of psychotherapy and the array of approaches can certainly be confusing to students and consumers.

C. Although psychotherapies can be classified in various ways according to historical traditions, goals of treatment, theoretical orientations, and stated principles of method, the organization in this chapter will be a descriptive one that is representative of the most widely used approaches.

   1. Psychoanalysis
   2. Expressive and insight-oriented psychodynamic therapies
   3. Supportive therapies
   4. Behavior therapies
   5. Cognitive therapies
   6. Humanistic therapies (phenomenological and existential)

D. Common elements in psychotherapy
   Marmor lists seven elements that are common to all forms of psychotherapy.

   1. Relationship (see therapist-patient relationship as discussed under IV.) Each person contributes something to the therapeutic experience.
      a) The patient has a perceived need to change. This must be accompanied by an element of motivation and expectancy of getting help.
      b) The therapist brings to the relationship knowledge (this includes adequate training, discipline, and the capability of "understanding"), objectivity (the "fair neutrality" that allows the patient to be himself or herself), empathy (warm understanding), and integrity.
   2. Emotional release (usually brought about by verbalizing).
   3. Cognitive learning (each psychotherapist, regardless of his or her orientation, conveys therapeutic objectives and in some way offers an explanation about how change is going to occur).
   4. Conditioning (all forms of therapy, regardless of orientation, have some element of conditioning, even if it is covert and implicit, e.g., the therapist conveys a certain set of values and what is "neurotic" and "nonneurotic").
   5. Identification (modeling or "social learning").
   6. Suggestion (persuasive and suggestive elements are either implicit or explicit in all forms of therapy).
   7. Reality testing (also referred to as "rehearsal," or "practicing" of the new ways of coping that are learned in therapy).

IV. **General characteristics of therapeutic relationships**
    Of the common elements in psychotherapy, the nature and quality of the therapist-patient relationship is often cited as of particular significance. While the special features of the therapeutic relationship may be identified by a variety of terms, the following psychodynamic concepts give an idea of its special nature.

A. Rapport
   1. *A Psychiatric Glossary* defines *rapport* as "the feeling of harmonious accord and mutual responsiveness that contributes to the patient's confidence in the therapist and willingness to work cooperatively. It is to be distinguished from *transference,* which is unconscious."[2]
   2. Rapport is important in any treatment relationship, regardless of whether the patient is being treated for an emotional or a physical illness.
   3. It is probably the single most effective therapeutic tool a physician has.
   4. Some therapists speak of the "therapeutic alliance," which involves the primarily conscious and rational aspects of the treatment relationship. It is an agreement to work toward a mutual therapeutic goal.
   5. Whatever treatment modality is used, *confidentiality* is an essential element of the relationship.
B. Transference—Countertransference
   1. *Transference* is the patient's unconscious attachment to the therapist (or others involved in the patient's treatment) of feelings and attitudes that were originally related to important figures (e.g., parents, siblings) in early life.
   2. Transference can become so intense that it leads to the development of a "transference neurosis," a state in which early feelings and attitudes make up the bulk of the patient's feelings toward the physician.
   3. *Countertransference* is the therapist's unconscious or conscious emotional reaction to the patient.
      a) Feelings arising from the therapist's unresolved underlying conflicts may at times become intense and interfere with an understanding of the patient.
      b) It is especially important that a therapist recognize any underlying negative countertransference.
      c) Sometimes countertransference can be used diagnostically and therapeutically. For example, irritability or hostility in a therapist may be induced by fear in the patient; if the therapist is aware of the countertransference, he or she may more directly and correctly help the patient identify the underlying conflicts, recognize the fear, and resolve the issues behind it.
   4. Both positive and negative feelings are involved in transference and countertransference.

2. American Psychiatric Association, *A Psychiatric Glossary,* 6th ed. (Washington, D.C., 1988).

C. Resistance
   1. Resistance arises from the conscious or unconscious psychological forces in the patient that oppose bringing repressed (unconscious) material into consciousness.
   2. Resistance is encountered in all forms of therapy, but is especially noted in individual psychotherapy.
   3. It represents a mobilization of underlying defenses to resist treatment.
   4. In any given situation, the physician must decide whether to leave the patient's resistance intact or to try to reduce it.
D. Many variables may affect outcomes in psychotherapy but the personality of the individual psychotherapist as it influences the relationship must be considered an important determinant.

V. Psychoanalysis
A. As noted in the chapter, "Psychodynamic Concepts," *psychoanalysis* means a theory of personality development, a method of research, and a system of treatment. It was originally developed by Sigmund Freud.
B. As a treatment technique, it is defined in *A Psychiatric Glossary* as follows: "Through analysis of *free associations* and *interpretation* of dreams, emotions and behavior are traced to the influence of *repressed instinctual drives* and *defenses against them in the unconscious*."[3]
C. Because it involves a large expenditure of time, feeling, and money, psychoanalysis has only a limited place in the treatment of most mental disorders. However, the insights gained from it have been extremely helpful in the other forms of psychotherapy.
D. Characteristics of psychoanalytic therapy
   1. As used by psychoanalysts, uncovering involves the exploration of the unconscious, chiefly through free association, which *A Psychiatric Glossary* defines as "the spontaneous uncensored verbalizations by the patient of whatever comes to mind."[4]
   2. Dream material is often evaluated for clues to unconscious feelings, and interpretations are made to the patient.
   3. Resistance (see above) must be recognized and dealt with.
   4. Of major importance in this type of therapy is the therapist's ability to be a meaningful listener.
   5. Interpretation is an integral part of this type of therapy. Interpretations may be made either of currently operating psychodynamic factors or of psychogenic forces. (The latter is focused on the relationship between current reactive states and past emotion.) Interpretation also helps to reduce resistance.

---

3. American Psychiatric Association, *A Psychiatric Glossary,* 6th ed. (Washington, D.C., 1988).
4. Ibid.

6. The interpretation and analysis of transference provides a substantial framework on which psychoanalytic therapy is developed.
7. Correlation (reconstruction) is also employed to help relate past, repressed conflicts to current situations.
8. "Working through" follows the development of insight and comprises a major portion of the treatment time. It includes repeated exploration of the insight gained through interpretation.

VI. Psychodynamic psychotherapy

A. Psychoanalytic theory has influenced the procedures of many psychotherapists who themselves are not practitioners of psychoanalysis.
B. The general purpose of psychodynamic therapy is to produce insight by uncovering emotional conflicts, chiefly unconscious, so that they can be dealt with in a way that does not hamper current relationships and activities.
C. Psychodynamic psychotherapy is based on assumptions that are derived from psychoanalytic theory.
1. Patients' symptoms are expressions in current relationships of neurotic conflicts.
2. Current conflicts are manifestations of patterns of conflict established in childhood.
3. Recognition of the conflict and its childhood relevance is difficult because of unconscious factors.
4. Therapeutic change occurs as a result of insight into the connections between current maladaptive behaviors and their relation to neurotic conflict.
5. Interpretation of transference and resistance is an important contributor to progress in treatment.
D. The following three case examples illustrate some of the features of psychodynamic therapy.

1. A forty-five-year-old widower complained of impotence. After three interviews, it became obvious that his symptom resulted from two important factors: (a) his guilt over having rejected his wife because she was physically unattractive; (b) the guilt was reactivated when he was sexually aroused.

His impotence was a protection against a second marriage to a woman he was dating but did not wish to marry. In this case, the conflicts were relatively superficial and readily accessible to the therapist. His symptom cleared up when he recognized the dynamic factors and broke off his relationship with the woman.

2. A twenty-five-year-old man had consulted many physicians for palpitation, tachycardia, precordial pain, and apprehension. Each time, physical and laboratory examinations revealed no evidence of cardiac disease. Although he worried about his heart, his symptoms were typical of anxiety disorder.

During the first interview, it became apparent that his symptoms were related to his feelings about his father, but it was not until he had been seen for twelve sessions that he was able to see the relationship between his own symptoms and his father's heart attack a year earlier. When he did see that the onset of his own symptoms followed his father's heart attack and that his anxiety was being perpetuated by his guilt over his unconscious wish for his father's death, his symptoms disappeared.

3. A thirty-year-old housewife had repeated episodes of parthesias, dizziness, and pains in her arms. These had begun shortly after marriage and seriously handicapped her. After about fifty hours of psychotherapy, she was able to recognize that these symptoms always developed when she felt rejected by her husband. This rejection awakened the underlying feelings that she had had when her father rejected her. When she recognized this, her symptoms cleared up.

The conflict here was unconscious and hence not as immediately available. Uncovering therapy brought the conflict to light.

VII. Supportive psychotherapy

A. Supportive psychotherapy deals predominantly with conscious material and is centered chiefly on bolstering the individual's strength and assets (enhancing self-esteem and ego-strength). It reinforces healthy defenses (enhances the patient's defensive functioning) and is based primarily on the therapist-patient relationship (thus, it fosters and maintains a positive transference), including the therapeutic alliance. Unlike uncovering psychotherapy, the focus tends to be on current problems; probing into the unconscious past is avoided. It usually requires an active "giving of self" by the therapist (e.g., it may require extra time, availability, and the giving of advice). As a matter of fact, many patients receiving supportive therapy have had such extreme difficulty with interpersonal relationships that the therapist must be more of a "real object" and less of an anonymous neutral figure as it necessary in more intensive or interpretative therapies.

B. The treatment objectives are usually limited. It is usually indicated for patients with acute emotional upheavals (e.g., anxiety disorders, depressive disorders) or for patients with acute psychotic decompensation, or it is often appropriate for chronically severely ill patients (especially those who are trying to live in the community and especially for those with prominent, primitive defense mechanisms of projection and denial).

C. Techniques include reassurance, unburdening, environmental modification, persuasion, and clarification. Interpretations are usually avoided.

1. Reassurance
   Reassurance is the imparting or restoration of confidence and freeing the patient from fear and anxiety. It does not mean false reassurance. Reassurance cannot be imparted if the therapist is not herself or himself assured.

a) Physical, laboratory, and X-ray examinations may relieve a person's anxiety about significant organic illness, and hence be reassuring.

b) Examples of psychological reassurance include assuring panicky or obsessive-ruminative persons who fear serious mental breakdown that they will not lose their minds; assuring parents that the hostile and aggressive feelings they occasionally have about their children are not abnormal and will not lead to physical abuse; explaining to acutely depressed persons that their illness will be resolved.

2. Unburdening

a) *Unburdening* is the therapeutic release of feelings through conscious, free expression. This is "getting it off the chest." It is also called *ventilation* and *catharsis*.

b) It serves two purposes: sharing, which helps "dilute" the feelings; and self-punishment, by revealing oneself.

c) For example, a sixty-year-old woman was finally able to tell the doctor how she had been emotionally clutching onto her thirty-five-year-old married daughter. After unburdening herself of this fact, which she had never before been able to verbalize, she was able to take the first major steps to release the hold on her daughter.

3. Environmental modification

a) *Environmental modification,* also called, *environmental intervention* or *environmental manipulation,* means altering the environment so as to relieve the patient's symptoms and distress.

b) Caution must be exercised lest this type of treatment be misused.

c) Examples are providing a temporary homemaker or housekeeper for an anxious or depressed mother whose symptoms are aggravated by her responsibility for her young children; placing a patient in the relatively neutral environment of a hospital; placing a runaway child in a foster home until the parents can work out the marital conflicts that contributed to the running away; advising a vacation for a widower whose grief has been unduly prolonged.

4. Persuasion

a) *Persuasion* is direct suggestion, inducement, or entreatment in an effort to influence a patient's behavior.

b) Examples include asking a person who seems to be becoming psychologically dependent on alcohol for relaxation to try jogging, bicycling, or some other kind of physical exercise; asking a spouse to modify his or her behavior and attitudes if the patient for some reason is unable to do this (this example also includes the element of environmental modification).

5. Clarification
   a) *Clarification* is a process by which the physician helps patients to understand their feelings and behavior and to gain a clearer picture of reality.
   b) Examples include pointing out to an agitated and depressed patient that a period of hospitalization will not worsen the condition; showing a paranoid patient how he or she is projecting; pointing out to a married person the rejecting behavior of a spouse who is really seeking a dissolution of the marriage.

VIII. Behavior therapy

Behavior therapy has a specific meaning when used by some writers, but it will be used here as a general term that refers to all therapy that is derived from principles of learning (see the chapter, "Behavioral and Cognitive Concepts").

A. Background
   1. Pavlov, late in his career, attempted to give an account of human psychiatric disorders in terms of excitation and inhibition, the concepts that had so successfully accounted for data from his animal laboratory. His clinical interpretations were less successful, but he did stimulate other experimental scientists of learning to apply their analyses to clinical disorders.
   2. Watson (1920) and Jones (1924) demonstrated how a focal fear or phobia could be learned and extinguished by classical conditioning, but these demonstrations had no significant impact on the practice or theory of clinical psychiatry.
   3. Psychologists working with children with poor "habits" (e.g., nail biting, bed-wetting, temper tantrums) during the 1920s and 1930s developed practical techniques that are now viewed as forms of behavior therapy (Dunlop, 1930).
   4. Learning theorists such as O. H. Mowrer (1950), Neal Miller and John Dollard (1950), attempted to interpret psychoanalytic theory and therapy in terms of the systematic learning theory of Clark Hull (1943); their writings renewed the interest of some experimental psychologists in psychiatric problems.
   5. B. F. Skinner and his student, Ogden Lindsley (1954), applied operant analysis of learning to the behavior of schizophrenics, and this incursion into the realm of psychiatric disorder was rapidly followed by the application of the same methods to treatment or, in operant conditioning terminology, behavior modification.
   6. The publication by Joseph Wolpe in 1958 of his book *Psychotherapy by Reciprocal Inhibition* attracted widespread attention to developments in therapy in several countries and signaled the beginning of the modern era of behavior therapy.

7. Hans Eysenck (1958) encouraged a systematic approach to the theory and practice of behavior therapy by emphasizing the main points of difference from traditional psychotherapy.

B. General principles

1. Behavior therapy can be defined as the modification of responses through the application of experimentally established principles of learning.

2. Maladaptive behavior is viewed as either deficient or excessive. Thus, therapy involves increasing the incidence of appropriate behavior and decreasing behavior that is inappropriate in frequency, duration, or place of occurrence.

3. Maladaptive responses may be covert as well as overt. Thus, such traditional cognitive symptoms as hallucinations, delusions, and fantasies are not, in principle, recalcitrant to behavior therapy.

4. Psychiatric disorders are viewed primarily, though not exclusively, as the result of faulty learning.

5. Treatment is directed toward the removal of the inappropriate behavior (symptoms) and toward learning new, more effective patterns of behavior.

6. Emphasis in treatment is placed particularly on the social environment as a source of stimuli that support symptoms but that can also support changes in behavior.

7. The experimental study of learning and the clinical practice of behavior therapy are viewed as mutually supporting activities that together can contribute to a unified understanding of learned behavior.

C. Types of behavior therapy

There are many variants of behavior therapy, but the examples that follow typify the most widely used techniques.

1. Systematic desensitization

a) This technique was developed by Joseph Wolpe as a means of associating anxiety-eliciting stimuli with relaxation.

b) Since anxiety and relaxation are incompatible reactions, the increase in the strength of relaxation responses will inhibit the anxious responses to the same stimuli.

c) Wolpe's approach consists of three stages.

(1) Relaxation training similar to the procedures introduced by Jacobson in 1938, in which the subject is taught to identify and control localized tension and relaxation of muscle groups.

(2) Construction of hierarchies of anxiety-producing stimuli by the subject; these threatening stimuli or events in the subject's life are ranked by the reactions they produce, from the weakest to strongest.

(3) Desensitization proper. The subject, in a deep state of relaxation, is presented with a stimulus from the weak end of the hierarchy and then with successively stronger ones as he or she is able to maintain relaxation.

d) Variations of this "gradual-approach" method have been used to rehearse adequate behavior in an anxiety-inhibiting context (e.g., assertiveness training).

2. Aversion therapy

a) This is the oldest of the three procedures outlined in this section, but it was used for many years with little systematic attention to the principles of learning that were applied.

b) This therapy is based on straightforward classical (Pavlovian) conditioning procedures. Stimuli are associated with some strong, unacceptable responses such as nausea, pain, or extreme disgust.

c) The noxious stimuli that are used to produce the response of aversion may be chemical (e.g., apomorphine), electrical, or visual (including imaginal).

d) Aversion therapy has most often been used in the treatment of habitual excesses (e.g., overuse of alcohol) and compulsive unacceptable or criminal social behavior (e.g., shoplifting, exhibitionism).

e) Considerable controversy has been generated both about the effectiveness of aversion therapy and the social appropriateness of aversive control of socially deviant behavior. (The novel and movie *A Clockwork Orange* provide examples of the social concern about aversive control of behavior.)

f) Both operant conditioning analyses of the effect of aversive stimuli and the exploration of the effect of aversive imagery are attempts to find less unpleasant and more socially acceptable alternatives to aversion therapy.

3. Behavior modification

a) *Behavior modification* is conducted by the application of operant conditioning principles to the interpretation and management of behavior problems.

b) The basic principle of behavior modification is the control of the reinforcing consequences of behavior. *Reinforcing consequences* range from physical reinforcers (e.g., food) to social reinforcers (e.g., approval, tokens of exchange).

c) Behavior modification has been used in a variety of institutional settings and on a great variety of problems. Striking examples include language training of autistic children, self-care training of intellectually retarded children and adults, and socialization of regressed psychotic patients.

d) Some chronic wards of psychiatric hospitals, some training schools and institutions for mentally retarded children and adults, and increasing numbers of day-care and residential programs for mentally ill and mentally retarded adults are managed according to operant conditioning principles in a "token economy." That is, appropriate changes in behavior are rewarded with tokens that can be exchanged for food, activities, and privileges.

e) Operant principles, combining rehearsal and modeling with reinforcement, have been used not only to modify maladaptive behaviors in chronic mentally ill individuals but also to train social skills toward a level of improved social skills toward a level of improved social adequacy and appropriateness.

f) Self-regulation techniques, by which patients learn to distinguish the environmental stimuli that evoke their maladaptive behavior and to manage their own reinforcing consequences, have grown in popularity among behavior therapists and have become a significant part of the popular literature of self-treatment (e.g., weight regulation, reduction of smoking, etc.).

g) Biofeedback techniques are a form of self-regulation based on operant methods. The subjects monitor their own physiological processes (muscle tension, brain waves) and, using the information they receive (feedback), learn to control them within limits.

h) Behavior modification is the most active, rapidly expanding, and enthusiastically professed learning approach to therapy.

4. Evaluation
   a) Although behavior therapy was initially developed for and applied in the treatment of phobias and compulsions, it does not appear to be limited to reactions (symptoms) that obviously fit a learning interpretation.
   b) Since the emphasis in treatment is on modification of symptoms, the question of substitution has been raised by some critics (i.e., the removal of one symptom may lead to another if the underlying cause is not also treated). However, according to proponents of the therapy, substitution does not usually occur.

c) Some enthusiastic supporters of behavior therapy, such as Hans Eysenck, claim that their evaluations show behavior therapy to be clearly superior to other forms of psychotherapy, particularly psychoanalysis.

d) More moderate and well-controlled evaluations indicate that behavior therapy is useful, that it is at least as effective as traditional psychotherapy, and that it may have particular benefits.

e) Since experimental investigations of learning and clinical applications of behavior therapy make use of similar concepts and sources of evidence, a consistent association between laboratory and clinic is maintained in this approach to treatment.

IX. Cognitive therapy

A. Early approaches to behavior therapy minimized or excluded from consideration such cognitive or mental variables as images, thoughts, expectations, or beliefs.

B. Many practitioners of behavior therapy, however, now assume that self-statements provide a basis for inferences about cognition and accept the idea that the beliefs and expectations that mediate much maladaptive behavior can be modified by behavior therapy.

C. Albert Ellis

1. Ellis names his approach "rational-emotive therapy."

2. This approach assumes that patients are maladaptive in their behavior because they act on irrational beliefs about themselves, about others, and the relationship between activating events on experiences and their consequences.

3. The goal of therapy is to eliminate or reduce the "irrational consequences" of irrational belief systems, which in turn reduces anxiety and hostility.

4. Through confrontation and active interpretation the patient is helped to restructure behavior by adopting more rational beliefs.

D. Aaron Beck

1. Beck (1967), in his cognitive therapy, also assigns major importance to correcting the faulty thinking about oneself and about the rewarding opportunities in one's present or future environment.

2. The approach focuses on helping the patient overcome faulty perceptions, distortions in self-concept, and false judgments about relationships in the world.

3. The therapist may begin at a behavioral level of working toward reduction of abnormal symptoms but the underlying distorted attitudes must also be identified and challenged.

4. Active testing of assumptions through a variety of problem-oriented tasks leads to engaging in new activities based on cognitive modification.

E. Donald Meichenbaum
  1. Meichenbaum developed his cognitive approach to behavior modification by treating cognitions as internal verbalizations and images that in distressed persons may interfere with performance.
  2. In treatment patients learn to identify and then replace the self-statements and self-instructions that are maladaptive.
  3. Treatment is also directed toward providing means of desensitizing tension-producing conditions and producing more successful coping behavior through reinforcing self-comments and reassuring imagery.
  4. As in the other cognitive therapies a cognitive restructuring is the desired outcome of treatment.
F. Evaluation
  1. As with behavioral therapies, cognitive therapies are most frequently applied where problems and desired outcomes can be specified.
  2. Evaluation of cognitive therapies has been associated with positive outcomes.
  3. Beck's procedures have been shown to be effective with depression when compared with other treatment approaches.
  4. Behavioral and cognitive approaches, by specifying methods of application, are seen as accessible and more possible to be applied in a uniform way.
  5. To some practitioners the integration of cognitive and behavior treatment modes is still controversial because they believe that concern with inferred mental states reduces the effectiveness of direct manipulation of the environment.

X. **Humanistic therapy**
A number of therapeutic approaches characterized by their phenomenological or existential assumptions about human experiences or by their opposition to traditional psychoanalysis or behavior therapy have come to be loosely referred to as "humanistic" therapy. While *humanistic* is a word with many connotations, it is used here merely as a conventional label for these approaches. (See the section on humanistic perspectives on personality in the chapter "Psychodynamic Concepts.")
A. Principles
  1. A person's world is a product of individual perceptions. Therefore, what one says about one's personal world should be accepted as subjective truth.
  2. Each person is unique. Therefore, individual dignity must not be affronted by the attempt to label, categorize, or reduce a person to some set of generalizations about human character or behavior.

3. Individuals are processes, rather than products of influences. Thus, each person has, in principle, the capacity to realize his or her potentialities and to live the life suited to those potentialities.
4. Individuals are free, capable of choice, and responsible for the choices, fulfilling or unfulfilling, that they make.
5. The goals of treatment are those that the patients choose freely and that are congruent with their understanding of themselves and their interests.
6. The role of the therapist is to provide a supportive, understanding, and accepting context for the exploration of opportunities for personal growth and development.

B. Variants

There are many variants of humanistic therapy, both individual and group. The following have achieved wide recognition.

1. Client-centered therapy
   a) The chief proponent of client-centered therapy is Carl Rogers.
   b) Rogers believes that there is a strong innate tendency to develop and realize one's potentialities. Nevertheless, a person may adopt a set of values or attitudes that limits experience or blocks development.
   c) The therapist offers total acceptance, which is the necessary condition of change.
   d) The therapist uses techniques of recognition and clarification of the client's feelings, and encourages honesty in communication.
   e) In a therapeutic context of this kind, the client can reassess his or her self-perceptions and make constructive choices.

2. Existential analysis
   a) Exponents include Medard Boss, Viktor Frankl, and Rollo May.
   b) They believe that people define themselves in terms of interpersonal relationships and that the relationships must be honest and open (authentic) to give existence its value and meaning.
   c) Patients' symptoms reflect evasions of responsibility for their own choices, for their dysphoria, or for their unstable or incoherent set of values (meaninglessness).
   d) The therapist encourages the patient to accept responsibility for symptoms as self-chosen and to decide on ways of dealing with life that are active, authentic, and meaningful.
   e) Since individuals (and therapists) are unique, no particular techniques and procedures can be formulated as general principles.

3. Gestalt therapy
   a) Fritz Perls is the leading proponent of gestalt therapy.
   b) Disordered behavior is viewed as the result of unresolved past conflicts, but its resolution occurs in the action and decisions of the here-and-now.
   c) Emphasis is placed on the identification and acceptance of one's needs and one's personal responsibility for meeting them by selecting effective strategies.
   d) Gestalt therapy is more technique-oriented than the other two humanistic therapies, using reenactment of dreams, role-played conversations with one's own feelings or with other persons or objects, cathartic "acting-out," and interpersonal confrontation in groups.
   e) The gestalt therapist is also more direct and manipulative in treatment sessions, but the patient is responsible for defining the changes to be made and for exploring change.
   f) The goal of gestalt therapy (the German word *gestalt* means "whole") is the unification of feeling and action into a new configuration of decisive and fulfilling experience.
C. Evaluation
   1. There has been little evaluation of humanistic therapy by practitioners. Evaluation is viewed as a violation of the humanistic emphasis on the uniqueness and integrity of the individual. Carl Rogers' research program is an exception.
   2. Concern with individual responsibility and choice is not the exclusive domain of humanistic approaches, though these approaches have led to a reevaluation of the role of self-determination in other types of therapy.
   3. It is doubtful that any therapeutic situation is as free from the therapist's influence as the humanistic therapists claim theirs are.
   4. The humanistic perspective is viewed by some critics as reflecting an unscientific and even antiscientific approach to the understanding and treatment of human problems.
   5. Nevertheless, humanistic therapy has achieved popular acceptance and has had a major role in the development of alternatives to traditional psychiatric and psychological treatment.

XI. **The assessment of therapeutic outcomes**
A. In the past, much treatment has been evaluated only in clinical reports and case histories or in studies lacking appropriate comparison groups.
B. The proper evaluation of psychotherapy is very difficult because there are so many patient, therapist, and method variables to sort out and control.

C. Also, no clearly reliable measures of improvement exist, so various subjective patient and observer judgments must be used.

D. Procedures of behavior therapies and cognitive therapies, when directed toward fairly specific outcomes, are easier to evaluate and show a reasonable rate of successful outcomes.

E. Cognitive therapy of depression has been shown to be effective in comparison to and in conjunction with pharmacological treatment.

F. It is hard to draw conclusions about the benefits of one therapy compared to another because most achieve similar rates of reported success with general patient groups.

G. However, it can be said with assurance that studies comparing psychotherapy with no treatment show benefits of psychotherapy.

XII. The future of psychotherapy

A. For many decades psychotherapy was based on Freudian psychoanalytic theory. It was basically a medical treatment performed by psychiatric physicians.

B. It was frequently the "core treatment" for the emotionally disordered and was the central focus of residency training programs in psychiatry.

C. With the advent of biologic psychiatry, the growth in and research focused on biological determinants, and the development of psychotropic drugs in the 1950s, there has been a simultaneous shift away from the practice of psychotherapy by psychiatrists.

D. As nonmedical practitioners (including psychologists, social workers, family and marriage counselors, nurse practitioners) began doing psychotherapy, they at first adhered to the psychodynamic model but ultimately developed treatment techniques based on their own training and experience.

E. For many decades psychotherapy was paid for primarily by the patient ("out-of-pocket"). Psychiatric treatment, especially outpatient psychotherapy was not covered by health insurance plans. Even now the health-care providers often place limits on the amount of coverage they will provide and often have a dollar limit on what they will cover. Since health insurance is usually provided by employers, governmental bodies, or welfare agencies, the practice of psychotherapy has become increasingly driven by the marketplace with the (1) increased external influence of clinical practices by the control of third party reimbursement, (2) the shifting of costs to the consumer (patient) through higher deductible, higher coinsurance and top dollar limits, (3) the availability of an ever-increasing array of different therapeutic options, and (4) an explosive increase in the number of nonmedically trained mental health professionals practicing psychotherapy.

F. Psychotherapy is now affected—for better or for worse—by the economics of the overall health care system.

References

Beck, A. T. *Depression: Clinical, Experimental, and Theoretical Aspects.* New York: Harper & Row, 1967.

Bellack, A. S., M. Hensen, and A. E. Kazdin, eds. *International Handbook of Behavior Modification and Therapy.* New York: Plenum Press, 1982.

Bergin, A. E., and S. L. Garfield. *Handbook of Psychotherapy and Behavior Change: An Empirical Analysis.* New York: John Wiley & Sons, 1971.

Boss, M. *Psychoanalysis and Daseinsanalysis.* New York: Basic Books, Inc., Publishers, 1967.

Calhoun, J. F. et al. *Abnormal Psychology: Current Perspectives.* 2d ed. New York: CRM/Random House, 1977.

Davison, G. C., and J. M. Neale. *Abnormal Psychology.* 3d ed. New York: John Wiley & Sons, 1982.

Dollard, J., and N. E. Miller. *Personality and Psychotherapy.* New York: McGraw-Hill, 1950.

Dunlop, K. *Habits: Their Making and Unmaking.* New York: Liveright, 1952.

Ellis, A. *Reason and Emotion in Psychotherapy.* New York: Lyle Stuart, Inc., 1962.

Eyesenck, H. J. "The Effects of Psychotherapy: An Evaluation." *Journal of Consulting Psychology* 16 (1952): 319–24.

Frankl, V. E. *Psychotherapy and Existentialism.* New York: Washington Square Press, 1967.

Freedman, D., and J. Dyruds eds. *American Handbook of Psychiatry.* 2d ed. Vol. 5. New York: Basic Books, 1975.

Gibson, R. W. "The Future of the Practice of Psychotherapy.", *The Psychiatric Hospital* 16 (4):155–59 (October 1984).

Gibson, R. W. "The Future of Psychotherapy." *The Psychiatric Times.* 3(7): 1 (July 1986).

Jacoboson, E. *Progressive Relaxation.* Chicago: University of Chicago Press, 1938.

Kaplan, H. I., and B. J. Sadock. *Comprehensive Textbook of Psychiatry.* 4th ed. Baltimore: Williams & Wilkins 1985.

Kolb, L. C. and H. K. H. Brodie. *Modern Clinical Psychiatry.* 10th ed. Philadelphia: W. B. Saunders Co. 1982.

Leitenberg, H., ed. *Handbook of Behavior Modification and Behavior Therapy.* Englewood Cliffs, NJ: Prentice-Hall, 1976.

Lindsley, O. R. "Operant Conditioning Methods Applied to Research in Chronic Schizophrenia." *Psychiatric Research Reports* 5 (1956): 118–39.

May R. "Contributions of Existential Psychotherapy." In *Existence: A New Dimension in Psychiatry and Psychology,* edited by R. May, F. Angel, and H. F. Ellenberger. New York: Basic Books, Inc., Publishers, 1958a.

Mowrer, O. H. *Learning Theory and Personality Dynamics.* New York: The Ronald Press Company, 1950.

Nicholi, A. M., Jr., ed. *The Harvard Guide to Modern Psychiatry.* Cambridge: Belknap Press of Harvard University Press, 1978.

Perls, F. S. "Four Lectures." In *Gestalt Therapy Now: Therapy, Techniques, Applications.* J. Fagan and I. L. Shepherd, Palo Alto, Calif.: Science and Behavior Books, 1970.

Rogers, C. R. *On Becoming a Person.* Boston: Houghton Mifflin Co., 1961.

Sipe, A. W. R., and C. J. Rowe, ed., *Psychiatry, Ministry and Pastoral Counseling.* Collegeville, Minn.: St. John's University Press, 1984.

Stuart, R. B., ed. *Behavioral Self-Management: Strategies, Techniques and Outcomes.* New York: Brunner/Mazel, 1977.

Wolpe, J. *Psychotherapy by Reciprocal Inhibition.* Stanford, Calif.: Stanford University Press, 1958.

Zeig, J., ed. *The Evolution of Psychotherapy.* New York: Brunner/Mazel, 1987.

All happy families resemble one another, each unhappy family is unhappy in its own way.

Leo Tolsoy (1828-1910):
Anna Karenina

Treatment in Psychiatry: Group, Family, and Adjunctive Therapies

Disorders of behavior, experience, and relationship develop and are expressed in a social context. All psychotherapeutic approaches recognize this obvious point but some therapeutic strategies emphasize the social environment as the source of opportunities to initiate and reinforce change. The techniques described in this chapter all have in common a concern for the network of human relations in which people live and attempt to mobilize and use group processes in promoting therapeutic change.

I. **Group psychotherapy**
   A. *Group psychotherapy* is defined in *A Psychiatric Glossary* as the "application of psychotherapeutic techniques to a group, including utilization of interactions of members of the group."[1]
   B. Although it is sometimes used as the sole psychotherapeutic modality, it is most commonly used in conjunction with individual psychotherapy and other types of psychiatric treatment.
   C. The groups are usually composed of one therapist and six or eight patients, who may be homogeneous in some way or heterogeneous. The sessions last about ninety minutes.
   D. This type of psychotherapy has its origins in observations made by Sigmund Freud (in 1919) of the dynamics of the interplay between individuals in a group setting. There is a definite pattern of interaction between the various members of a group that facilitates the therapeutic process. The group provides an opportunity for developing personal insights as well as testing out new methods of coping and relating in a controlled type of environment.
   E. The group process
      Three stages characterize the life of the group, bringing specific issues into focus and dominating group interaction.
      1. In the first phase, the patient is concerned about whether she or he will be accepted as a part of the group.
      2. In the second phase, the patient is concerned with issues of autonomy, that is, becoming an independent person within the group.
      3. In the third stage, the patient deals with the issues of sharing and equality.
   F. There was a time when group psychotherapy was considered an expedient, a way to involve a greater number of patients, but this is no longer felt to be true.
      1. For many patients, it is superior to individual psychotherapy.
      2. The techniques used closely parallel those used in individual psychotherapy, and they vary with the aims of the therapist and the type of patient. Some group therapists are relatively nonparticipating and mostly summarize what is going on in the group; others are very active and confrontive, suggesting subject material, making interpretations, setting up role-playing situations,

---

1. American Psychiatric Association, *A Psychiatric Glossary,* 6th ed. (Washington, D.C., 1988)

and so forth. Patients who have fragmented into psychosis need more supportive, reality-oriented therapy whereas those with greater ego-strength may use more insight-oriented therapy.

G. Factors that induce therapeutic change in groups
   1. Groups can develop a sense of cohesiveness and provide an experience of social solidarity and belonging.
   2. Group membership can have important motivational consequences by supporting and encouraging (rewarding) some kinds of behavior and by implicitly or explicitly developing rules and standards of conduct within the group.
   3. In a cohesive and supportive group a member may be able to experience, express, and release strong feelings and beliefs.
   4. A group provides a basis for self-definition both by defining a social reality for members and by affirming insights and improvements.

H. There are many types of groups that vary in goals of participation, role of therapist, and assumptions about the nature of problems. Almost every variant of individual psychotherapy has a counterpart in group therapy.
   1. Since 1960, a number of variations of group therapy have emerged. They emphasize the usefulness of social processes in increasing self-understanding, improving relationships, and developing human potentialities; such procedures can be used adjunct to psychiatric treatment.
   2. However, the variety of group procedures that is available may be confusing to many people; no "consumer's guide" is available and care must be exercised in evaluating the appropriateness of a group for oneself.

I. Self-help groups
   1. *Self-help* or support groups without professionally trained leaders, in which the group experience does not uncover basic conflicts but does offer new shared experiences to the patient.
   2. Alcoholics Anonymous (AA) and the substance abusers group are effective self-help groups, as are groups for persons and families of persons living with chronic or fatal illness.

II. Family therapy

A. Description
   1. Family therapy is a form of group therapy, wherein the nuclear family is the unit, that has developed during the past three or four decades.
   2. Family therapists view the family as a behavioral system with unique properties. Emotional disturbances of individual members are therefore regarded as outgrowths of conflicts between family members.

3. One or more therapists deal with an entire family unit (or sometimes with a part of the family) during the therapeutic sessions. The goal of treatment is to resolve or reduce the pathogenic conflicts and anxiety within the unit.

4. Forms of family therapy vary in the same characteristics as do other group therapies and individual psychotherapies.

B. Scope

1. In the past, in certain experimental situations, entire family units were hospitalized so that the genesis of schizophrenia and other emotional disorders could be studied.

2. Family therapy may be used as the sole treatment, or it may be used in conjunction with other types of therapy.

3. It has been recommended for marital conflict and child-parent conflicts.

C. Difficulties

1. The therapist often finds it difficult to keep the family group intact for sessons (siblings resist, parents have to work, and so forth).

2. Another difficulty is keeping the focus on the family process and related to the family as a functioning unit rather than shifting to individual members.

III. **Adjunctive therapies** (therapies used in psychiatric inpatient, day treatment, and partial hospital programs)

A. A wide spectrum of therapies is available for use in psychiatric and outpatient settings. These therapies can be classified into three groups: activity therapies, expressive (or creative arts) therapies, and verbal therapies.

1. Activity therapies include occupational therapy and therapeutic recreation.

a) History

Concerned observers of the institutionalized mentally ill in the nineteenth century recognized the value of structured activity in reducing maladaptive behavior. Industrial and/or agricultural activities were developed in most state hospitals. During World War I, the reconstruction aides demonstrated their effectiveness through activity programs and were the immediate forerunners of occupational therapy. After World War II, therapeutic recreation developed out of occupational therapy and physical education.

b) Definition

Activity therapies are concerned with the adaptation of the individual in the community. They provide evaluation and treatment of the patient's independent living skills, for example, physical and psychological skills, work and play-leisure skills, and the sensorimotor, cognitive, and psychosocial components that influence these skills.

c) Philosophy

The assumption is made that through structured activities persons can learn a range of interpersonal attitudes and behaviors as well as new skills that will help them in coping with life tasks, in controlling their own resources, and in maintaining increased self-esteem.

d) Treatment

Activity therapists provide here-and-now experiences in which individuals can acquire and practice skills, learn how their behavior affects not only the task, recreational event, or activity, but also the members of the participating group and, consequently, how it affects their roles in the community. Occupational therapists and therapeutic recreation professionals are trained in activity analysis and group process. They adapt activities to meet the needs of the patients involved and provide feedback to the treatment team.

(1) The occupational therapist evaluates the patient's performance and plans treatment to remediate deficits in independent living skills and/or performance components. Techniques used may be individual or group craft activities, task groups, homemaking or child/parenting sessions, or prevocational skill development. In addition, for the more severely impaired, self-care activities, such as use of public transportation, budgeting and check writing, and time organization, may be utilized to increase functional independence.

(2) The therapeutic recreation professional uses recreation to promote personal growth and development. Some examples are the use of such activities as volleyball or creative writing to promote opportunities for the expression and release of feelings; the use of individual or group recreation to facilitate the development of leadership, self-confidence, cooperation, and social skills; the use of programs to facilitate and practice behavior changes (feeling charades for the appropriate expression of affect); leisure education to aid in the development of new interests and to provide balance in the patient's daily life; and training in the use of recreation for relaxation and anxiety reduction.

e) Credentials

Occupational therapy has the longest history and is the most widely accepted and utilized of all the therapies in inpatient settings. Both occupational therapy and therapeutic recreation have specific educational curricula and internship programs leading to certification. Both fields have well-developed, articulated standards and codes of ethics.

2. Expressive (creative arts) therapies include music therapy, art therapy, and movement (or dance) therapy.

 a) History

 Expressive therapies have emerged over the past two decades. The roots of each therapy are in the arts (e.g., music, art, or dance) from which it has developed and in the field of special education. Teachers of emotionally disturbed children discovered that the arts often provided a way of communicating and provided information that could not be obtained in structured activities or in attempts at verbal exchanges. The expressive therapies are growing rapidly as professions and are predicted by some to become major therapies in psychiatric settings in the 1980s.

 b) Definition

 Expressive therapists are concerned with maximizing the possibilities of communicating and the media through which persons can express and communicate their feelings, conflicts, personal characteristics, and creative potential. Expressive therapists provide evaluation of these expressions and give feedback to patients, the patients' primary therapists, and the treatment teams.

 c) Philosophy

 The assumption is made that through participation in creative processes and using a variety of media, materials, instruments, tools, and body motions, persons can express themselves in ways that provide information, communication possibilities, and a sense of personal productivity that leads to the reduction of disturbing symptoms, increased trust in interpersonal relationships, and raised self-esteem.

 d) Treatment

 Each of the expressive therapies uses materials and methods associated with the art from which it has developed.

 (1) In art therapy, a patient provided with clay may construct figures and place them in positions in relationship to one another that reveal information about family dynamics and his or her relationship to them. This may lead to communication with the therapist and provide information that can also be utilized by other members of the treatment team.

 (2) In music therapy, an anxious patient may learn to relax and experience increased comfort through listening to music or by participating in the making of music.

(3) In movement therapy, body language that a person uses in movement in interactions with others (movements that may express resistance, withdrawal, manipulation, etc.) becomes apparent to other members of the group and to the therapist and is noted and processed by the therapist, patient, and group members.

e) Credentials

Since the expressive therapies are relatively new, the educational, internship, and credentialing process is not as completely developed as it is for these activity therapies. There is, however, now an American Art Therapy Association, a National Association of Music Therapy, and an American Dance Therapy Association. These groups are working to professionalize their disciplines, have established some criteria for training and credentialing, and are in the process of developing professional standards and ethics.

3. Verbal therapies include individual psychotherapy, group therapy, and family therapy.

a) Most patients in psychiatric hospitals or treatment programs have a primary therapist, usually a psychiatrist, but sometimes a psychologist, social worker, or nurse, who works in collaboration with a psychiatrist. The primary therapist provides individual psychotherapy for his or her patients and usually is the head of the treatment team and responsible for taking leadership in the development of the treatment plan. Other members of the treatment staff may also provide individual psychotherapy. It is, for example, usual for patients to have one-to-one sessions with members of the nursing and therapy staff. Often these sessions are of a supportive nature but sometimes are directed toward a particular problem identified in the treatment plan.

b) Group and family therapy have already been presented (see pages 340–342) and are essentially the same in inpatient and outpatient settings. For the more disturbed patients in inpatient settings, group therapy should be supportive and reality oriented.

c) Group and family therapists come from a variety of educational and professional backgrounds, including psychiatry, psychology, social work, and psychiatric nursing. In order to function as group and family therapists, such persons should have special training in group and family therapy. Unfortunately, no credentialing programs are in existence at this time. This means that institutions employing these therapists must be responsible for setting up educational and training requirements that are appropriate for their settings.

B. Treatment

Each of the above adjunctive therapists makes an evaluation of the patient, which is the basis for the setting of goals or the suggesting of interventions. These are then presented to the treatment team, which is under the leadership of a psychiatrist. Often, the patient attends the treatment plan review and participates in the development of the treatment plan. At any rate, the treatment *team* formulates an overall treatment plan for the patient.

References

Kaplan, H. I. and B. J. Sadock. *Comprehensive Textbook of Psychiatry/ IV.* Baltimore: Williams & Wilkins, 1985.

L'Abate, L., ed. *The Handbook of Family Psychology and Therapy.* Vol. 1. Homewood, Ill.: Dorsey Press, 1985.

Nicholi, A. M., Jr., ed. *The Harvard Guide to Modern Psychiatry.* Cambridge: Belknap Press of Harvard University Press, 1978.

Canst thou not minister to a mind diseas'd;
Pluck from the memory a rooted sorrow;
Raze out the written troubles of the brain;
And, with some sweet oblivious antidote,
Cleanse the staff'd bosom of that perilous matter
Which weighs upon the heart?

Shakespeare: *Macbeth,* **Act V (c. 1606)**

Treatment in Psychiatry: Pharmacological and Somatic Treatment

I. Introduction

A. Relation to the somatogenic hypothesis

  1. It is assumed, in the treatment of psychiatric disorders by pharmacotherapy, that the effectiveness of the drug is achieved by action on the central nervous system; in turn, it is implied that at least some psychiatric disorders, especially psychoses, involve defective functioning of the central nervous system.

  2. Although the effectiveness of pharmacotherapy and somatic therapies in relieving symptoms of psychiatric disorders may be taken as support of the somatogenic hypothesis, the relation between effects of drug treatment and underlying pathology is not clear for most conditions.

B. History of drug treatment

  1. Historically, attempts have been made to use chemical or medicinal means to modify abnormal behavior and emotional pain. Alcohol and opiates have been used for many centuries.

  2. Prior to the early 1950s, drug treatment in psychiatry consisted primarily of attempts to sedate excited and overactive patients or to stimulate withdrawn or underactive patients.

  3. The history of drug treatment in psychiatry has been dated from 1949, when the antimanic effects of lithium were discovered, or, to 1952 when reserpine was isolated and chlorpromazine (Thorazine) was discovered.

  4. Additionally, the history of drug treatment reveals many examples of initially promising effects that did not persist. In some cases the drugs themselves produced additional problems of dependency and misuse (e.g., opium, cocaine, barbiturates).

  5. In the early 1950s new groups of drugs were introduced in the treatment of psychiatric disorders and the outcome has been characterized as the "third psychiatric revolution" (the freeing of patients from prisonlike conditions—removing their chains and using "moral" treatment by French physician Phillipe Pinel at the Bicetre in 1793; and the development of psychoanalytic theory and psychotherapy by Sigmund Freud are the other two "revolutions").

  6. Developments in pharmacological therapy and research into underlying neural mechanisms have transformed institutional treatment and pointed the way to a much more sophisticated but still incomplete understanding of brain functions in mental illness.

II. Principles of psychopharmacology

A. The nervous system can be influenced in many ways, but direct effects are mediated by two categories of *neuroactive* substances.

1. *Neurotransmitters* are released from activated axons of neurons (and from some dendrites) and communicate across synapses with other neurons.

    a) The effect of most neurotransmitters on other neurons is relatively short-acting with a time course of one millisecond to a second or more.

    b) Some neurotransmitters, however, may facilitate or depress activity in other neurons for many minutes or even hours.

2. *Neuropeptides* are hormonelike substances that are secreted from *neuroendocrine cells* or from some neurons. Neuropeptides may have effects lasting from seconds to days.

B. *Neuromodulation* is the action of neuroactive substances that tends to amplify or dampen the degree of neurotransmitter action.

C. Typical sequence of neurotransmitter activity

1. Neurotransmitters are synthesized and stored within neurons.

2. Release of neurotransmitters occurs when neurons are stimulated to the point of "firing."

3. Some neurotransmitters stimulate other neurons; others inhibit the neurons they affect.

4. Neurotransmitter substances in the synapse are inactivated by metabolic processes and by reabsorption into the neuron.

5. The synthesis and inactivation of neurotransmitters are complex chemical processes that can be influenced by other substances, including neuroactive drugs that may stimulate the release of neurotransmitters or may block the synthesis, release, synaptic activity, or inactivation of neurotransmitters.

D. Examples of neuroactive substances

1. Several neurotransmitter substances have been identified and established as active in the central nervous system, and others are under investigation.

2. The neurotransmitters about which most is known are

    a) Acetylcholine (ACh)

    b) Norepinephrine (NE)

    c) Dopamine (DA)

    d) Serotonin (5HT)

    e) Gamma Amino Butyric Acid (GABA)

    f) Glycine (Gly)

    g) Glutamic acid

3. Over twenty neuropeptides are currently being vigorously investigated with special attention given to opioid (opiumlike in effect) peptides, endorphins, and enkephalins, which modulate response to pain and emotional distress.

E. Current biochemical hypotheses
   1. The biogenic amines are the neurotransmitters that have been implicated as having roles in schizophrenia and affective disorders.
   2. The biogenic amines include (1) serotonin, which is an indoleamine; and (2) norepinephrine and dopamine, which are catecholamines.
   3. The biogenic amines theory of depression
      a) Depression is assumed to reflect a reduced effective level of biogenic amines in brain systems.
      b) Reserpine is a drug that reduces the level of serotonin, norepinephrine, and dopamine in patients and, in some cases, produces an accompanying clinical depression.
      c) The major category of antidepressants, the tricyclics, block the "reuptake" of biogenic amine neurotransmitters from synapses, thus increasing the concentration of the neurotransmitters in the synapses.
      d) The other category of antidepressants, the monoamine oxidase inhibitors (MAOI) prevent the inactivation of biogenic amines by the enzyme MAO, thereby increasing the potentiating effects of available neurotransmitters. Clinically effective MAOI antidepressants reverse the effect of reserpine-induced depression.
      e) Mood elevators like amphetamine and cocaine stimulate the release of catecholamines (but do not effectively alter mood in depressed patients).
      f) Pharmacological studies have suggested that some depressions may be related to a norepinephrine deficiency, and some others to a serotonin deficiency.
   4. The dopamine theory of schizophrenia
      a) Schizophrenia is assumed to reflect a defect in dopamine-mediated brain systems.
      b) Amphetamine, which stimulates the release of catecholamines, can produce, in some persons, psychotic symptoms that resemble schizophrenia, and it can also exacerbate psychotic symptoms in acute schizophrenia.
      c) The antipsychotic drugs, the phenothiazines, thioxanthenes and butyrophenones, act to inhibit dopamine-mediated neurotransmission by blocking dopamine receptor sites.
      d) There are different dopamine receptor subtypes and the clinical effects of antipsychotic drugs are related to the blocking of a specific subtype (D2).

    e) The use of antipsychotics sometimes produces motor system symptoms like those of Parkinson's disease, which is caused by a dopamine deficiency. This observation further implicates dopamine transmission in the treatment and possible cause of schizophrenia.

    5. No current biochemical hypothesis is free from conflicting findings and internal contradictions, but the combination of precise diagnosis, pharmacological analysis of drug effects, and investigation of the operation of neuroregulators will extend our knowledge of the nervous system correlates of the psychoses.

III. Major classes of psychoactive drugs

A. Reasonably safe and effective medical treatment is available for most of the major mental disorders.

B. A limitation to developing uniquely specific therapeutic agents is the lack of knowledge of the biological basis of most major mental disorders.

C. There have been few fundamentally new agents since the 1950s.

D. Psychoactive drugs used in psychiatric practice
1. Antipsychotics (neuroleptics)
2. Mood modifiers (antidepressants, lithium)
3. Antianxiety agents

E. Other psychoactive drugs not used primarily in psychiatric practice
1. Opiates
2. Stimulants
3. Sedative-hypnotics
4. Psychedelics

IV. Antipsychotic agents

A. There are a large number of these agents, whose effects are characterized more by their similarity than by their differences.
1. They produce emotional calmness and mental relaxation.
2. They effectively control symptoms of both acutely and chronically disturbed psychotic patients.
3. They are capable of producing the reversible "extrapyramidal syndrome" (rigidity, tremors, drooling).
4. Although they produce a relatively high incidence of annoying side reactions, the reactions are not dangerous.
5. They create little, if any, habituation or dependency.
6. They have revolutionized the pattern of treating psychiatric patients. With the advent of the antipsychotic agents, most psychotic patients can be managed with reduced periods of hospitalization or as outpatients.

B. Indications
1. They are more efficacious for patients with acute illness and the best prognosis.

2. The symptoms that respond best to these agents include tension, hyperactivity, hostility, combativeness, negativism, acute delusions, hallucinations, poor self-care, anorexia, sleep disturbance, sociability, and sometimes seclusiveness.
C. Toxicity and side reactions
   1. In general, these agents are very safe.
   2. Side effects include certain mild anticholinergic autonomic effects (e.g., dry mouth and blurred vision; feelings of sluggishness); the extrapyramidal syndrome (Parkinson's syndrome); occasionally, acute dystonia (including chronic contractions of muscles in the neck, mouth, tongue, and "restless legs").
   3. Tardive dyskinesia is a late-appearing extrapyramidal symptom that can be troublesome. It is a choreiform, ticlike involuntary or semivoluntary muscular movement, classically involving the tongue, face, and neck muscles (oral lingual dyskinesia or buccal lingual masticatory dyskinesia). Although originally considered a rare symptom, estimates now range from 10 percent to 40 percent, depending upon the narrowness or looseness of the definition. Additionally, some symptoms that had been considered to be tardive dyskinesia are probably manifestations of movement disturbances associated with other conditions: for example, schizophrenia or senile disorders.
      Continued use of antipsychotics is frequently necessary despite tardive dyskinesia if the patient is to remain free of disabling psychotic symptoms.
   4. Treatment of side effects
      a) Most of the extrapyramidal symptoms respond to anti-Parkinson's drugs (e.g., benztropine mesylate, marketed under the trade name of Cogentin; diphenhydramine hydrochloride, marketed under the trade name of Benadryl; trihexyphenidyl HCI, marketed under the trade name Artane; biperiden, marketed under the trade name of Akineton).
      b) There is no adequate treatment of tardive dyskinesia. Lithium carbonate, diazepam (Valium) may help. Reducing the drug may worsen the symptoms.
D. Types of antipsychotic agents
   1. Among the commonly used antipsychotic agents are
      a) Phenothiazines
         (1) Aliphatic
            These are chlorpromazine (Thorazine) and triflupromazine hydrochloride (Vesprin)
         (2) Piperidines
            These are mesoridazine besylate (Serentil); piperacetazine (Quide); and thioridazine HCL (Mellaril)

(3) Piperazines

These are acetophenazine maleate (Tindal); butaperazine (Repoise); carphenazine maleate (Proketazine); fluphenazine hydrochloride (Prolixin and Permitil); perphenazine (Trilafon); and trifluoperazine hydrochloride (Stelazine).

b) Thioxanthenes
   (1) Chlorprothixene (Taractan)
   (2) Thiothixene (Navane)
c) Dibenzazepines
   (1) Loxapine succinate (Loxitane, Daxolin)
   (2) Clozapine (Leponex, experimental)—not available in the U.S.
d) Butyrophenones
   (1) Haloperidol (Haldol)
   (2) Other butyrophenones: trifluperiodol, droperidol
e) Diphenylbutyrylpiperidines—a new family of drugs resulting from slight modification of the butyrophenone structure. Not available in the U.S.
f) Oxoindoles (tetrahydrooxoindole)
g) Indolones: molindone hydrochloride (Moban; Lidone)

This antipsychotic has the unique property of being effective without associated weight gain but with weight reduction.

2. Drugs that had originally been developed for other therapeutic purposes have recently been found to be helpful in treatment of some of the psychotic illnesses. Among the classes of drugs that have been studied are the anticonvulsants and the calcium channel blockers.

a) Carbamazepine (Tegretol) is an anticonvulsant drug used for the treatment of psychomotor and grand mal seizures. It also works well in trigeminal neuralgia and other paroxysmal pain syndromes.

This drug has been found to have antimanic effects. It probably does not act by blocking dopamine receptors as has been the case for the neuroleptics—and it does not produce acute Parkinsonian side effects or induce tardive dyskinesia. It is an important treatment for alternative or supplemental treatment of the lithium nonresponsive patient with manic or schizoaffective symptoms. It seems to work especially well with rapid or continuous manic depressive cycles (four or more cycles per year). The combination of carbamazepine and lithium seems particularly beneficial to manic episodes and also for its prophylactic effects.

b) Clonazepam

This is reported to have antimanic effects by some investigators. It also may have antidepressant and prophylactic effects in the treatment of bipolar disorder.

3. Calcium channel blocking agents

Verapamil is a calcium channel blocker that had been used primarily for the treatment of cardiac arrhythmias, hypertension, and other cardiac conditions. Recent reports suggest a possible role for it (and other calcium channel blockers) in the treatment of both acute mania and the maintenance phase of bipolar disorder. (Manic episodes have been associated with transient increases of serum calcium.)

4. Clorgyline, a selected inhibitor of monoamine oxidase type A alone or in combination with lithium carbonate, has been found to prolong the duration and lessen the severity of mood cycles in bipolar patients. May be both an anticycling and an antidepressant drug in patients with rapid-cycling bipolar illness who respond poorly to conventional treatments.

E. The rauwolfia alkaloids, forms of reserpine (e.g., Serpasil), once part of the "third revolution" are rarely used, at least by themselves, for the treatment of psychotic disorders now because they are clearly less effective as antipsychotics. Among the side effects are drug-induced depression.

V. Mood modifiers

A. Antidepressant Agents

1. Antidepressant agents can be divided into the following groups:
   a) Stimulants
   b) Tricyclic antidepressants (TCA)
   c) Monoamine oxidase inhibitors (MAOI)
   d) Tetracyclics
   e) New antidepressants

2. Stimulants
   a) Stimulants, for example, dextroamphetamines (Dexedrine); methamphetamines (Methedrine and Desoxyn); and methylphenidate (Ritalin) have limited place in the current treatment of serious depressive disorders.
   b) However, Ritalin is often prescribed for *mild* depressions.
   c) Some recent studies suggest stimulants may be viewed as having a place in the treatment of depression.

3. Tricyclic antidepressants
   a) These are the most commonly employed agents in the treatment of depression.
   b) They act by blocking the neuronal uptake of amines into the presynaptic nerve endings (see "Principles of psychopharmacology" at the beginning of this section).
   c) The overall improvement they achieve is about 70 percent.

d) There are several effective tricyclic antidepressants. Although there are more similarities than differences among them, there is variation in some of the side effects (e.g., some are more stimulating and less sedative; others are more sedative and less stimulating). Among these are:
  (1) Amitriptyline (Elavil, Endep)
  (2) Desipramine hydrochloride (Norpramin, Pertofrane)
  (3) Doxepin HCL (Sinequan, Adapin)
  (4) Imipramine HCL (Tofranil, also available in generic form)
  (5) Nortriptyline HCL (Aventyl, Pamelor)
  (6) Protriptyline HCL (Vivactil)

4. Monoamine oxidase inhibitors
  a) The clinical efficacy is less than that of tricyclic antidepressants in most controlled studies of endogenous depression.
  b) However, they are clearly effective in certain atypical depressions.
  c) The MAO inhibitors still in use
    (1) Tranylcypromine sulfate (Parnate)
    (2) Phenelzine sulfate (Nardil)
  d) MAOI drugs deserve consideration for the treatment of depressions refractory to usual tricyclic treatment, regardless of subtype.
  e) The major role appears to be in the large heterogeneous group of ambulatory depressions with features of both anxiety and depression.

5. Tetracyclics
Maprotiline HCI (Ludiomil) is the only tetracyclic marketed in the United States at the present time. It is thought to produce fewer anticholinergic side effects and to be less cardiotoxic.

6. New antidepressants
Among the recently released antidepressants are:
  a) Amoxapine (Asendin)
  This drug produces a more rapid improvement in the symptoms of depression than tricyclic antidepressants.
  b) Trazodone HCI (Desyrel)
  This antidepressant has fewer anticholinergic side effects than tricyclic antidepressants and also has more rapid action on depressive symptoms.
  c) Fluoxetine hydrochloride (Prozac) is chemically unrelated to any of the above antidepressants, and is said to block serotonin uptake.

    d) Nomifensine maleate (Merital) was introduced in the United States as an antidepressant, and was considered to be more activating and less sedating. It was subsequently withdrawn from the market.

7. Toxicity and side reactions of antidepressant agents

    a) The tricyclic and MAO inhibitors often have the anticholinergic side effects listed under the antipsychotic agents (dry mouth, sweating, blurred vision, constipation, etc.) Central nervous system effects include drowsiness, occasionally agitation, or fine tremor. They rarely may precipitate hallucinations and delusions in patients who appear depressed but are latently psychotic.

    b) The changeover to MAO inhibitors after using tricyclics was thought to require a waiting period of one to two weeks in order to avoid the rare but serious side reactions that were said to ensue (e.g., hyperprexia, convulsions). However, recent reports indicate that these serious reactions were rare or exaggerated and that the two may actually be used simultaneously.

    c) An important caution for people who are using MAOI inhibitors (Parnate and Nardil) is that they must avoid foods that have a high tyramine content and certain other drugs that contain sympathominetic amines, since there is danger of a "hypertensive crisis."

B. Lithium carbonate

1. This drug is marketed under the trade names of Lithane, Lithonate, Eskalith, and Lithobid (this last one is a slow-release compound that can be given twice a day instead of three or four times a day, as with the other forms).

2. The mechanism of action is via catecholamine or electrolyte metabolism. It blocks the release and stimulates reuptake of norepinephrine.

3. Indications

    a) Acute mania and hypomania. It is effective in 80 percent of acute manias in one to two weeks. There is a lithium lag period of four to ten days, during which time one should administer a phenothiazine, butyrophenone or thioxanthene.

    b) It can be used prophylactically to prevent recurrent attacks of mania in bipolar affective disorders.

    c) Some schizoaffective patients respond to lithium, but less well than manias.

    d) Some investigators speak of "lithium responders" and report that certain schizophrenics also respond to lithium. Why

this is so is not known. Perhaps it is a reflection of diagnostic confusion (patients who really are schizoaffective or manic-depressive erroneously diagnosed as schizophrenics).
- e) Currently it is often used in combination with other antipsychotic agents or anticonvulsive drugs or calcium channel blockers (refer to the previous section under the newer drugs listed under the antipsychotic agents).

4. Summary
- a) Although lithium is a specific form of treatment for manic and hypomanic episodes, it is often necessary, because there is a delay in its action, to use another antipsychotic agent initially (e.g., chlorpromazine, thioridazine, or haloperidol) to control the disturbed behavior.
- b) Its main limitation is the narrowness between the therapeutic range and the toxic range.
- c) It seems most promising because of its prophylactic effect in reducing the frequency and severity of episodes in bipolar disorders.
- d) It is used in combination with other agents to treat refractory, continuous, and rapid-cycling mood disorders.

VI. Antianxiety agents

A. Introduction
1. For many centuries alcohol was used in many cultures as a nonspecific tranquilizer.
2. In the early twentieth century, bromides were used as sedatives but often produced toxic deliria.
3. Subsequently, barbiturates replaced the bromides as sedatives.
4. Meprobamate largely replaced the barbiturates.
5. Benzodiazepines are the currently popular anxiolytic agents.

B. Characteristics of antianxiety agents
1. They produce calmness and relaxation, but of a different quality than the antipsychotic agents.
2. They are not useful in ameliorating disturbed psychotic reactions but are helpful in relieving anxiety and tension.
3. They have little effect on autonomic functions (except for the antihistamines).
4. All have depressant effects on the central nervous system.
5. Many also have muscle relaxant and anticonvulsant properties.

C. Toxicity and side reactions
1. Annoying side reactions are relatively rare.
2. They do not produce extrapyramidal phenomena.
3. There is some risk of abuse, habituation, and addiction with these agents.
4. Their effect is potentiated by alcohol and other central nervous system depressants.

D. Indications
   1. The chief use of antianxiety agents is in the treatment of disabling forms of anxiety. Generally, they should be used for short periods of time (although there are exceptions to this).
   2. They are commonly employed as preoperative sedatives and in the management of pain syndromes, especially those accompanied by muscular tension.
E. List of commonly used antianxiety agents
   1. Meprobamate (Equanil, Miltown) is listed here because of its historical importance. It is not commonly used at present.
   2. Antihistamines have sedative side effects.
      a) Diphenhydramine hydrochloride (Benadryl)
      b) Hydroxyzine hydrochloride (Atarax)
      c) Hydroxyzine pamoate (Vistaril)
   3. Benzodiazepines are effective antianxiety agents. All have roughly similar anxiolytic sedative, hypnotic, and anticonvulsive properties.
      a) Chlordiazepoxide (Librium)
      b) Diazepam (Valium)
         (1) This was for a long time the most commonly prescribed of all drugs.
         (2) It became a popularly abused drug because it acted rapidly and tended to produce euphoria. As a consequence, it received more negative publicity than any of the other antianxiety agents (much of it undeserved).
      c) Oxazepam (Serax)
      d) Lorezapam (Ativan)
      e) Clorazepate dipotassium (Tranxene)
      f) Clorazepate monopotassium (Azene)
      g) Prazepam (Verstran)
      h) Halazepam (Paxiapam)
      i) Alprazolam (Xanax) This benzodiazepine in higher doses (approximately 4 mg/day) is said to be effective in treating depression. (Some recent studies have reported serious side effects.)
   4. Buspirone (BuSpar) is a new agent that is not a benzodiazepine and is not a sedative drug. It is relatively free of side effects and is considered nonaddictive.
VII. **Evaluation of pharmacological treatment**
A. Assessment of the effectiveness of drugs in the treatment of psychiatric disorders requires special research designs.
B. The response of patients to drug therapy is influenced by a number of variables only some of which are related to the pharmacological properties of the drug.

1. Taking a drug is a complex social behavior and social suggestion may operate to produce the so-called "placebo" effect.
2. Researchers, physicians, and hospital or clinic staff also have expectations and hopes about the benefits of drugs, which may affect their observations.
3. To control for patient and observer expectations that might bias results the *double-blind* research design is used, which controls for placebo effects in the patient and expectation effects of the researchers by hiding the identity of who is given the active drug from participants.

C. The results of careful double-blind research together with research into the mechanisms of drug action have established the effectiveness of antipsychotic, mood modifying, and antianxiety drugs in relieving the symptoms of many patients.

D. A continuing problem in the evaluation of drugs, however, is the lack of diagnostic precision in identifying treatment groups for research purposes.

E. A "boot-straps" effect may be occurring, however, in which diagnostic classification may be improved by paying attention to which patients respond to which drugs.

VIII. Somatic therapy

A. Electroconvulsive therapy

1. Since the introduction of the antipsychotic and antidepressant drugs in the late 1950s and early 1960s, the use of electroconvulsive therapy (ECT) as a treatment for schizophrenic disorders has declined, but it remains a treatment for severe affective illness.

2. It is known that convulsive activity is necessary for effectiveness. Recent neurobiological research suggests that ECT
   a) Increases the serotonin levels.
   b) Increases the turnover rate of norepinephrine.
   c) Improves the sodium transport system in the red blood cells.
   d) Decreases serum calcium concentration.

3. It is an empirical treatment, in use for fifty years, that relieves symptoms. Many theories have been proposed yet no satisfactory explanations of why convulsive seizures elicit behavioral improvement has been accepted. Recent neurobiological research suggests that ECT may alter amine metabolism in the central nervous system. (Some researchers have found increased serotonin levels, others have noted a decrease in norepinephrine.) Such a theory seems plausible in light of studies that indicate that catecholamines play a role in affective illnesses. Amnesia is the principal risk, and this usually dissolves rapidly.

4. Techniques
   a) Sufficient electrical current is passed through electrodes applied to both temporal areas of the head to produce a grand mal seizure. A series of such treatments is given, the average being six to twelve.
   b) Regressive electroshock, a more intensive course of ECT than the standard one, was employed for a brief period of time about twenty years ago. In this treatment, two or three grand mal convulsions were induced daily until regression had occurred (marked confusion, memory loss, disorganization, lack of verbal spontaneity, slurring of speech, and apathy; in other words, the patient behaved like a helpless infant, with bowel and bladder incontinence and a need to be fed). This was thought to be effective in cases of schizophrenic disorder that had been refractory to other forms of treatment.
   c) In recent years, electrodes have been applied over the nondominant temporal hemisphere. This unipolar technique was thought to produce less postseizure confusion and memory loss. Although at first it was claimed to be as effective as bilateral ECT, this claim has now been questioned. The recent study of the American Psychiatric Association's task force found that 70 to 80 percent of all psychiatrists questioned still used the bilateral technique.
   d) Certain medications are given in conjunction with the treatment to minimize apprehension and physical risk. These are usually administered and monitored by a trained anesthesiologist. The following drugs are given intravenously.
      (1) Atropine, to reduce salivation and inhibit vagal action
      (2) Succinylcholine chloride (Anectine), to modify the muscular contractions of the convulsive seizures
      (3) Sedatives, usually pentothal sodium or brevital to put the patient to sleep just prior to the treatment. (Some physicians use oral barbiturates instead of intravenous pentothal prior to the treatment.) Thus, the patient is put under light general anesthesia for a brief period of time.
   e) During the procedure, the patient receives oxygen under pressure.

5. Indications
   a) According to a task force of the American Psychiatric Association,
      (1) ECT is an effective treatment for
         (a) Severe depression, when the risk of suicide is high, the patient is not taking adequate food or fluids, and when the use of drugs or other therapy is very risky or will take an unacceptably long time.
         (b) Severe psychoses characterized by behavior that threatens the safety and well-being of the patient or others, that cannot be controlled by drugs or other means, or for which drugs cannot be employed because of adverse reactions or because of the risk entailed.
         (c) Severe catatonia that has not responded to drugs, when the patient is not taking food or fluids, or when drug or other therapy entails unacceptable risk.
         (d) Severe mania, when the use of drug therapy entails unacceptable risk or when coexisting medical problems (e.g., recent myocardial infarction) either require prompt resolution of the mania or make the use of drug therapy unacceptable.
      (2) ECT is probably effective for
         (a) Depressions, particularly those characterized by vegetative or endogenous symptoms, that have not responded satisfactorily to an adequate course of therapy with antidepressant drugs.
         (b) Depressions, particularly those with vegetative or endogenous elements, when drug therapy is contraindicated.
         (c) Psychoses, particularly those with an endogenous affective component, that have not responded to an adequate trial of antipsychotic drugs or when drugs cannot be used because of adverse reactions.
         (d) It is important to remember that ECT does not ensure against relapse.
         (e) It should be kept in mind that most depressions respond to ECT. Also, studies comparing ECT and antidepressants indicate that ECT is more effective than both tricyclics and MAOI drugs.

   (f) Maintenance ECT—there are occasional cases of recurrent affective disorders that respond to maintenance (or preventive) ECT given at intervals of a few to several weeks. This is less commonly employed now since the introduction of lithium in bipolar disorders or the tricyclic antidepressants in recurrent unipolar disorders.

 6. Contraindications

  a) The physical risk is extremely small, particularly when given with the medications listed under Techniques on p. 360.

  b) There are many physical conditions that were thought to increase the risk of the treatment but, as experience with ECT has increased, the number of physical conditions that contraindicate it has dwindled to a bare minimum (e.g., the presence of a brain tumor with its accompanying increased intracranial pressure; an acute myocardial infarction; abdominal aneurysm).

  c) Cases must be judged individually, however, weighing the possibility of psychiatric recovery against the possible physical risk.

B. Psychosurgery

 1. Although it is usually regarded as beginning in 1936 by Egas Moniz, a psychiatrist collaborating with a neurosurgeon, a Swiss psychiatrist had reported on a small series of cases fifty years earlier (ablation of sensory and parietal cortex). They operated on the frontal lobes of the brain to relieve various symptoms of mental illness.

 2. Techniques

 Various procedures are directed at selected areas of the brain, depending upon the type of disabling symptoms present.

 3. Indications

  a) Patients for whom psychosurgery has been recommended generally have had crippling mental disorders (unusually crippling obsessive-compulsive disorder) that have not responded to adequate trials of other treatment modalities and that have a poor prognosis.

  b) The results of modern surgery on such carefully selected cases vary with the series; in general, more than 50 percent of the patients show major improvement and a few are made worse by the procedure.

c) It should be kept in mind that psychosurgery is radical therapy and is used only as a last resort when other methods have failed.

d) It is performed infrequently in the United States at the present time.

4. Although this is a radical treatment, it would be premature to abandon it until further evaluation has been made.

References

American Psychiatric Association. *A Psychiatric Glossary*. 6th ed. Washington, D.C., 1988.

———. *Electroconvulsive Therapy*. Task Report No. 14. Washington, D.C., 1978.

Baldessarini, R. J. *Chemotherapy in Psychiatry*. 2d ed. Cambridge: Harvard University Press, 1985.

Barchas, J. D., P. A. Bergen, R. D. Ciaranello, and G. R. Elliott, eds. *Psychopharmacology: From Theory to Practice*. New York: Oxford University Press, 1977.

Benson, W. M., and B. C. Schiele. *Tranquilizing and Antidepressive Drugs*. Springfield, Ill.: Charles C. Thomas, Publisher, 1962.

Fink, M. *Convulsive Therapy: Theory and Practice*. New York: Raven Press, 2nd printing, 1985.

Kalinowsky, L. B., and P. H. Hoch. *Somatic Treatment in Psychiatry*. New York: Grune & Stratton, 1961.

Kaplan, H. I., and B. J. Sadock. *Comprehensive Textbook of Psychiatry/ IV*. 4th ed. Baltimore: Williams & Wilkins, 1985.

Kolb, L. C., and H. K. H. Brodie. *Modern Clinical Psychiatry*. 10th ed. Philadelphia: W. B. Saunders Co., 1982.

Synder, S. *Drugs and the Brain*. New York: Scientific American Books, 1986.

GLOSSARY

Acrophobia   Fear of heights.

Acting out   A mechanism in which a person acts without reflection or apparent regard for negative consequences.

Activity therapies   Therapies concerned with the adaptation of the individual in the community.

Actual self   The sum total of an individual's experiences.

Actualizing tendency   Striving to maintain and enhance the experiencing person.

Adjunctive therapies   Therapies used in psychiatric inpatient, day treatment, and partial hospital programs.

Adjustment disorder   A maladaptive reaction to an identifiable psychosocial stressor or stressors that occurs within three months after onset of the stressor and has persisted for no longer than six months.

Agitated-retarded dichotomy   A subdivision of depression, based on whether or not the symptoms include uneasiness, mental perturbation, and motor restlessness (agitation), and slowing down of mental and physical activity (retardation).

Agnosia   A failure to recognize or identify objects, despite intact sensory function.

Agoraphobia   The fear of being in places or situations from which escape might be difficult (or embarassing) or in which help might not be available in the event of a panic attack.

Alcohol amnestic syndrome (Korsakoff's syndrome)   A disorder in which there is an amnestic syndrome (demonstrable evidence of impairment in both short and long term memory), apparently due to the vitamin deficiency associated with prolonged, heavy ingestion of alcohol.

Alcohol hallucinosis   A disorder in which there is an organic hallucinosis, where vivid and persistent hallucinations develop shortly (usually within 48 hours) after cessation of or reduction in alcohol ingestion by a person who apparently has alcohol dependence.

Alcohol idiosyncratic intoxication (pathological intoxication)   A disorder with a marked behavioral change, usually to aggressiveness, due to the recent ingestion of an amount of alcohol insufficient to induce intoxication in most people.

Alcohol intoxication   A disorder in which there are maladaptive behavioral changes due to recent ingestion of alcohol.

Alcohol withdrawal delirium   A disorder in which there are delirium, disorganized thinking, as indicated by rambling, irrelevant, or incoherent speech, and at least two of the following: reduced level of consciousness; perceptual disturbances; misinterpretations, illusions, or hallucinations; disturbances of sleep-wake cycles, with insomnia or daytime sleepiness; increased or decreased psychomotor activity; disorientation to time, place, or person; memory impairment.

Alcoholics   Excessive drinkers whose dependence upon alcohol has attained such a degree that it causes a noticeable mental disturbance or interferes with their bodily and mental health, their interpersonal relationships, or their smooth and economic functioning.

Alcoholics Anonymous   An informal worldwide fellowship of groups of alcoholics, who help each other to stay sober and to remain abstinent.

Alcoholism   A disorder characterized by excessive use of alcohol to the point of habituation, overdependence, or addiction.

Alexithymic   Persons who define their emotions only in terms of somatic sensations or in behavioral reactions rather than relating them to accompanying thoughts.

Algolagnia, active   Sadism.

Algolagnia, passive   Masochism.

Alpha alcoholism (problem drinking or thymogenic drinking)   A purely psychological, continual dependence upon the effects of alcohol, which is used to relieve bodily or emotional pain.

Alzheimer's disease   A progressive dementia occurring in late life.

Anal phase   The period from the eighteenth month until the end of the third year, in which the infant's attention is centered on excretory functions.

Analgesia   Diminished sense of pain.

Anankastic personality (anal character)   An individual who needs to feel in control of himself or herself and of the environment. (Obsessive compulsive personality.)

Ambivalence   The coexistence of two opposing feelings toward the same individual or object.

Anesthesia   Absence of feeling.

Anima   The true inner self, or soul.

Anima   The female component of the male personality.

Animus   The masculine component of the female personality.

Anorexia   A disorder marked by loss of appetite and loss of weight.

Anorexia nervosa   A disorder in which the essential features are refusal to maintain body weight over a minimal normal weight for age and height; intense fear of gaining weight or becoming fat, even though underweight; a distorted body image; and amenorrhea in females.

Antisocial personality disorder (character disorder, character neurosis)   A disorder in which there is a pattern of irresponsible and antisocial behavior, beginning in childhood or early adolescence and continuing into adulthood.

Anxiety   A diffuse, unpleasant uneasiness, apprehension, or fearfulness stemming from anticipated danger, the source of which is uncertain or unidentifiable.

Anxiety disorders   Disorders in which the essential features are symptoms of anxiety and avoidance behavior.

Aphasia   A disorder of language.

Aphonia   An inability to produce normal speech.

Apraxia   An inability to carry out motor activities despite intact comprehension and motor function.

Asexual   A person who denies having had strong sexual feelings.

Atypical depression   A depressive syndrome responsive to a monoamine oxidase inhibitor (MAOI).

Autistic fantasy   A mechanism in which a person substitutes excessive daydreaming for pursuits of human relationships or the more direct and effective action of problem solving.

Autochthonous ideas   Ideas originating within the psyche without external stimuli.

Aversion therapy   A form of therapy based on straightforward classical (Pavlovian) conditioning procedures, whereby stimuli are associated with some strong unacceptable responses, such as nausea, pain, or extreme disgust.

Avoidant personality disorder   A disorder in which there is a pervasive pattern of social discomfort, fear of negative evaluation, and timidity, beginning by early adulthood and present in a variety of contexts.

Behavior modification   The application of operant conditioning principles to the interpretation and management of behavior problems.

Behavior therapy   The modification of responses through the application of experimentally established principles of learning.

Behaviorism   John B. Watson's definition for the methodological position in psychology.

Bereavement   A normal, appropriate, affective sadness in response to a recognizable external loss.

Beta alcoholism (somatophathic)   Similar to alpha, with the added complication of physiological derangements, such as gastritis, neuritis, liver and vascular disease.

Bipolar disorder   A disorder in which the essential feature is the presence of one or more manic or hypomanic episodes (usually with a history of major depressive episodes).

Birth trauma   Primal anxiety, in response to feelings of helplessness, produced by birth.

Body dysmorphic disorder (dysmorphophobia)   A disorder in which there is preoccupation with some imagined defect in appearance in a normal appearing person.

Borderline personality disorder   A pervasive pattern of instability of self-image, interpersonal relationships, and mood, beginning by early adulthood and present in a variety of contexts.

Brief reactive psychosis   A disorder in which the essential feature is sudden onset of psychotic symptoms of at least a few hours, but no more than one month's duration, with eventual return to premorbid level of functioning.

Bulimia   Increased appetite.

Bulimia nervosa   A disorder in which there are recurrent episodes of binge eating.

Castration anxiety   Anxiety that results from the boy's fear of damage to or loss of his genitals.

Catatonic excitement   A disorder characterized by excited motor activity, apparently purposeless and not influenced by external stimuli.

Catatonic negativism A disorder characterized by an apparently motiveless resistance to all instructions or attempts to be moved.

Catatonic posturing A disorder characterized by voluntary assumptions of inappropriate or bizarre posture.

Catatonic schizophrenia A disorder in which the essential feature is marked psychomotor disturbance, which may involve stupor, negativism, rigidity, excitement, or posturing.

Catatonic stupor or mutism A disorder characterized by marked decrease in reactivity to environment, reduction of spontaneous movements or activity, or mutism.

Cathexis The process by which the unconscious primitive drives are vested with psychic energy.

Character neurosis Impulses and ideas are acceptable to the ego as consonant and compatible with its principles.

Clarification A process by which the physician helps patients to understand their feelings and behavior and to gain a clearer picture of reality.

Claustrophobia Fear of closed spaces.

Collective unconscious (racial or archaic unconscious) An inheritance of primitive racial ideas and impulses.

Commonsense psychiatry Understanding the patient in the simplest terms possible.

Compensation A conscious or unconscious attempt to overcome real or fancied inferiorities.

Compulsions Repetitive, purposeful, and intentional behaviors that are performed in response to an obsession, according to certain rules, or in a stereotyped fashion.

Conscience The conscious part of the superego.

Conscious Composes ideas, feelings, drives, and urges of which a person is aware.

Constructional difficulty Inability to copy three-dimensional figures, assemble blocks, or arrange sticks in specific designs.

Consultation liaison psychiatry A subspeciality of psychiatry that is concerned with clinical service teaching and research at the borderline of psychiatry and medicine.

Continuous amnesia Failure to recall events, subsequent to a specific time and up to, and including, the present.

Conversion disorder A disorder in which there is an alteration or loss of physical functioning that suggests physical disorder, but instead is apparently an expression of a psychological conflict or need.

Coping mechanisms Conscious efforts to control anxiety.

Coprophilia A pathological sexual interest in excretions.

Cosmic consciousness (or illumination) A fabulous sense of joy or well-being, sometimes produced by hallucinogenic drugs.

Countercathexis The opposition of ego energy to id energy.

Countertransference The therapist's unconscious or conscious emotional reaction to the patient.

Cyclothymia A disorder in which there are numerous hypomanic episodes and numerous periods with depressive symptoms.

Defense mechanisms (mental mechanisms, mental dynamisms, ego-defense mechanisms) Specific, unconscious, intrapsychic adjustments that come into play to resolve emotional conflict and reduce the individual's anxiety.

Déjà vu A subjective sensation that an experience that is really happening for the first time occurred on a previous occasion.

Delusional (paranoid) disorder A disorder in which there is the presence of a persistent, nonbizarre delusion that is not due to any other mental disorder.

Dementia associated with alcoholism A disorder in which there is the development of a dementia, following a prolonged and heavy ingestion of alcohol, for which all other causes of dementia have been excluded.

Dementia praecox A type of reaction to environmental experiences (parergastic reaction).

Denial (negation) The unconscious disavowal of a thought, feeling, wish, need, or reality that is consciously unacceptable.

Dependent personality disorder A disorder in which there is a pervasive pattern of dependent and submissive behavior beginning by early adulthood and present in a variety of contexts.

Depersonalization A sense of estrangement from oneself.

Depersonalization disorder A disorder in which the person has feelings of unreality, altered personality, or altered identity, and might deny his or her own existence along with that of his environment.

Depression The emotion of feeling sad, blue, or unhappy (dysthymia).

Derealization A feeling that the environment has changed.

Diathesis-stress factor Views mental disorders as the product of a predisposition toward the development of a particular disorder (diathesis), and conditions operating on the person that require an adjustive response.

Displacement The redirection of an emotion from the original object to a more acceptable substitute.

Disorganized schizophrenia A disorder in which the essential features are marked incoherence, marked loosening of associations, or grossly disorganized behavior, flat or grossly inappropriate affect, fragmentary, unsystematized delusions or hallucinations with an incoherent theme.

Dissociation The unconscious detachment of certain behavior from the normal or usual conscious behavior patterns of an individual, which then function alone (compartmentalization).

Dissociative disorders (or hysterical neuroses, dissociative type) Disorders in which there is a disturbance or alteration in the normally integrative functions of identity, memory, or consciousness.

Dissociative disorder not otherwise specified A dissociative symptoms that does not meet the criteria for a specific dissociative disorder.

Dizygotic twins Fraternal twins.

Dynamic unconscious Certain significant desires and drives that are repressed.

Dyspareunia A disorder in which there is recurrent or persistent genital pain in either a male or female, before, during, or after sexual intercourse.

Dysthymia A disorder in which there is chronic disturbance of mood involving depressed mood (or possibly an irritable mood in children or adolescents), for most of the day, more days than not, for at least two years (one year for children and adolescents).

Ego   The part of the personality that meets and interacts with the outside world; the "integrator" or "mediator" of the personality.

Ego-dystonic homosexuality   A disorder in which there are a desire to acquire or increase heterosexual arousal, so that heterosexual relationships can be initiated or maintained, and a sustained pattern of overt homosexual arousal, which the individual explicitly states has been unwanted and a persistent source of distress.

Ego ideal   The part of the ego devoted to the development of parental substitutes, (parental images).

Ego ideal   The nonpunitive, positive aspect of the superego.

Empathy   The capacity for participating in, or vicariously experiencing another's feelings, volitions, or ideas.

Endogenous-reactive dichotomy   A subdivision of depression based on whether or not the depression seemed to develop "from within" (endogenous) or was related to life events (reactive).

Environmental modification (environmental intervention, environmental manipulation)   Altering the environment so as to relieve the patient's symptoms and distress.

Epigenesis   The stages of ego and social development.

Epsilon alcoholism (periodic drinking, dipsomania)   Alcoholism characterized by paroxysmal drinking bouts, during which the alcoholic drinks for varying periods of time, ranging from days to weeks.

Eros   The creative forces, the life instinct.

Erotomanic delusion   An erotic delusion that one is loved by another, usually of a higher status, such as a famous person or a superior at work.

Essential alcoholism (addictive drinking, compulsive drinking, alcoholism simplex)   Alcoholism in which a person drifts across the line from social drinking, and alcoholism simplex.

Exhibitionism   A disorder in which there are recurrent, intense sexual urges and sexually arousing fantasies, of at least six months' duration, involving the exposure of one's genitals to a stranger.

Existential psychoanalysis   Stresses the here and now rather than the past in the evaluation of personality disorder.

Expressive therapies   Therapies concerned with maximizing the possibilities of communicating and the media through which persons can express and communicate their feelings, conflicts, personal characteristics, and creative potential.

Extroversion   Outwardly directed libido.

Factitious disorder   A disorder that is characterized by physical or psychological symptoms that are intentionally produced or feigned.

Factitious disorder not otherwise specified   A disorder that cannot be classified in any other specific category.

Factitious disorder with physical symptoms   A disorder in which there is the intentional production of physical symptoms.

Factitious disorder with psychological symptoms   A disorder in which there is intentional production or feigning of psychological (often psychotic) symptoms, suggestive of mental disorder.

Family therapy   A form of group therapy, wherein the nuclear family is the unit, which has developed during the past three or four decades.

Fantasy A fabricated series of mental pictures or sequence of events; daydreaming.

Fascination (or fixation) A trancelike state induced in individuals who are compelled to focus on a given object for long periods of time.

Feelings of derealization Feelings that the environment has changed.

Feelings of estrangement A sense of detachment from people, the environment, or concepts.

Feelings of unreality Feelings that one is unreal.

Female sexual arousal disorder A disorder in which there is persistent or recurrent partial or complete failure to attain or maintain the lubrication-swelling response of sexual excitement until the completion of the sexual activity; and the persistent or recurrent lack of a subjective sense of sexual excitement and pleasure in a female during sexual activity.

Fetishism A disorder in which there are recurrent, intense sexual urges and sexually arousing fantasies, of at least six months' duration, involving the use of nonliving objects.

Fixation The arrest of maturation at an immature level of psychosexual development.

Flagellation Erotic whipping.

Free association The spontaneous uncensored verbalizations by the patient of whatever comes to mind.

Frotteurism A disorder in which there are recurrent, intense sexual urges and sexually arousing fantasies, of at least six months' duration, involving touching and rubbing against a nonconsenting person.

Gamma alcoholism (essential alcoholism) Alcoholism characterized by the traditional pharmacological criterion of addiction, including both tolerance (a diminished effect with repeated use) and dependency.

Ganser's syndrome (nonsense syndrome, prison psychosis) "The syndrome of appropriate answers" to questions, commonly associated with other symptoms such as amnesia, disorientation, perceptual disturbances, fugue, and conversion.

Gender identity The inner conviction that one is either male, female, ambivalent, or neutral.

Gender identity disorder A disorder in which the essential feature is an incongruence between assigned sex (i.e., the sex that is recorded on the birth certificate) and gender identity.

Gender identity disorder of adolescence or adulthood, nontranssexual type A disorder in which there are persistent or recurrent discomfort and sense of inappropriateness about one's assigned sex, and persistent or recurrent cross-dressing in the role of the other sex, either in fantasy or in actuality.

Gender identity disorder of childhood A disorder in which the essential feature is persistent and intense distress in a child about his or her assigned sex and the desire to be, or insistence that he or she is, of the other sex.

Gender role The behavior and appearance that one presents in terms of what the culture considers to be "masculine" or "feminine."

Generalized amnesia Failure to recall the individual's entire life.

Generalized anxiety disorder A disorder in which there are unrealistic or excessive anxiety and worry about two or more life circumstances.

Genital phase   The final stage of psychosexual development.

Grandiose delusions   Delusions that are centered around the person's conviction that he or she possesses great unrecognized talent or insight or has made some important discovery.

Group psychotherapy   Application of psychotherapeutic techniques to a group, including utilization of interactions of members of the group.

Hebephrenia   A progressive psychotic illness of rapid onset in adolescence.

Histrionic personality disorder   A disorder in which there is a pervasive pattern of excessive emotionality and attention-seeking, beginning by early adulthood and present in a variety of contexts.

Holism (holistic approach)   The understanding of the individual personality based on the interplay of his inherited structure, his uniqueness, and the cultural pattern in which he lives.

Homeostasis   The individual's tendency to maintain a relatively stable psychological condition with respect to contending drives, motivations, and other psychodynamic forces.

Homosexual   A person whose object choice has been the same anatomic sex.

Homosexuality   A preferential *erotic* attraction for members of the same sex.

Hostile identification   Internalization of undesirable personality traits of parents or authority figures.

Humanistic psychology   The study of the experiencing person.

Humanistic therapy   A number of therapeutic approaches characterized by their phenomenological or existential assumptions about human experiences or by their opposition to traditional psychoanalysis or behavior therapy.

Huntington's chorea   A disorder characterized by progressive intellectual loss and motor dysfunction.

Hypersomnia   Excessive sleep.

Hypnagogic hallucinations   The mental images that occur just before sleep.

Hypnopompic hallucinations   Images seen in dreams that persist on awakening.

Hypoactive sexual desire disorder   A disorder in which there are persistent or recurrent, deficient or absent sexual fantasies and desire for sexual activity.

Hypochondriasis (Hypochondriacal neurosis)   The fear of having, or the belief that one has a serious disease, based on the person's interpretation of physical signs or sensations as evidence of physical illness.

Hypoxyphilia   Sexual arousal by oxygen deprivation.

Hysterical personality   See histrionic personality.

Id   The unconscious reservoir of primitive drives (instincts).

Idealization   The overestimation of admired qualities of another person or desired object.

Idealized self   A glorified self-image, closely related to the current concept of narcissism.

Identification   The unconscious, wishful adaption, or internalization of the personality characteristics or identity of another individual, generally one possessing attributes that the subject envies or admires.

Identification with the aggressor   The unconscious internalization of the characteristics of a frustrating or feared person.

Identity   An inner sense of sameness that perseveres, despite external changes.

Identity crisis   The inability of the adolescent to accept a role he or she believes to be expected by society.

Imitation   A conscious mimicking of the behavior of others.

Incorporation   A primitive defense mechanism in which the psychic image of another person is wholly or partially assimilated into an individual's personality.

Induced psychotic disorder   A disorder in which the essential feature is a delusional system that develops in a second person as a result of a close relationship with another person who already has a psychotic disorder with prominent delusions.

Infantilism   A desire to be treated as a helpless infant and clothed in diapers.

Inferiority complex   The conflict, partly conscious and partly unconscious, that impels the individual to attempt to overcome the distress accompanying feelings of inferiority.

Inhibited female orgasm   A disorder in which there is persistent or recurrent delay in, or absence of, orgasm in a female following a normal sexual excitement phase during sexual activity that the clinician judges to be adequate in focus, intensity, and duration.

Inhibited male orgasm   A disorder in which there is persistent or recurrent delay in, or absence of, orgasm in a male following a normal heterosexual excitement phase during sexual activity that the clinician, taking into account the person's age, judges to be adequate in focus, intensity, and duration.

Initial insomnia   Difficulty falling asleep.

Intellectualization   The overuse of intellectual concepts and words to avoid affective experience or expressions of feelings.

Intoxication   Development of a substance-specific syndrome due to recent ingestion of a psychoactive substance.

Intrapsychic   That which occurs within the personality.

Introjection   The symbolic internalization of assimilation (taking into oneself) of a loved or hated person or external object.

Introversion   Inwardly directed libido, reflected in the tendency to be preoccupied with oneself.

Involutional melancholia   A depression of initial onset occurring during the involutional years (40–55 in women and 50–65 in men), with symptoms of marked anxiety, agitation, restlessness, somatic concerns, hypochondriasis, occasional somatic or nihilistic delusions, insomnia, anorexia and weight loss.

Isolation   The separation of an unacceptable impulse, act, or idea from its memory origin, thereby removing the emotional charge associated with the original memory.

Klismophilia   The love of enemas and a dependence on their use for sexual arousal.

La belle indifference   Indifference to an illness.

Late luteal phase dysphoric disorder   A disorder in which a pattern of clinically significant emotional and behavioral symptoms occur during the last week of the luteal phase and remit within a few days after the onset of the follicular phase.

Latency   The stage between the Oedipal period and the adolescent years.

Libido   The emotional energy broadly derived from the underlying instincts (psychosexual energy) and presumably present at birth.

Litigious delusions   Delusions that produce disputatiousness, contentiousness, fondness for litigation, or proneness to engage in lawsuits.

Localization theory   Mental and emotional life is dependent on the brain.

Localized (circumscribed) amnesia   Failure to recall all events during a circumscribed period of time, usually the first few hours following a profoundly disturbing event.

Logo therapy   Psychotherapy, based on a system of spiritual values, that stresses the search for the meaning of human existence.

Major depression, recurrent or major depression, single   A disorder in which there are one or more major depressive episodes without a history of either a manic episode or unequivocal hypomanic episode (unipolar depression).

Major depressive episode   A major depressive syndrome in which it cannot be established that an organic factor initiated and maintained the disturbance and the presence of a nonmood psychotic disorder has been ruled out.

Major depressive episode, melancholic type   A severe depression that includes anhedonia (loss of pleasure), lack of reactivity to usually pleasurable stimuli, depression regularly worse in the morning, early morning awakening (terminal insomnia), psychomotor retardation or agitation, significant anorexia, weight loss, no significant personality disturbance before the first major depressive episode, one or more previous major depressive episodes, followed by complete or nearly complete recovery and previous good responses to specific and adequate somatic antidepressive therapy.

Major depressive syndrome   A depressed mood or loss of interest of at least two weeks' duration accompanied by several associated symptoms (such as weight loss and difficulty concentrating).

Male erectile disorder   A disorder with persistent or recurrent partial or complete failure in a male to attain or maintain erection until completion of the sexual activity.

Malingering   A conscious simulation of illness in order to avoid an unpleasant or intolerable alternative.

Mania   A disorder in which there is elevated euphoric, expansive, or irritable mood.

Masculine protest   The individual's (male-female) attempt to escape from the feminine submissive role.

Mental-status examination   A special form of assessment often conducted in conjunction with the history-taking interview.

Middle insomnia   Difficulty remaining asleep.

Minnesota Multiphasic Personality Inventory (MMPI)   The most widely used objective personality test in psychiatric practice in the United States, consisting of 566 true-false items.

Monozygotic twins   Identical twins.

Mood episode (major depressive, manic, or hypomanic)   A mood syndrome that is not due to a known organic factor and is not part of a nonmood psychotic disorder.

Mood syndrome (depressive or manic)   A group of mood and associated symptoms that occur together for a minimal period of time.

Moral masochism   The seeking of humiliation and failure rather than physical pain.

Multiple personality   A disorder in which there is the existence within the person of two or more distinct personalities or personality states.

Münchausen   A chronic form of factitious disorder, in which a person's plausible presentation of factitious physical symptoms is associated with multiple hospitalizations.

Narcissistic or pregenital phase   The oral and anal phases considered together.

Narcissistic personality disorder   A disorder in which there is a pervasive pattern of grandiosity (in fantasy or behavior), hypersensitivity to the evaluation of others, and lack of empathy that begins by early adulthood and is present in a variety of contexts.

Necrophilia   The deriving of sexual gratification from corpses.

Neuroendocrine   The chief hormone adrenaline or epinephrine, secreted by the medulla of the adrenal glands.

Neuromodulation   The action of neuroactive substances that tends to amplify or dampen the degree of neurotransmitter action.

Neuropeptides   Hormonelike substances that are secreted from neuroendocrine cells or from some neurons.

Neurotic disorder   A mental disorder in which the predominant disturbance is a symptom or group of symptoms that is distressing to the individual and is recognized by the individual as unacceptable and alien (ego-dystonic).

Neurotransmitters   Substances released from activated axons of neurons (and from some dendrites) that communicate across synapses with other neurons.

Nicotine dependence   A disorder associated with the inhalation of cigarette smoke.

Nicotine withdrawal   A disorder in which there is a characteristic withdrawal syndrome due to the abrupt cessation of or reduction in the use of nicotine-containing substances that have been at least moderate in duration and amount.

Nocturnal anxiety   The infant's fear of the dark.

Normotensive hydrocephalus   A nonabsorptive communicating type of hydrocephalus that develops in the absence of a demonstrable lesion.

Object libido   The libido that is directed outward toward another person or thing.

Obsessions   Persistent ideas, thoughts, impulses, or images that are experienced, at least initially, as intrusive and senseless.

Obsessive-compulsive disorders   A disorder in which there are recurrent obsessions or compulsions sufficiently severe to cause marked distress because they are time-consuming or significantly interfere with the person's normal routine, occupational functioning, or usual social activities or relationships.

Obsessive-compulsive personality disorder   A disorder in which there is a pervasive pattern of perfectionism and inflexibility, beginning by early adulthood and present in a variety of contexts.

Oedipus complex   The attachment of the child to the parent of the opposite sex, accompanied by envious and aggressive feelings toward the parent of the same sex.

Operant conditioning   Reinforcing or not reinforcing the consequences of an act, so that it tends to be repeated or extinguished.

Oral phase The first twelve to eighteen months of life, characterized chiefly by preoccupation with feeding.

Organic anxiety syndrome Prominent, recurrent panic attacks or generalized anxiety.

Organic hallucinosis Persistent or recurrent hallucinations in a state of full wakefulness and alertness.

Organic mental disorder A particular organic mental syndrome in which the etiology is known or presumed.

Organic mental syndrome A constellation of psychological or behavioral signs and symptoms without reference to etiology.

Organic mental syndrome not otherwise specified Syndromes that do not meet the criteria for any of the other organic mental syndromes, and in which there are maladaptive changes during the waking state with evidence from either physical examination, laboratory tests, or history of a specific organic factor that is judged to be etiologically related to the disturbance.

Organic mood syndrome A disorder in which there is a prominent and persistent depressed, elevated, or expansive mood, resembling either a manic episode or a major depressive episode, that is due to a specific organic factor.

Organic personality syndrome A persistent personality disturbance, either lifelong or representing a change or accentuation of a previous characteristic trait.

Panic disorder with or without agoraphobia A disorder in which there are recurrent panic attacks, which typically begin with the sudden onset of intense apprehension, fear, or terror.

Paramnesia A distortion or falsification of memory in which the individual confuses reality and fantasy.

Paranoid personality disorder A disorder in which there is a pervasive and unwarranted tendency, beginning by early adulthood and present in a variety of contexts, to interpret the actions of people as deliberately demeaning or threatening.

Paranoid schizophrenia A disorder in which there is preoccupation with one or more systematized delusions or with frequent auditory hallucinations related to a single theme.

Paraphilias Disorders characterized by arousal and response to sexual objects or situations that are not part of normative arousal activity patterns, which in varying degrees may interfere with the capacity for reciprocal, affectionate sexual activity.

Parataxic distortions Attitudes toward other persons that are based on distorted evaluations of them or on an identification of such persons with figures from one's past life.

Paresis Muscular weakness.

Paresthesia Tingling feeling.

Passive-aggression A mechanism in which a person indirectly and unassertively expresses aggression toward others.

Passive-aggressive personality disorder A disorder in which there is a pervasive pattern of passive resistance to demands for adequate social and occupational performance, beginning by early adulthood and present in a variety of contexts.

Pedophilia   A disorder in which there are recurrent, intense sexual urges and sexually arousing fantasies, of at least six months' duration, involving sexual activity with a prepubescent child.

Penis envy   The girl's desire to possess a penis and, thus, to become masculine.

Periodic catatonia   A rare form of episodic catatonia that is related to shifts in an individual's metabolic nitrogen balance.

Persecutory delusion   A delusion in which a person feels conspired against, cheated and spied upon, followed, poisoned, or drugged, maliciously maligned, harassed, or obstructed in the pursuit of long-term goals.

Persona   The social facade assumed by an individual (so named from the mask worn by actors in ancient Greek drama, which characterized the mood portrayed).

Personality   The sum total of a person's internal and external patterns of adjustment to life.

Personality   The characteristic way in which a person thinks, feels, and behaves; the ingrained pattern of behavior that each person evolves both consciously and unconsciously as the style or way of being in adapting to the environment.

Personality disorders   Disorders that develop when personality traits are inflexible and maladaptive and cause either significant functional impairment or subjective distress.

Personality traits   Enduring patterns of perceiving, relating to, and thinking about the environment and oneself, which are exhibited in a wide range of important social and personal contexts.

Persuasion   Direct suggestion, inducement, or entreatment in an effort to influence a patient's behavior.

Phallic phase   Period extending from the end of the third year to the seventh year.

Phenomenological reality   Subjective, personal interpretation of experience rather than physical reality, which determines behavior.

Pick's disease   A presenile focal degenerative disease of the brain affecting the cerebral cortex, particularly the frontal lobe.

Pleasure principle   The seeking of pleasure and the avoidance of pain.

Post-traumatic stress disorder   A disorder in which an event is experienced that is outside the range of usual human experience and that would be markedly distressing to almost anyone.

Preconscious   Comprises feelings, ideas, drives and urges that are out of the individual's immediate awareness, but that can be readily recalled.

Premature ejaculation   A disorder in which there is persistent or recurrent ejaculation, with minimal sexual stimulation, before, upon, or shortly after penetration and before the person wishes it.

Primary affective disorder   A disorder that occurs in persons who have never had an episode before or whose only previous psychiatric illnesses were episodes of depression or mania.

Primary narcissism   The original state of the newborn.

Primary processes   The psychological expressions of the underlying basic drives.

Primordial images   A phylogenetic memory heavily laden with mythological references.

Projection   The attributing to another person or object, the thoughts, feelings, motives, or desires that are really one's own disavowed and unacceptable traits.

Projective identification   The association of uncomfortable aspects of one's own personality with their projection onto another person, resulting in identification with the other person.

Pseudodementia   Exaggerated indifference to one's surroundings, without actual mental impairment, and reversible decline of mental functioning that occurs in depression.

Psychic manifestation of anxiety   The sensation of apprehension and the cortical perception of discomfort.

Psychoactive substance-induced organic mental disorders   Disorders caused by the direct, acute, or chronic effect of substances on the central nervous system.

Psychoactive substance use disorders   Disorders with the symptoms and maladaptive behavioral changes associated with more or less regular use of psychoactive substances that affect the central nervous system.

Psychoanalysis   A theory of personality development, a method of research, and a system of treatment.

Psychobiology   The study not only of the person as a whole, as a unit, but also the whole man.

Psychodynamic therapy   Therapy that produces insight by uncovering emotional conflicts, chiefly unconscious, so that they can be dealt with in a way that does not hamper current relationships and activities.

Psychodynamics   The study, explanation, or interpretation of behavior or mental states in terms of mental or emotional forces or processes.

Psychogenic amnesia   A disorder in which there is sudden inability to recall important personal information, an inability not due to an organic mental disorder.

Psychogenic fugue   Sudden, unexpected travel away from home or customary work locale with assumption of a new identity and an inability to recall one's previous identity.

Psychogenic hypothesis   A hypothesis that regards mental disorder as the effect of environmental factors that affect the psychological integration and social adequacy of the individual, particularly the effectiveness of the management of individual needs in relation to the demands of the world.

Psychosocial stressors   The usual stresses of life.

Psychotherapy   A process in which a person who wishes to relieve symptoms or resolve problems in living or in seeking personal growth enters into an implicit or explicit contract to interact in a prescribed way with the psychotherapist.

Rapport   The feeling of harmonious accord and mutual responsiveness that contributes to the patient's confidence in the therapist and willingness to work cooperatively.

Rationalization   The ascribing of acceptable or worthwhile motives to one's own thoughts, feelings, or behavior that really have unrecognized motives.

Reaction formation   The direction of overt behavior or attitudes in precisely the opposite direction of the individual's underlying, unacceptable conscious or unconscious impulses.

Reactive drinking   Drinking in response to some particular emotional stress, such as the death of a loved one.

Real self   The unique total force and sense of integration found in each person.

Reassurance   The imparting or restoration of confidence and freeing the patient from fear and anxiety.

Regression   The unconscious return to an earlier level of emotional adjustment at which gratification was assured.

Repression   The involuntary, automatic banishment of unacceptable ideas, impulses, or feelings into the unconscious (motivated unconscious forgetting).

Residual schizophrenia   A disorder in which the clinical picture is without permanent psychotic symptoms, though signs of the illness persist.

Resistance   The conscious or unconscious psychological forces in the patient that oppose bringing repressed (unconscious) material into consciousness.

Restitution   The supplanting of a highly valued object that has been lost through rejection by, or death or departure of, another object.

Rorschach Test   The best known and most widely used of the projective techniques.

Sadistic personality disorder   A disorder in which there is a pervasive pattern of cruel, demeaning, and aggressive behavior directed toward other people, beginning by early adulthood.

Sado-masochism   The occurrence of sadism and masochism in the same person.

Schizoid personality disorder (introverted personality)   A disorder in which there are a pervasive pattern of indifference to social relationships, and a restricted range of emotional experience and expression, beginning by early adulthood and present in a variety of contexts.

Schizophrenia   A large group of disorders, usually of psychotic proportion, manifested by characteristic disturbances of language and communication, thought, perception, affect, and behavior, which last longer than six months.

Schizophreniform disorder   A disorder in which the essential features are identical with those of schizophrenia, with the exception that the duration, including prodromal, active, and residual phases, is less than six months.

Schizotypal personality disorder   A disorder in which there is a pervasive pattern of peculiarities of ideation, appearance, and behavior and deficits in interpersonal relatedness, beginning by early adulthood and present in a variety of contexts, which are not severe enough to meet the criteria for schizophrenia.

Seasonal affective disorder   A disorder in which there is a regular temporal relationship between the onset of an episode of bipolar disorder or recurrent major depression and a particular sixty-day period of the year.

Secondary affective disorder   A disorder that occurs in persons who have had other psychiatric illnesses (i.e., schizophrenia or alcoholism), or who have suffered an affective disorder related to a medical condition.

Secondary processes   The reasonable and acceptable ways in which the underlying basic drives are controlled and permitted expression according to the demands of the outside world.

Selective amnesia   Failure to recall some, but not all, of the events occurring during a circumscribed period of time.

Self-defeating personality disorder   A disorder in which there is a pervasive pattern of self-defeating behavior, beginning by early adulthood and present in a variety of contexts.

Self-help groups   Groups without professionally trained leaders, in which the group experience does not uncover basic conflicts, but does offer new shared experiences to the patient.

Sexual aversion disorder   A disorder in which there is persistent or recurrent extreme aversion to and avoidance of, all or almost all, genital sexual contact with a sexual partner.

Sexual dysfunction   A disorder in which the essential feature is inhibition in the appetite or psychophysiologic changes that characterize the complete sexual response cycle.

Sexual masochism   A disorder in which there are recurrent, intense sexual urges and sexually arousing fantasies, of at least six months' duration, involving the act (real, not similated) of being humiliated, beaten, bound, or otherwise made to suffer.

Sexual sadism   A disorder in which there are recurrent, intense, sexual urges and sexually arousing fantasies, of at least six months' duration, involving acts (real, not simulated) in which the psychological or physical suffering (including humiliation) of the victim is sexually exciting.

Shadow   The objective counterpart of the underlying personal unconscious and collective unconscious.

Simple phobia   A disorder in which there is persistent fear of a circumscribed stimulus other than fear of having a panic attack or of humiliation or embarrassment in certain social situations.

Somatic delusions   Delusions that can take one of several forms: most common ones involve belief that the person emits a foul odor from his or her skin, mouth, rectum, or vagina, or that there's an infestation of insects on his or her skin, or that he or she has an internal parasite, or certain parts of the body are misshapen or ugly, or that certain parts of the body are not functioning.

Somatic (or motor-visceral) manifestations of anxiety   The result of the physiological responses of the various bodily systems to the increased secretion of epinephrine.

Somatization disorder   A disorder with recurrent and multiple somatic complaints, of several years' duration for which medical attention has been sought, but that apparently are not due to any physical disorder.

Somatoform disorders   A group of disorders with physical symptoms suggesting physical disorder for which there are no demonstrable organic findings or known physiological mechanism and for which there is positive evidence or strong presumption that the symptoms are linked to psychological factors or conflicts.

Somatoform pain disorder   A disorder in which there is preoccupation with pain in the absence of adequate physical findings to account for the pain or its intensity.

Somatogenic hypothesis   A hypothesis that regards mental illness as resulting from the malfunction of the central nervous system in a way that effects cognitive, emotional, and expressive processes.

Somnambulism   Sleepwalking.

Splitting   The inability to unite and integrate the hating and loving aspects of both one's self-image and one's image of another person.

Stanford-Binet (New Revised)   Individually administered intelligence test for children and for the assessment of mental retardation.

Stranger anxiety   The apprehension noted in infants when they are approached by strangers.

Stress   Conditions that are extremely unpleasant, noxious, or demanding, which produce both the experience of stress (often characterized as anxiety) and effects on the behavior and physiological state of the individual.

Strong-Campbell Interest Inventory (SCII)   The most commonly used vocational interest test for adults.

Sublimation   The diversion of unacceptable instinctual drives into socially sanctioned channels.

Substitution   An unconscious replacement of a highly valued, but unattainable or unacceptable emotional goal or object by one that is attainable or acceptable.

Successful defenses   Defenses that eliminate the need for immediate gratification or provide substitute socially acceptable gratification.

Superego   The censoring force of the personality.

Supportive psychotherapy   A therapy that deals predominantly with conscious material and is centered chiefly on bolstering the individual's strengths and assets.

Suppression   The voluntary, intentional relegation of unacceptable ideas or impulses to the foreconscious (volitional exclusion or conscious forgetting).

Symbolization   The unconscious mechanism by which a neutral idea or object is used to represent another idea or object that has a forbidden aspect.

Symptom neurosis   The stimuli from any source are rejected by the ego or are prevented from reaching the ego for consideration.

Symptomatic alcoholism   Alcoholism in which the drinking is a symptom of a serious emotional disorder such as anxiety disorder, affective disorder, or schizophrenic disorder.

Systematic desensitization   A means of associating anxiety-eliciting stimuli with relaxation.

Tardive dyskinesia   A choreiform, ticlike involuntary or semivoluntary muscular movement, classically involving the tongue, face, and neck muscles (oral lingual dyskinesia or buccal lingual masticatory dyskinesia).

Telephone scatologia (lewdness)   A sexual gratification, derived usually by men who telephone women, make obscene remarks, and suggest that the woman meet them and engage in sexual activity.

Terminal insomnia   Early morning awakening.

Thanatos   The aggressive, destructive, or death forces.

Thematic Apperception Test (TAT)   A test consisting of twenty illustrations, in which the patient is asked to tell a story about the content of each picture.

Trance state   A psychological stupor characterized by immobility and unresponsiveness to the environment.

Trancelike state   A similiar experience, ordinarily induced in normal individuals by prolonged and unusual concentration on a task or object.

Transference   The displacement of feelings for significant people in one's earlier life onto the physician or therapist.

Transference neurosis   A state in which early feelings and attitudes make up the bulk of the patient's feelings toward the physician.

Transsexualism   A disorder in which there are persistent discomfort and a sense of inappropriateness about one's assigned sex in a person who has reached puberty.

Transvestic fetishism   A disorder in which there are recurrent, intense sexual urges and sexually arousing fantasies, of at least six months' duration, involving cross-dressing.

Unburdening (ventilation; catharsis)   The therapeutic release of feelings through conscious, free expression.

Uncomplicated alcohol withdrawal   A disorder in which there are certain characteristic symptoms such as a coarse tremor of hands, tongue, or eyelids; nausea or vomiting; malaise or weakness; autonomic hyperactivity; anxiety, depressed mood, or irritability; transient hallucinations or illusions; headache; and insomnia.

Unconscious   The drives, feelings, ideas, and urges that are outside of the individual's awareness.

Uncovering therapy   The exploration of the unconscious, chiefly through free association.

Undifferentiated schizophrenia   A disorder in which there are permanent psychotic symptoms (delusions, hallucinations, incoherence, or grossly disorganized behavior), which cannot be classified as catatonic, disorganized, or paranoid.

Undifferentiated somatoform disorder   A disorder in which there is difficulty swallowing (globus hystericus), or commonly, multiple physical complaints, such as fatigue, loss of appetite, and gastrointestinal problems.

Undoing (symbolic atonement)   A primitive defense mechanism in which some unacceptable past behavior is symbolically acted out in reverse, usually repetitiously.

Unsuccessful defenses   Defenses that do not resolve the conflict and the continuing need for the defense.

Urophilia   A pathological love for, or interest in, urine.

Vaginismus   A disorder in which there is a recurrent or persistent involuntary spasm of the musculature of the outer third of the vagina that interferes with coitus.

Voyeurism   A disorder in which there are recurrent, intense sexual urges and sexually arousing fantasies, of at least six months' duration, involving the act of observing unsuspecting people, usually strangers, who are either naked, in the process of disrobing, or engaging in sexual activity.

Wechsler Adult Intelligence Scale (WAIS)   Individually administered intelligence test for adults and the standard against which other adult intelligence tests are compared.

Wechsler Intelligence Scale for Children (WISC-R)   Designed for children ages five to fifteen and is the most widely used intelligence test for children.

Wernicke's disease   A rare disorder of central nervous system metabolism associated with a thiamine deficiency and seen chiefly in chronic alcoholics.

Wide Range Achievement Test (WRAT)   An achievement test for psychiatric assessment.

Withdrawal   Development of a substance-specific syndrome that follows the cessation of, or reduction in, intake of a psychoactive substance that the person previously used regularly.

Zoophilia (beastiality)   A disorder in which there is the use of animals as a repeatedly preferred or exclusive method of achieving sexual excitement.

INDEX

Counterwill, 22
Creative arts therapies, 344
Cyclothymia, 245, 257

Defenses, 60
  Successful, 64
  Unsuccessful, 65
Déjà vu, 45, 121
Delirium, 46
  Tremens, 47
Delusional (Paranoid) disorder, 286
Delusions, 49
  Erotomanic, 286
  Grandiose, 49, 286
  Influential, 50
  Jealous, 286
  Litigious, 286
  Nihilistic, 50
  Persecutory, 49, 286
  Referential, 49
  Self-accusatory, 50
  Somatic, 49, 287
Demence precoce, 268
Dementia, 46, 268
  Associated with alcoholism, 226
  Praecox, 268
  Pseudo, 253
Denial, 72
Depersonalization, 44, 121
  Disorder, 120
  Neurosis, 120
Depression, 43
  Atypical, 249
  Major, 245, 256
Depressive disorders
  Recurrent, 256
  Single, 256
Depressive neurosis, 256
Derealization, 44
Dereism, 51
Deterioration, 46
Diathesis-stress factor, 3
Differential Personality Inventory (DFI), 313
Dipsomania, 218
Discrimination, 35, 37
Disorders of impulse control, 166
Disorientation, 46
Displacement, 73
Dissociation, 74
Dissociative disorders, 115
  Not otherwise specified, 122
Distractibility, 53
Dizygotic twins, 271
Dollard, John, 329
Dopamine theory, 350
Double insanity, 291
Dream state, 46

Drinking
  Addictive, 223
  Compulsive, 223
  Periodic, 218
  Problem, 218
  Reactive, 223
  Thymogenic, 218
Dunlop, 329
Dupont, R. L., 202
Dyskinesia
  Buccal lingual masticatory, 352
  Oral lingual, 352
Dysmorphophobia, 102
Dysthymia, 245, 256

Echolalia, 52
Echopraxis, 52
Ecstasy, 43
Ego, 16
  Defense mechanisms, 64
  Dystonic, 78
  Ideal, 17
  Psychology, 27
Eidetic imagery, 48
Elation, 43
Electra complex, 18
Electroconvulsive therapy, 359, 360, 361, 362
Ellis, Albert, 333
Empathy, 67
Endogenous-reactive dichotomy, 247
Environmental
  Intervention, 328
  Manipulation, 328
  Modification, 328
Epigenesis, 25
Erikson, Erik, 7, 25, 26, 158
Eros, 16
Etiology, 2
Euphoria, 43
Exaltation, 43
Exhibitionism, 179
Exner, J. E., 313
Expressive therapies, 344
Expulsive phase, 18
Extinction, 35, 37
Extrapsychic, 60
Extroversion, 20
Eysench, Hans, 330

Faberow, 251
Factitious disorder, 103, 124
  Not otherwise specified, 128
  With physical symptoms, 124
  With psychological symptoms, 126
Falret, J., 291
Family therapy, 341
Fantasy, 49, 75
  Autistic, 76